Rickets, Race and Reproduction

ALSO OF INTEREST
AND FROM MCFARLAND

The Story of a Forest: Growth, Destruction and Renewal in the Upper Delaware Valley (Robert Kuhn McGregor, 2018)

A Wider View of the Universe: Henry Thoreau's Study of Nature (Robert Kuhn McGregor, revised edition, 2017)

A Calculus of Color: The Integration of Baseball's American League (Robert Kuhn McGregor, 2015)

Rickets, Race and Reproduction

*Contracted Pelvis and
the American Way of Birth*

DEBORAH KUHN MCGREGOR
WITH ROBERT KUHN MCGREGOR

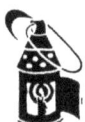

McFarland & Company, Inc., Publishers
Jefferson, North Carolina

ISBN (print) 978-1-4766-9371-2
ISBN (ebook) 978-1-4766-5104-0

LIBRARY OF CONGRESS AND BRITISH LIBRARY
CATALOGUING DATA ARE AVAILABLE

Library of Congress Control Number 2023046252

© 2023 Robert Kuhn McGregor. All rights reserved

No part of this book may be reproduced or transmitted in any form or by any means, electronic or mechanical, including photocopying or recording, or by any information storage and retrieval system, without permission in writing from the publisher.

Front cover image: children and old home on badly eroded land near Wadesboro, North Carolina, Marion Post Wolcott, 1938 (Library of Congress)

Printed in the United States of America

*McFarland & Company, Inc., Publishers
Box 611, Jefferson, North Carolina 28640
www.mcfarlandpub.com*

Contents

Coauthor's Note by Robert Kuhn McGregor — vii
Preface by Robert Kuhn McGregor — 1
Introduction. Considering the Contracted Pelvis — 5

Part I. The Problem — 11
ONE—The Lens of the Female Pelvis — 13
TWO—The Riddle of Rickets — 31
THREE—The Impediment of Race — 50
FOUR—Science Reloads — 63
FIVE—American Research Impaired — 78
SIX—Combating a Riddle Unresolved — 95

Part II. Resolution — 113
SEVEN—Johns Hopkins to the Fore — 115
EIGHT—Intervention in Childbirth — 127
NINE—Pediatricians' Progress — 146
TEN—Case Records at the OOS — 161
ELEVEN—An Obstetrical Definition of Race — 178
TWELVE—The Learning Curve of Alfred F. Hess — 188
THIRTEEN—Control of American Birth — 200
FOURTEEN—Solving the Riddle of Rickets — 220

Conclusion. The Sum of the Equation — 241
Chapter Notes — 251
Bibliography — 283
Index — 295

Coauthor's Note

by Robert Kuhn McGregor

Deborah Kuhn McGregor devoted her academic life to the study of medicine, examining the history of reproduction from a feminist perspective. Rather than focus on "heroic" pioneer physicians, she sought to examine the experience of patients, especially the subjects of medical experimentation, those exploited because of race or ethnic origin. After publishing *From Midwives to Medicine*—a study of the origins of gynecology—in 1998, she immediately began gathering materials pertinent to the experience of birth as practiced in twentieth-century America. Why did the incidence of rickets lead to hospital supervision of birth?

Deborah was a most careful, cautious, and thorough researcher; her approach to writing was much the same. She wrote and rewrote for sixteen years, reworking, re-examining, thinking anew. It is difficult to say how far she intended to carry the research; she was nowhere close to completion when her health began to fail. Parkinson's disease. She soldiered on as long as she could, determined to see the project completed. Deborah died on March 14, 2020, leaving behind a library of books, file cabinets stuffed to bursting, a computer overrun with files. Deborah never erased a file, even after reconsidering, rewriting. The result was a welter of chapters in various stages of completion, with little in the way of indication as to which was preferred or what the organization was to be.

She and I were graduate students working on doctoral dissertations when we married in 1982. We achieved positions at the same university, retired as full professors. Always we shared our work, assisting one another in finding materials, reading one another's drafts, discussing ideas. Essentially, we served as one another's research assistant. This was very fortunate. I understood the intent of her research fully, saw her interpretations unfold, was familiar with the content of her writing. Faced with more than forty computer files in various stages of completeness after her death, I chose to take on the task of completing her work. Her voice was stilled, but the words, the thought-provoking ideas should live. I needed to honor her memory, but more importantly, to share her knowledge.

Rickets, Race and Reproduction is the product of Deborah's devotion and research skill, her nuanced analysis of medical research. It is also in some small degree the result of my organizational choices, my editing, and, occasionally, my writing. I suspect her book would have been fifty to one hundred pages longer had she lived to complete her task; I was forced to develop a sensible point at which to conclude the narrative, given the material at hand. A new introduction detailing the construction became a necessity; the fourteen chapters to follow are largely Deborah. The work's conclusion attempts to capture the essence of her perspective; the words on the page are largely mine. This is Deborah's book; I am the midwife, assisting delivery while intruding in the product as little as possible.

I wish to acknowledge the contributions of our children to the completion of this work. Leaf and Janna offered continued and valuable support; Bran and Blueberry read and commented on portions of the manuscript; Molly provided a medical perspective in addition to reading chapters. This was in many ways a family project, a tribute to Deborah's memory, a legacy in recognition of her formidable scholarship. Deborah Kuhn McGregor was a passionate historian, and also a compassionate one. This book was the work of her life.

Preface

BY ROBERT KUHN MCGREGOR

A question posed at the Berkshire Women's History Conference in 1984 germinated the seed destined to grow into the work before the reader. Undertaking research for her doctoral dissertation, Deborah Kuhn McGregor presented a paper outlining the surgical experimentation performed on Black slaves by Doctor J. Marion Sims, regarded as the "father of gynecology." Sims sought a cure for a condition known as vesico-vaginal fistula—a tearing of the vaginal wall, incurred most often in childbirth. A member of the audience wondered why Black women in the American South suffered from such a condition. Deborah thought about the question for a moment before responding. The answer, quite possibly, was rickets. The disease could contract the pelvis, impeding birth, resulting in deadened tissues and eventual tearing.

Deborah spent several years researching the career of Marion Sims, publishing *From Midwives to Medicine: The Birth of American Gynecology* in 1998. Rather than focus the interpretation on the work of Sims, the book explored the experiences of his patients—his experimental subjects. Their numbers included Black women of the South, Irish immigrants in New York City, and, eventually, highborn women in Europe. Moral ambiguity lay at the heart of such pioneering research: to what extent were helpless women exploited to advance the science of medicine? Was the experimentation justified? In what manner did Sims's efforts shape the course of modern medicine, making medical doctors—almost exclusively male—authoritarian figures in the province of women's health?

Upon completion of the book, Deborah immediately took up the question asked so many years before: what was the significance of rickets in the history of women's reproductive health? Females faced a double jeopardy from the disease: weakened bones and possible death as a child, a contracted pelvis and difficult birth in maturity. Where did the disease come from? What were the effects? How did researchers—European and

American—comprehend the condition? What resulted? One question led inevitably to another. An inquiry into the etiology of rickets grew into a voyage of discovery extended over twenty years.

Discussions of rickets and contracted pelvis appeared in European works devoted to midwifery and childbirth as early as the seventeenth century, necessitating research in an increasingly complicated history of medicine. Germ theory. Surgical intervention. Anesthesia. The list grew long. A "science" of anthropology appeared, advancing theories of hierarchical differences among races, built on dubious measures of intelligence and physical difference. The study of pelvimetry—measurement of the female pelvis to identify abnormalities—entered the picture.

Shifting the focus to American practice made race and racism essential aspects of the study. Physicians and anthropologists evaluated the physiology and health of Blacks through a lens of a "scientific" racism, painting them as physical and mental inferiors, prone to rickets. Black women became the subjects of experimental surgery. The history assumed fundamental importance in Deborah's work—the conditions of slavery, the impact of abolition, the Great Migration, the unrelenting discrimination weighed heavily in medical efforts to understand and treat rickets. In America, the disease was generally viewed as a condition limited to Blacks, a sign of racial weakness and disintegration. A wave of new immigrants from southern and eastern Europe complicated the picture.

The "Progressive Era," designated to have begun around 1890, ushered in widespread efforts to reform American culture through the intervention of social science. America would be run by experts—social technicians intent on transforming health care, the home, motherhood itself. American medicine was more than willing to cooperate, employing pelvimetry to justify medical supervision of birth, save the mothers and babies. Midwifery, common at the beginning of the twentieth century, slowly but steadily vanished under the vicious attacks of medical reformers. Birth became a cold, clinical, hospital experience. Treated as a sick person, the expectant mother surrendered control of her body to an obstetrician, almost certainly male. At its heinous worst, elements of the medical profession promoted and supported the advance of eugenics—the pseudoscience contending that the state had a duty to advance the race by eliminating the weak through sterilization. While America embarked on that dangerous course, rickets grew to epidemic proportions as researchers sought an answer and the use of Caesarean section grew.

Contracted pelvis. Rickets, race, reproduction. Anthropology. Medicine. Health. Science. Progressivism. Childhood. Womanhood. One theme built on another, reflected in the impressively large library of volumes lining the bookcases in Deborah's study. The work here is constructed on a foundation of research and evaluation wrought by a vast array of scholars. The history of American birth has been examined and debated thoroughly; Deborah relied heavily on Irvine Loudon's *Death in Childbirth*, Judith Leavitt's *Brought to Bed*, and Robbie Davis-Floyd's *Birth as an American Rite of Passage*, among many, many others. Michel Foucault's *The Birth of the Clinic* informed her understanding of the history of medicine, supplemented by Roy Porter's *The Greatest Benefit to Mankind*. Historians such as Rima Apple and Barbara Ehrenreich added perspective. The scholarship of race is especially rich and compelling; the works of Kenneth Kiple, Todd Savitt, and Robert Wald Sussman proved especially helpful; Evelyn Brooks Higginbotham's "African American History and the Metalanguage of Race" was essential to the development of her interpretation. Turning to the "science" of racism, Stephen Jay Gould's *The Mismeasure of Man* and Nell Irvin Painter's *The History of White People* were pivotal. Considering the experience of experimental patients, Deborah found Harriet Washington's *Medical Apartheid* and Deidre Cooper Owens' *Medical Bondage* especially supportive of her point of view. For the nightmare aspects of the American Progressive movement, she turned to Robert Wiebe's *The Search for Order*, along with works on eugenics including *Illiberal Reformers* by Thomas C. Leonard, Edwin Black's *War Against the Weak*, and *Better for All the World* by Harry Brunius.

The scholarship of rickets is scattered; no recent book examines the subject historically. Vitamin D, the cure for rickets, became widely understood and available almost a century ago; only recently has the disease become a problem once more. Recent works, such as Michael F. Holick's *The Vitamin D Solution*, address the reasons behind the current outbreak, but discuss the etiology of the disease sketchily at best. Nor is there much discussion of contracted pelvis; the condition has become increasingly rare, even as the number of Caesarean sections has continued to increase.

Deborah's commitment to the study of contracted pelvis was both intellectual and personal. As a scholar, she determined to place the history of the disorder, the resultant interpretation and treatments before the world of scholarship. As a birthing mother, she sought to establish a framework in which women could reassert their right to a meaningful birth experience. The book before you is testimony to that commitment.

Introduction

Considering the Contracted Pelvis

The binding drawing together the three subject matters explored in these pages—rickets, race, and reproduction—is a condition perhaps most commonly recognized as the contracted pelvis. The disorder is a complaint easily defined: a pelvis contracted is a hip structure smaller than normal, perhaps abnormally shaped. Such a definition begs the larger question—what shape and size of pelvis is to be considered normal? This was an issue hotly contested among Western scientists for long decades stretching back to at least the seventeenth century. Identification of contracted pelvis was a matter of undeniable import; a woman so afflicted could experience grave or mortal difficulty bearing a child.

Each in its own way, rickets, race, and reproduction bore essentially on the investigation into contracted pelves. The three themes are not to be regarded separately; each was an integral influence on the other two. Explored extensively, taken together, they become the essential components of a history chronicling the story of birth as experienced in modern America and, to a certain extent, the entire world. Was contracted pelvis a pathological condition? In what way did its presumed existence shape medical practice? How did contracted pelvis affect the experience of birth and early infancy? There are no easy answers to these questions. Seeking perspective, the chapters to follow trace the etiology of rickets, the role of racially biased perception, the efforts of science to control reproduction—a human experience extending back at least five hundred thousand years. Racism, poverty, and malnutrition affected the body's susceptibility to development of contracted pelvis. This work argues that conceptions of pelvic "normalcy" emerged over several centuries in Europe and the United States shaped the development of health care, medical treatment, and reproduction for individuals exhibiting a contracted pelvis.

Rickets is a disease disrupting the normal formation of bone, leading to weakening, bending and contortion, especially in the limbs. Most common in infancy and childhood, rachitic disease may result in bowed legs, flat feet, malformed ribs, weak teeth. In extreme cases, skeletal infirmity could result in death. The disease holds a two-fold threat to females: the damage to growth in childhood and the dangers later posed by pelvic contraction. Though many scientists looked elsewhere for the cause, rachitic disease was a major source of pelvic disproportion.

Rickets affected rich and poor, often in inexplicable circumstances, defying treatment. It was once thought to be an unfortunate byproduct of modern civilization, but archaeological investigations demonstrate the presence of rickets in pre-industrial societies. Frequency grew to epidemic proportions as Europe industrialized; American physicians long denied a parallel occurrence with the advent of urban growth. By the early 1900s, American physicians had encountered enough cases to make rickets significant in their practices. As the incidence of contracted pelvis mounted, rickets became one of the great mysteries of medical science, variously attributed to environmental conditions, nutritional lack, unhygienic practice, and racial inheritance. Cultural subjectivities heavily influenced the frame of reference.

English medical historian Irvine Loudon argues that childbed fever killed many more women in the nineteenth and twentieth centuries than rickets, that rachitic disease has a lesser significance in the history of childbirth.[1] On the contrary, in addition to the harm rendered by rickets and the difficulties doctors experienced assessing the disease, the perceived threat to childbirth posed by a deformed or contracted pelvis dramatically altered the practice of obstetrics over the course of three centuries. By the early 1900s, contracted pelvis, the product of rickets, had become an international context for routine surgical intervention. The cognizance and experience of birth fundamentally altered. Why does the history of childbirth and midwifery have so little to say about this disease?

"Scientific" racism essentially influenced both the understanding of rickets and perceptions of birth. Growing out of European philosophical concepts embodied in the Great Chain of Being, race science hypothesized a hierarchy of human races based on superficial characteristics, skin color the most obvious. Whites occupied the highest rung, the "lower races" to follow, each supposedly endowed with a lesser physical prowess, a meaner intelligence. These were thought to be heritable qualities; many sicknesses, including rickets, were considered the consequence of racial susceptibility. While Europeans clearly saw that rickets was endemic among whites, American researchers allowed racial assumptions to obscure study of the disease, maintaining that rickets was largely an affliction of African Americans and darker-skinned European immigrants. Journal publications and discussions at professional meetings document an approach flawed by presupposition. Encountering pelvic disproportion among white women, American physicians tended to attribute the cause to factors other than rickets.

Needless to say, issues of race were omnipresent in the United States of America. Leaders of the Progressive Era (1890–1920) warned continually of "race suicide"—the notion that African Americans and immigrants were about to overwhelm the white population. That fear actually fueled the obstetrical revolution; doctors sought to make birth safer and easier for white women in the hope of raising the birth rate. Again, racial considerations obscured the effort; the "lower races" were believed to experience easier births. Gaining obstetrical experience attending Black deliveries at hospital dispensaries, physicians applied the knowledge acquired to advance their science. Cases of contracted pelvis were often attributed to inter-racial mixing.

The Progressive Era saw the beginning of fundamental change in American birth. In 1900, the vast majority of births took place not in a hospital but the home, where a midwife generally attended. A physician's presence was limited largely to cases of obstruction—the consequence of contracted pelvis. Just how many such cases occurred was a matter of vigorous debate. With the growing incidence of rickets, the numbers undoubtedly rose; the estimate of actual numbers depended entirely on definition of the condition. Firmly wedded to the scientific method, researchers sought the answer in statistical analyses—actual measurements of the size and shape of the female pelvis.

Pelvimetry as a science developed in Europe in the nineteenth century, both as a means to measure pelvic proportion and as a method to define race—racial types were deemed to exhibit differing pelvic structures. The practice was imported to America, where race continued as a factor in measurement and the statistical definition of deformity steadily inflated. By the early years of the twentieth century, leading obstetrical practitioners insisted on the necessity of pelvic measurement for all expectant women. Record keeping became imperative. Based on measures invasive and uncomfortable, doctors determined a growing number of women required hospitalization to give birth. The hospital provided ready access to interventions ranging from surgical forceps to Caesarean section, to say nothing of anesthesia. Debating the results of pelvimetric measure, some doctors maintained that contracted pelvis occurred in as many as one American woman in five.

The social trends of the Progressive Era sustained the changes in medicine taking place. Falling birth rates among whites inspired efforts to promote children's welfare—the "save the child" movement. Committed to collective action, reform organizations government and private engaged scientific solutions to reduce infant and child mortality. Efforts to improve nutrition and hygiene in the home accentuated a concept of "scientific motherhood."

Medicine itself underwent enormous change. Hospitals became research institutions; knowledge grew as patients endured experimental procedures. Often the subjects were the underprivileged and defenseless: African Americans or Irish immigrants. With the burgeoning growth of knowledge wrought by laboratory research and the advent of germ theory, the field of medicine grew too large for any one person to encompass. Specialization became unavoidable. Ongoing study of the experience of childbirth led to the development of three separate yet related specialties. Gynecology appeared first, based on surgical techniques to repair injuries to the reproductive organs. Obstetrics emerged as a science dedicated to the actual process of birth, a devotion grown more surgical with time. Following birth, care of the child fell to the pediatrician, who addressed the health and afflictions of the early years.

The divisions resulted in an odd bifurcation of the understanding and treatment of contracted pelvis. Obstetricians assumed control of definition and medical response to the condition, seeking methods to screen for deformity, alleviate the potential danger. Should pelvic distortion cause injury in birth, the gynecologist stepped in. Rickets, the root cause of the contraction, was a disease of childhood, therefore the province of the pediatrician. Pediatric studies inquiring into the efficacy of cod liver oil and ultraviolet light would lead eventually to the identification of vitamin D, the cure for the disease. By then the authoritative qualities of medical practice were firmly entrenched. Midwifery steadily diminished, home birth became a peculiar memory of a distant and relatively uncivilized past.

Rickets, Race and Reproduction is divided into two portions. The first, titled "The Problem," encompasses six chapters, beginning with a consideration of the female pelvis, the anatomy of childbirth, early efforts to address the problem of pelvic disproportion, cultural perceptions of birth. Subsequent chapters explore the science of rachitic disease, the development of a biology defined by race, the rise of empirical science, the eventual impact on reproduction. "The Problem" spans the years from the Early Modern Era to the close of the nineteenth century. The focus is international; much of early medical science developed in Europe, to be followed closely in America. Scientific racism too was a European concept, though Americans made their own peculiar contributions.

Part II, eight chapters in length, is simply labeled "Resolution," a title implying both a solution of the riddle of rickets and the development of a medical regimen governing childbirth. These chapters dwell largely (though not exclusively) on developments in the United States over the period lasting from 1890 to 1930—the "Age of Reform," when the people of the United States embraced the social sciences, worried about public health, intensified racial discrimination, sought to regulate every aspect of human behavior, including birth. Again, the three subject matters overlap, each conditioning comprehension of the others.

Racism, sexism, and poverty shaped the identities of countless women suffering from contracted pelvis. Such women too often became the unwilling subjects of medical practitioners determined to advance their careers, shape their disciplines. The contracted pelvis became the means to establish a standardized definition of the female body as well as an institutional form of birth based in a hospital setting. In sum, the pages to follow seek to weave the strands of rickets and childbirth into a multifaceted context, showing race and sex to be central to the history of medicine.

Part I

The Problem

Medical investigations of rachitic disease and the condition known as contracted pelvis began to appear in the seventeenth century. The timing was by no means accidental or unusual; European civilization was undergoing profound intellectual change, renewing long neglected efforts to comprehend the human condition, the world surrounding. What would become known as the "Scientific Revolution" was underway, inspiring disciplined research into fields as disparate as astronomy, physics, geology, biology, anthropology, chemistry. And medicine. At the heart of the endeavor was the now so familiar scientific method: the investigator focused on a specific problem, posing a carefully defined question, identifying a repeatable procedure to perform tests, analyzing the results, trying again. Mathematics became very important. Sir Francis Bacon summarized the methodology in an essay titled "Novum Organum" in 1620; the essentials of that process define scientific inquiry to this day. Most importantly, to be useful, the investigation must be without bias, value neutral. The scientist asks an unprejudiced question, seeks an answer utilizing untainted methodology.

Science is value neutral; scientists are not. Scientists are human beings, subject to all manner of dubious influences, inbred assumptions, moral suasion. A few are cheats. More than once a study has been shaped to arrive at a pre-ordained outcome. Nowhere is this more plain than in the myriad investigations into the cause of rickets, the resulting contracted pelves, the subsequent course of treatments. Physicians set out with the best of intentions, determined to alleviate human suffering, find a cure for the disease, facilitate safer human birth. At every step, biased assumptions clouded the process, creating false paths, impeding advance. Racism was worst of these. As the "Age of Enlightenment" embraced the pathways of science, dawning anthropology ranked the human races—white Europeans at the top of the chain, Black Africans at the bottom. Measurements of bone structure sought to "prove" racial difference, racial superiority. Pelvimetry—one such measurement—became a tool to define pelvic contraction, believed to vary from race to race. The prejudice inherent in the practice distorted interpretation of the condition.

Investigation into the cause of rickets suffered similar analytic distortion, understandable given the peculiar nature of the disease. Researchers advanced interpretations based on the observation of patients, experiments with animals, comparison of statistical incidence among populations spread across the globe. A seemingly contradictory host of results suggested a variety of cures, each with hopeful advocates, skeptical detractors. Rickets was variously described as a product of industrialization, poor diet, lack of exercise, poverty, insufficient sunshine, racial vulnerability, neglectful motherhood. A mountain of statistics supported each and every interpretation, lending credibility. Entrenched in competing comprehensions, treatments differed, solutions came and went. Cod liver oil was variously seen as a cure for rachitic disease or a useless offense to the taste buds. While physicians armed with selective evidence stood firm in their positions, incidence of rickets grew to epidemic proportions in western Europe and the United States. Some children died, many grew to adulthood with distorted limbs, weakened constitutions. Pelvic disproportion resulted in obstructed births. Competing solutions to that special problem inspired another mountain of statistics, shaped to support whatever treatment the analyst envisioned. Medical intervention in birth was much the preferred result.

Science is a very powerful tool. Much depends on the practitioners wielding such power. By the eighteenth century, medicine had become a science, conducted by very human scientists. All the attributes of science, the good and bad, the inspired and prejudiced, combined to shape the modern experience of birth. The history is complicated.

One

The Lens of the Female Pelvis

She was known to medical authorities as Mrs. H, described as "a large, strong, apparently well built Irish woman." Mrs. H was in labor for the fifth time—a variety of experiences had accompanied the four previous birth experiences: "two forceps deliveries; one craniotomy; one spontaneous delivery, child living." The woman's difficulties were grounded in "a case of flat rachitic pelvis"—her birth canal was too narrow to insure an untroubled delivery. Begun in Chicago at 9 p.m. on November 9, 1896, this latest confinement would present a still different and grave issue. The umbilical cord was prolapsed, appearing in advance of the infant's head.

Mrs. H. may have been a strong woman, but the previous birth experiences left their mark. "Internally—perineum torn deeply at some previous labor, cervix thick, os admits the hand easily, old scar in the vagina, head movable above the inlet…. Pelvis roomy below and at the sides, contracted in the conjugate diameter." Medical intervention, necessitated by that conjugate contraction, had wrought some damage. Now the medical men would intervene yet again, first to address the problem of the prolapsed cord, secondly to see the child delivered. Working together, two doctors undertook a complicated "version" (manual manipulation) to restore the umbilicus to proper position. Then came the birth. The child's head "was arrested at the inlet." More version, followed by an intense use of traction (essentially a pulley system) and external pressure to deliver the trunk—"the arms were thrown up alongside the head." The climax proved much happier than many such experiences. The little girl, seven and a half pounds, was born alive. Mrs. H survived as well.[1]

A horrific story, rooted in a misshapen female pelvis. An emblematic story, in the fact that cases such as this opened the door to fundamental change in the perception, the comprehension, the ministration of birth in America. This history hinges entirely on the anatomy of the female pelvis: its structure, its shape, its function. The female pelvis is a critical element in the history of science, deserving further exploration.

* * *

The unique human physiology of birth evolved over 4.5 million years. The first significant source of change came with standing up, or becoming bipedal. Upright posture changed the pelvic shape, the anatomy of the legs and feet and the spine. The pre-hominid fossil Australopithecus afarensis, known as Lucy, discovered in Kenya in the late 1970s, opened discussion of birth. Anthropologists for the first time had a complete enough female pelvis (the complete sacrum and left innominate bone) to interpret changes in the mechanisms of birth and labor beginning several million years ago. Here they found morphology that reflected both bipedal upright posture and quadrupedal activities. Seemingly encephalization (enlargement of the fetal head) had not yet developed.[2] Encephalization began with the appearance of Homo habilis roughly 2.8 million years ago; brain size grew larger than the chimpanzee. Specimens again found in Kenya demonstrate that by the time Homo erectus walked the earth 1.9 million years ago, infants were born far more dependent and less mature than other mammals.[3] Enlargement of the brain and consequent growth of the skull dictated that birth come sooner, before the head grew too large. Pelvic size dictated a boundary for the size of the fetal brain. At this time, the human fetus developed a secondary altricial characteristic, so that babies were born with less developed brains than other primates, hence more dependence on nurturance following birth—the helplessness of newborns. The evolutionary trend continued for another 1.3 million years, down to the appearance of Homo sapiens. Fully modern human beings emerged perhaps as many as 550,000 years ago, nurturing their helpless infants as they spread across the globe.[4]

Often overlooked in the evolution of the much celebrated human brain—eighty-one cubic inches, three times the size of the great apes—is the parallel evolution of the female pelvis. Human understanding of this aspect of evolutionary change is a very recent development.[5] The ratio of the size of the fetal skull to the size of the birth canal, known among physicians as the cephalo-pelvic proportion, has been crucial to the evolution of human birth. To accommodate the larger human head, the female pelvis had to widen. This characteristic of the species was accompanied by the development of the radical turns and rotations which came to be required of the fetus as it moved from the inlet to the outlet during birth. No matter whether or not a birth is normal, the fetus must follow a sharply turning birth canal and rotate its head and shoulders to be born. The birth canal changes and encephalization made labor and birth more difficult for humans because of the possibility of large fetal heads or stuck shoulders, otherwise known as dystocia. The human birth canal complicates getting born. The occasional severe complication would, in the modern world, prompt determined investigation.[6]

One. The Lens of the Female Pelvis   15

* * *

To understand how late nineteenth-century and early twentieth-century American obstetrics viewed the pelvis requires consideration of European antecedents. Beginning in the eighteenth century, ongoing research in medicine, anatomy and anthropology overlapped, seeking an understanding of pelvic form, function and variation, the process of childbirth, and why births sometimes went wrong. Questions about the human female pelvis touched directly on the process of birth.

Medieval European physicians had established anatomy as medical knowledge, at once drawing from and feeding the emergence of a scientific culture. In northern Italian cities as early as the mid-fourteenth and fifteenth centuries, physicians began to embrace dissection and the study of female anatomy as a basis for gynecology and obstetrics. Their curiosity about the generative qualities of female physiology combined with an interest in ancient texts and ideas of first cause posited by Aristotle, who argued for medical knowledge, based more on "abstract and intellectual understanding of cause" than the secrets of private lay knowledge shrouded in religious belief that had previously governed the study of women's bodies.[7] Italian physicians specifically excluded women midwives whose knowledge came out of the private lay order. The masterpiece of Andreas Vesalius (1514–1564), *De Humani Corporis Fabrica,* published in 1543, brought together the practice of ancient traditions with the experience of public anatomical dissection, foregrounding the book's content on the cover with a public dissection of the reproductive parts of an impoverished woman's cadaver.[8] By the eighteenth century, scientific interest in the "new anatomy" had spread across Europe.[9]

In 1774, William Hunter (1718–1783), an English obstetrician, brought a new focus to studies of physical reproduction. To that point, fetal representations had looked more like grown children or sometimes dolls. Hunter reproduced the nine months of pregnancy in life-like images of cross-sections of pregnant women and charted the hours of labor in the first, second and third stages. His work, substantively expressed in artistic plates, depicted the "gravid uterus" in relation to various parts of the body of a woman. Hunter's art derived from dissected corpses of women who had died during pregnancy and sometimes during birth itself.[10] The plates themselves seemed natural, fleshy and tangible. The text, *Anatoma Humani Gravidi,* expressed a kind of medical and artistic celebration of the physical reality of birth. Encapsulating changes that came with new medical authority in birth, both by portraying women who had died and in the name of future laboring women, gave authority to Hunter's work in a subtle way, turning obstetrics into a science. Over the next 150 years, Hunter's work helped obstetrics to slowly develop a system intended to divert death in childbirth. His drawings, despite naysayers, established a new image of birth, leading doctors to envision the internal process, to understand in some ways the meaning of pelvic measure, most importantly to see the procession of a regular or "normal" birth.[11]

Social factors influenced the history of obstetrics and childbirth. William Hunter's subjects, dead bodies of pregnant women, likely came from impoverished or at the very least lesser privileged walks of life; bodies available for autopsy, dissection and public exhibition usually were from less privileged social groups or possibly single women giving birth to children conceived out of wedlock.[12] In his rendering the images took on a different status, representing the cultural ideal, a transcending image of womanhood. The material and economic status of a woman greatly influenced the nature of her childbirth experience, perhaps even her death from childbirth, though medical work often glossed over her background. Racial diversity among patients, another important socially-defining factor, rarely appeared in textbooks. Medical writers in these years usually assumed that their medical insights were meant to apply to a white patient of European origin, married with a secure financial status. Many of the assumptions governing their anatomical presentation of the female pelvis persist to this day. Subjectivity enters when attempts are made to establish one female pelvis as representative of all women, a concept intended to define "normalcy" in textual and visual representations.[13]

* * *

Even as the science of obstetrics took shape in the late eighteenth century, a new order in sexual and gender relations began to evolve. Sex and the subjectification of women became part of the political and economic development of the early modern and modern periods in western history. Science and rationalism found expression in the Enlightenment and brought with them a hierarchy of gender relations based on an assumption of women as subordinate. The era brought a vision of the environment as shaping each individual. Women and men assumed a new partnership, a gender system based on sexual complementarity. A myriad of social, political, economic, and ideological changes influenced the development of the scientific intellectual framework.[14]

In the medieval period, gender roles eclipsed physical identity, becoming a flowing one-sex continuum where masculinity and femininity overlapped. A woman was simply a lesser man—with her reproductive organs turned outside in. The eighteenth century came to define masculine and feminine as distinctly different; they became two sexes with different roles. According to the prevailing version of the social order, the difference between men and women ruled out the possibility of equality.

The classic dualities of submissive/aggressive, emotional/rational, nature/culture, weak/strong, culture/nature and more came to identify femininity and masculinity respectively, and women and men. Women, narrowly confined through their gender role, could not qualify to practice science and lost ground in their centuries-old practice of midwifery. In such a framework women's sexuality as well as reproductivity needed containment.[15]

Pelves became for many a measure of women's productiveness. By the nineteenth century, scientists and political economists, early anthropologists and anatomists came to view the skull as a measure of masculine prowess and pelves that of feminine strength. The wider the female pelvis, the higher the status of that skeleton in the hierarchy of humans. Medical interest, if traced simply through medical practitioners, suggested that measuring pelves was one step in the path of addressing complications of birth. This focus came out of a social context that subordinated and objectified women as the patient, not the practitioner, and that endeavored to limit women's roles to reproduction.[16] Though the ability to reproduce represented the potential singular female power of generativity, men as physicians and obstetricians acted upon reproducing women to measure their capabilities—in terms of birth and more.

* * *

By the nineteenth century, the medical approach *to* and understanding *of* childbirth had changed profoundly. From the seventeenth century onward, physicians looked more and more at birth as the product of female skeletal anatomy. Obstructed births, often tragic in their occurrence, were attributed to the condition labeled contracted pelvis. Increasingly, childbirth was perceived as a sickness. Scientific innovation offered new and what was for quite a while secret instrumental intervention in these obstructed or, as physicians then expressed it, "preternatural" (meaning unusually difficult) labors, offering hope for a good outcome where there had been none. Irregularities and possible complications of birth became more prominent in the eyes of medicine as physicians and midwives defined the new science of obstetrics.

Manual techniques appeared first. Hendrik van Deventer (1651–1724), a Dutch obstetrician, identified methods to intervene in obstructed labor by focusing on the gravid pelvis. Deventer helped to articulate the eventually commonplace idea that difficult births often resulted from the disproportion of the size of the pelvis of the mother relative to the size of the fetal head. The Dutch physician adopted the use of "version" (the turning and manipulation of the fetus within the uterus), coming to rely on such manual maneuvers to intervene in what he saw as stymied or prolonged labors. This was a practice common among midwives. Deventer's spouse was a midwife; together they confronted a number of such birth crises. They came to identify the central aspects of birthing, establishing a theory and practice of obstetrics. Deventer published *The New Light for Male and Female Midwives* in 1701, describing the introduction of the hand into the laboring woman's vagina with the palm facing forward and the back of the hand pressing on the coccyx, moving it backwards to bring the fetal head through the birth canal. His work identified the importance of bony structure and bone disease, likely providing the first description of pelvic deformity, which Deventer saw as the likely product of rickets. Now regarded as the first obstetrics manual, Deventer intended his work to be a practical support for midwives, providing valuable instructions for attending births ranging from the typical experience to the unusual challenge. Later physicians resorted to version frequently, but altered the practice to serve the use of instruments.[17]

By the time Deventer wrote his book, forceps had entered the medically-trained accoucheur's armamentarium. The Chamberlins, a Huguenot family forced to flee France for England in 1569, invented the tool and kept it under wraps throughout the seventeenth century. Two blades made up a pair of forceps, with traction established inside the woman's reproductive tract by the application of one, usually to the side of the fetal head and then locking the second blade to the other side. How this was done depended in part upon the fetal presentation, whether the woman's cervix was fully dilated, whether the head was engaged in the cervix or the degree to which the fetus had traveled down the birth canal, and the nature of the path to birth.[18]

When forceps became public knowledge, many were shocked by what seemed to be a moral depravity in the Chamberlin family's approach to medical practice. The family had kept secret a tool which could have helped physicians in obstructed births to bring forth a living child and prevent the death of the mother. The potential of forceps most importantly, it seemed at the time, was to save the life of the mother. No matter their mixed reviews, the new technology was a welcome alternative to stymied labors with no alternative but to either destroy the fetus or wait for both mother and child to die. Internationally reputed French obstetrician François Mauriceau (1637–1709), a contemporary of Hugh Chamberlin the elder (c. 1632–after 1720), like Deventer, refused to use forceps and resorted instead to hooks and crochets to extricate the infant body. Chamberlin translated Mauriceau's obstetrical text into English, providing an introduction in which he chided Mauriceau for choosing to kill the infant when forceps offered an alternative.[19]

Forceps stood as a milestone in the history of obstetrics and midwifery for more than one hundred years despite conflict over their best use. Retrospective measure of their utility presents a challenging question. Elizabeth Nihell (1723–1776), an eighteenth-century English midwife, published a text damning the use of forceps, as well as hooks, crochets and other destructive tools of medicine. The developing use of forceps underscored the growing separation of midwifery from scientific obstetrical practice.[20]

Reluctant to use the forceps, William Smellie (1697–1763) of London, a rival of Deventer, added to the treatment of contracted pelves during labor by being the first to prescribe pelvic measurement before labor set in. Smellie's method developed an internal measure of the pregnant woman's pelvis, using fingers to approximate the cephalo-pelvic proportion of the fetal head to the mother's pelvic opening. Smellie believed that rickets in childhood caused misshapen pelves in adulthood, resulting in difficult labors. He recognized the utility of forceps in such a labor and helped to introduce them to medical practice, but in his own practice he went back and forth regarding their employment, his lack of experience making him afraid of them. His momentary embrace of forceps in a treatise on obstetrics in 1871 linked his name with their use, masking the mutability of his practice.[21]

Smellie's actual system combined different aspects of obstetrics in his time. Smellie may have used Deventer's maneuver to guide the fetal head past the coccyx in obstructed births, especially in the periods when he shunned the use of forceps. From the writings of London man-midwife Frederick Ould published in 1742, Smellie learned that the rotation of the fetal head in a head presentation happened routinely in labor and found this knowledge useful in employing forceps. There was much in midwifery for Smellie to learn. Looking in a new direction, he helped to establish the British male medical dominance of obstetrics, keeping forceps out of the pockets of midwives.[22] Above all, Smellie treated birth as an entirely mechanical process, a view echoed by Angélique Marguerite Le Bousier du Coudray (c. 1712–1794), midwife in service to King Louis XV. Du Coudray created a "machine," as she called it, to represent birth and to teach fledgling midwives the process of birth and the role of the midwife.[23]

Samuel Bard (1742–1819) wrote the first American text in obstetrics, published in 1808. Arguing against the use of forceps, Bard wrote about deformed pelves and osteomalacia, an adult equivalent of rickets. Similar to many obstetricians in America who followed him, Bard argued that there were more deformed or rachitic pelves abroad than there were in America, hence negating the need for forceps.[24]

More than two centuries following their invention, American physician Charles Meigs (1792–1869) celebrated the mechanical basis of the forceps. "The great desideratum in Midwifery was a forceps that might seize the head and extract it, without inflicting a wound.... The blades became capable of grasping and firmly holding the oval-shaped head of the child, while still contained in the womb or vagina."[25] By the nineteenth century, physicians routinely denied women midwives the education needed to use forceps, in effect denying them access to instrumental intervention in an obstructed birth. Realizing midwives would have access to their texts, Hugh Chamberlin and Charles Meigs addressed these practitioners directly, insisting they make no attempt to employ forceps themselves. Midwives needed to know the instrument existed, that they should consult an obstetrician when labor reached a dangerous point.[26]

When obstructed labors did occur, physicians thought and wrote more about the best technique to use in such cases, less about what might produce the obstruction. Several operative interventions had emerged by the late nineteenth century, including craniotomy and Caesarean section. In 1871, Robert Harris of Philadelphia launched a mission to gather reports of all the American Caesarean sections for the nineteenth century. Because of a high rate of infection and little applicable knowledge of antiseptic procedure, Caesarean sections were very dangerous; incurring a high death rate, yet Harris expressed his intent to promote the practice. He compared American mortality rates with British statistics. From the beginning of his studies, Harris believed Caesarean section was more successful and safer in the United States. The patients he described included women with contracted pelves, dwarfs and others diagnosed with osteomalacia or childhood rickets. In 1871, Harris published his first article in a long series, analyzing fifty-nine American births over the nineteenth century, mostly cases of contracted pelves, and found a maternal mortality rate of 48 percent. Harris interpreted this percentage as better than most people expected. With his statistical collections, he hoped to demonstrate the viability of the surgery if performed early in the labor and under antiseptic conditions. Many doctors felt torn between the choice of craniotomy and Caesarean section. In the 1870s most chose craniotomies, a centuries-old procedure that persisted into the twentieth century.[27]

A craniotomy involved crushing the fetal cranium and extracting the contents in order to draw the deceased fetus through the pelvic opening. Although this sounds horrible, doctors felt the procedure relatively easy and could be done without threatening the mother's life. Physicians believed the fetus did not experience a sensation of pain.[28] Embryotomy was a similar procedure, but involved pulling apart the fetus piece by piece. Craniotomy was preferable, as saving the mother's life was the essential consideration.[29]

* * *

Moving beyond the immediacy of problematic birth, obstetrical science came to consider the underlying cause—a contracted pelvis. As far back as the early eighteenth century, Hendrik van Deventer considered the concept of an irregular pelvis—the narrowed, flattened pelvis found in some pregnant women—to explain difficult births, prolonged labors. A student of Renaissance anatomist Andreas Vesalius had first described the condition in the sixteenth century. Deventer now articulated the eventually common-place belief that difficult births often resulted from the disproportion of the size of the pelvis of the mother relative to the size of the fetal head. Building on the Dutchman's observations, European practitioners came to perceive a significant presence of contracted pelves among women in labor, impacting the historical experience of childbirth and the practice of medicine.[30]

Studies of disproportion compared the estimated measure of the fetal cranium to the maternal pelvic diameters, looking for situations where the fetal head apparently could not pass through the bony pelvis during birth. Physicians concluded disproportion of infant head to pelvic size to be a significant factor defining obstructed births, deriving the knowledge from dissection of cadavers and autopsies of disastrous births. In the case of a living birth, approximations were necessary because first, there was no way to measure the fetal head before birth, and second, measuring the pelvis of the woman in labor was difficult. Yet the issue seemed important. Physicians increasingly conceived of obstructed childbirth as a sickness originating in a contracted pelvis. Even with a name, the condition was vague enough to encompass a large component of the childbirth experience.

Jean-Louis Baudeloque, a Frenchman and contemporary of William Hunter, wrote on the science of childbirth in the 1780s, contributing substantially to the science of contracted pelves. His work established pelvimetry—the science of pelvic measurement—a method used for more than 150 years to assess the size of a woman's pelvis in the context of her pregnancy. The purpose of the measurement was to identify contracted pelves before labor. Pelvimetry established what was considered to be a standard for pelvic size; doubtless Baudeloque used both cadavers and living women to devise his technique. The measure allowed physicians to anticipate a complicated or obstructed birth, thereby building a context for the decision of when and if to engage obstetrical interventions or surgeries. Baudeloque employed a caliper to measure the size of the female pelvis externally—as pelvimetry became basic to obstetrics, external measure proved the acceptable method. Doctors struggled to measure a living pregnant woman's pelvis without disturbing her.[31]

Baudeloque recommended the physician take three diameters, the interspinous, intercristal, and external conjugate, from the pregnant patient's bony pelvis. The interspinous diameter measured the anterior or front distance between the superior iliac spines. The intercristal diameter measured the greatest distance between the widest points on the crests of the bony ridges. These two measures established the breadth of what was called the woman's bony false pelvis. In evaluating a possibly rachitic pelvis, the most meaningful use of the numbers was to compare the two previous measures with Baudeloque's conjugate diameter. The external conjugate, otherwise known as Baudeloque's diameter, measured from the spine of the last lumbar vertebra to the upper anterior edge of the symphysis pubis, and in turn measured the depth from front to back within the cavity of the true pelvis. Baudeloque's calculations sought to provide the smallest distance of each given measure before the pelvis became contracted. For the interspinous diameter, 8 inches, for the intercristal diameter, 10¾ inches and 10 inches for conjugate diameter (or respectively, 20, 27.5 and 25.5 centimeters). The combination of the measurements was meant to provide an informed estimation of the diameter of the true pelvic brim.[32]

Out of this standard, practitioners derived a somewhat crude measurement for a regular pelvis. Anything less was considered irregular. With time practitioners varied categories established by the measures, refining definition of irregular pelvic shape, sometimes linking the condition to different origins. Practitioners argued about where to set the standards, but recognized Baudeloque as the originator. He determined the measures that he thought ensured a progressive labor, one neither obstructed nor dependent upon the attendant's intervention.[33]

Baudeloque's research established a quantitative standard for the depth and width of the female pelvis. Along with the forceps, this innovation became part of the specialty of obstetrics over the next one hundred years. Baudeloque's name was and still is associated with his measures. Most discussions of contracted pelves considered his definitions while often amending them, sometimes referring simply to the technique of external pelvic measurement. Physicians realized they could quantify observations of a pregnant woman's pelvic area to assess possible future complications in birth. What is science without numbers?

Memories of eighteenth-century achievements in medical history would appear in nineteenth and twentieth-century essays and texts, commemorating the work of past leaders in medicine. Science emanating from the eighteenth-century fostered innovations and cloaked them with authority. Baudeloque's influence in the nineteenth century, along with that of Deventer, Smellie and Hunter, rendered what must have been sometimes emotional, sometimes desperate, sometimes deadly and often tedious labors into abstract numbers, providing a basis for continuing medical discussions of challenging obstetrical practice.[34]

Baudeloque, along with William Smellie, also practiced an internal measure, the *conjugata diagonalis,* also called the diagonal conjugate. Each determined this measure using his right hand inside the woman's vagina. Such an intrusion during labor called for extreme care. The middle-finger and the fore-finger passed into the vagina, pressing on the promontory of the sacrum while the fore-finger marked the lower margin of the subpubic ligament at the pubic symphysis. Withdrawing the hand while maintaining their position gave the diagonal conjugate. In other words, this internal measure, if done carefully and exactly, gave the distance between the front and the back of the woman's bony pelvic inlet. Four inches, or 11.5 centimeters marked the size of a regular, or subsequently termed, a "normal" pelvic brim. Anything less was irregular. Usually 3.5 inches or less declared a deformed pelvis. Baudeloque's diameter, variously called *conjugata vera*, could be estimated from *conjugata diagonalis,* but was deemed less accurate in succeeding generations. In this time, with no knowledge of bacteria or the benefits of antiseptic procedure, physicians practicing internal measurement most certainly brought disease to women in labor.[35]

Slowly, steadily, contracted pelves came into view for many medical practitioners. The work of German obstetrician Franz Karl Naegele early in the nineteenth century included studies of the "Obliquely Contracted Pelvis." Drawing on French studies, Naegele focused on one specific type, asymmetrically formed (hence oblique), originating more in spinal disease such as ankylosis, resulting in distortion of the bony pelvis.[36]

Identifying a specific female anatomical irregularity, the deformed pelvis, with an obstructed birth helped turn attention of patients and attending doctors to the small percent of laboring women who met their own demise from obstructed labor or whose infants died before, during or soon after birth. Imperfect in their ability to successfully intervene in obstructed labors and often the source of disease and injury, doctors were nonetheless gaining control of techniques of intervention. Their anatomical and cadaveric knowledge created a barrier between patients and death.[37]

Two pioneer physicians in Germany—a teacher and his student— most influenced the coming generations of medical men pursuing contracted pelves as a critical area of focus. Working in Kiel in the 1850s, Gustav Michaëlis (1796–1848) and his student, Carl Litzmann (1815–1890), built on the measurements proposed by Smellie and promoted the work of Baudeloque by enhancing its application. Together they established a system of classification for abnormal pelves while analyzing statistics on their incidence, thereby refining pelvimetry to clarify the different kinds of deformed pelves and how to treat them. Theirs was more an applied science, but they too relied on mortal anatomy and cadaveric study.

Michaëlis began his study of pelves at the University of Kiel, laying the groundwork for research and identification of pelvic deformities.[38] Unfortunately his career ended abruptly. After reading Ignaz Simmelweis's (1818–1865) theory that physicians' hands carried puerperal fever, Michaëlis grasped the implications, concluding that he had infected his cousin, who had died after giving birth with Michaëlis her attendant. Displaying perhaps the romantic influence of Sturm und Drang, Michaëlis took his role as obstetrician to a dramatic end, committing suicide.[39]

Carl Litzmann carried forth his research, publishing Michaëlis's important work on the pelvis, *Das Enge der Becken,* in a new edition, and going on to publish his own work in 1861.[40] His book was *Die Formen das Becken*—the "study of birth through a narrow pelvis." Litzmann's work treated "das Enge der Becken," or the contracted pelvis, as a "clinical diagnosis."[41]

Litzmann argued firmly that the contracted pelvis was the most frequent cause of obstructed birth, or dystocia. Measurement became the key to diagnosis. "Based on my research, I believe that a pelvic passage narrowed by ¼-inch can markedly increase the difficulty of a birth."[42]

Litzmann placed the *conjugata vera* at the center of pelvic measurement, and marked the abnormal or contracted pelvis as less than 3.5 inches. He defined this as the true measure of the pelvic inlet, the anteroposterior diameter, measured from the top of the pubic symphysis to the sacrovertebral angle. Physicians could obtain this number in cadavers but rarely living women before or during labor. By the early twentieth-century Litzmann's *conjugata vera* became the standard for the contracted pelvis.[43]

In his text Litzmann provided a drawing of side-views of three overlapping types of pelvic shape to illustrate the extreme variation in the depth of the pelvis.[44] These he identified as normal, rachitic, and osteomalacian. As rickets and osteomalacia are essentially the same disease, he used rickets to represent all abnormal pelves, showing the primacy of rickets (not universality) in the contracted pelvis.

Litzmann carefully derived a system of medical classification for abnormally-shaped pelves. Following the anthropological and predominant morphological emphasis already in place, Litzmann chose to analyze the shape of the pelvis rather than the etiology (causes of the deformities) as the basis for classification. Subordinately, a general reference to rickets appeared as a possible cause in several different categories and subcategories.

First were pelves of normal shape—generally contracted plus either too small or too large: justo minor or justo major, respectively. The second group were those with abnormal shape. This group comprised three types of the most common contracted pelvis, including the flat pelvis, sometimes produced by rickets. Beside the abnormally shaped pelves were the transversely contracted pelves, then the third group, the irregularly contracted pelves, including Naegele's obliquely contracted pelvis, and finally, a fourth group that included an assortment of deformities originating in spinal disease. In subcategories were several others, including osteomalacian pelves from adult rickets. Other classifications in sub-groups used the origin of deformity as defining of the sub-type. For instance, the loss of use of a leg caused a diagonally shifted pelvis. There were also such possibilities as "flat non-rickety" or "simple flat rickety."[45]

Relying on the methodology of clinical medicine, collecting statistics from his medical practice for analysis, Litzmann presented computations of incidence of contracted pelves he had measured himself.[46] His statistics compared his own cases with those of Michaëlis. Looking at maternal mortality, Michaëlis found 151 cases of contracted pelves in which ten mothers died (6.62 percent), while Litzmann had four deaths in 180 (2.22 percent). Of the same cases of Michaëlis, looking at fetal mortality, 153 babies were born, twenty-three born dead or dying (15.03 percent); Litzmann numbered 182 children born, with twenty-eight born dead or dying (15.38 percent).[47] Instrumental delivery (from forceps to craniotomies) characterized these births, a possible source of the injuries many women suffered during this period. These statistics spoke to Litzmann's belief that to diagnose a contracted pelvis before a birth could lead to a better outcome. Many American physicians in the late 1890s and early 1910s referred back to these statistics and others Litzmann presented, often re-presented them, and modeled their numerous studies of contracted pelves after his work, using evidence from their own practices.

Litzmann recognized that changes had begun in obstetrical practice in the late seventeenth century but felt he and his mentor created seachanges in the practice of obstetrics. They had clarified the significance of narrow or contracted pelves in birth. "Few writers have dealt until now … with the fundamental pelvic passage…. To my knowledge Michaëlis was the first to explore [it]."[48] The smallest degree of contraction could substantially impact a woman and her child's life and childbirth experience.

Why had contracted pelves as a cause of complicated births stayed hidden so long? Litzmann puzzled. "Michaëlis appropriately emphasized the reasons, which can explain some remarkable misjudgments though the truth lay so close…. One assumed wrongly that each birth must widen the pelvis and the opening, that the original design of the birth canal was too narrow, and that belief blocked better insights."[49] Michaëlis and Litzmann premised their idea of contracted pelvis on a permanently *narrowed* or abnormal bony structure making the birth canal simply impassable. According to Litzmann and many twentieth-century obstetricians, earlier folk medicine from the medieval period, represented mostly as false beliefs of midwives, had supposed that the bony pelvis moved apart during birth.[50]

Litzmann's work offered a new emphasis on the contracted pelvis as central to an obstructed birth—leaving attending physicians with new choices to make regarding how to proceed in a birth obstructed by a deformed pelvis. While William Smellie in the eighteenth century had assumed a hierarchy of humans in "castes and ranks," Litzmann and Michaëlis never broached issues of race or social class in their analyses.[51] While Litzmann's pelvic measurements offered a racially neutral definition of the contracted pelvis, by the 1870s several European authors quantified data from skulls and pelves out of various museum collections to represent differences by race and sex. At the Paris Museum of Natural History French anthropologist Paul Broca's forty instruments for anthropometric measurement further developed pelvimetric quantification. Drawing on European research to develop their own theories, American physicians increasingly employed statistical analyses as well.[52]

* * *

Philadelphia physician William DeWees (1768–1841) was an early American proponent of pelvimetry, urging instrumental intervention with forceps in problematic births. Dewees paid to have Baudeloque's text republished in translation in the United States in 1807.[53] Relying on the work, Dewees described misshapen pelves in three categories of contracted pelves. His "system of obstetrics" designated three interventions in birth, according to the measurement of the conjugata vera. Beginning with the least obstructive narrowing of the pelvis, the first intervention required forceps, the second craniotomy, and the third Caesarean section. This protocol strongly anticipates writings from a much later period.[54]

By the mid-nineteenth century, American physicians were developing profound interest in the subject. Thomas F. Cock, an attending physician at the Lying-In Asylum of Bellevue Hospital in New York City, wrote specifically about childbirth and "delayed labor," producing a textbook in obstetrics in 1853. Following Deventer and Smellie, Cock referred to "Labor Difficulty from Disproportion."[55] He defined trouble in labor as one in which the head had presented but no birth followed for twenty-four hours, a very long time to wait in what would likely have been the second stage of labor. Cock understood the origins of this stymied delivery as too small a pelvis and too large a fetal head, citing an incidence of one in thirty-six cases, or 2.8 percent.[56]

Cock meticulously described the differences in the bony structures of male and female pelves. Charts served his text, describing the dimensions of each pelvis. He made no judgmental distinctions, nor did he explicitly relate either prototype to sexual or reproductive functions. His description did demonstrate that the female pelvis was more suitable for childbirth in its shape by comparing the prototypes of the two pelves in the shapes and sizes of various bony parts and in the sizes of the pelvic inlet and the pelvic basin. Like most, he assumed a connection of form and function; Cock wanted to show that the female pelvis was different.[57]

Cock likewise discussed "Deformities of the Pelvis."[58] Here he directly connected complicated birth with rickets. Pelvic deformities were those too large in some proportion or too small (the more common determination). A pelvis too small was the consequence of rachitis, the medical term for rickets. Cock (and many others) denoted an enlarged pelvis as coming from "*malacosteon* (osteo-malacia, Mollities Ossium),"[59] conditions of softened bones. Medicine in the next century would consider osteomalacia as late rickets, though the symptoms were quite different. The third cause he saw were scars and deformities, incapabilities and asymmetries resulting from other diseases, past and present. He argued that "a true pelvis should have well rounded hips, and be of equal height."[60] In this description he conflated the anatomical definition of the true pelvis with the notion of a perfect pelvis of sorts, providing a singular aesthetic model of normalcy by which to judge all women with a glance of the eye.

Many practicing obstetricians considered pelvic structure at midcentury, but Charles Meigs of Philadelphia was especially prominent and articulate regarding contracted pelves. Meigs was a transitional figure in American medical science, one of the last to employ bloodletting, urging its use as routine during labor. If a woman was flushed during labor, he bled her until she fainted. Meigs thought of puerperal fever—by far the greatest cause of maternal mortality in eighteenth, nineteenth and early twentieth centuries in Europe and the United States—as inflammation that should be treated with bleeding and argued against the likelihood that physicians carried the disease. The plague of childbed fever and streptococcus infection followed physicians in lying-in hospital wards and asylums.[61]

Meigs's text, published in 1856, urged performance of destructive interventions such as craniotomy and hooks when necessary to save the mother. At the same time, Meigs was a proponent of the use of forceps and pelvic measurement. "The whole difficulty in delivering a child through so contracted a pelvis," Meigs said, "can scarcely be conceived by one who has not engaged in such an operation."[62] He connected contracted pelves to rickets, following much the same argument as Cock. Distortion in pelves came from either rickets or *mollities ossium*. Meigs argued that a woman with a "figure 8-shaped" pelvis (identification of the shape of the inlet as a figure 8 on its side which many saw as classically rachitic) immediately get an abortion to avoid a Caesarean section.[63]

Hugh Hodge, emeritus professor, practicing obstetrician and pediatrician at the University of Pennsylvania Hospital, wrote an obstetric text in 1866, a pivotal point in discussions of the deformed pelvis in the United States. The text's introduction included a lengthy rendering of obstetrical history, even as he laid the ground-work for an American obstetrics.[64]

Hodge deemed the idea of deformed pelves as key to obstetrical practice. Displaying his facility with contemporary medical writers and his ability to read German as well as English, Hodge's discussion of the pelves was based on European ideas of the unusual, deformed or contracted pelvis.[65] Hodge presented images of bony pelves, demonstrating the effect of various kinds of contractions. He resisted the idea that contraction of the pelvis itself was unusual. Rather, he enumerated three degrees of "irregular" pelvic contraction, drawing primarily from Baudeloque's external measurements but also from the practice of Smellie, as well as the work of his German contemporaries, Michaëlis and Litzmann. Hodge described how he used his hands and fingers to measure the pelvis through the vagina of a laboring woman (or possibly in the months just before the birth). Hodge articulated the details of a "standard" pelvis and urged that "any great departure from this standard may be regarded as a deformity, and may interfere to a greater or less degree, in proportion to this departure, with the natural process of parturition."[66]

Probing the idea of deformed or diseased pelves, Hodge further drew on the nineteenth-century pioneering work of the French pathologist Xavier Bichat (1771–1802), who referred to the equitable "diminution" (contraction) of the pelvis as opposed to an asymmetrical pelvic narrowing. Hodge showed that the issue of contracted pelves was puzzling and ambiguous in origin. Whatever caused pelvic distortion was not readily apparent or life-threatening until the time of giving birth. Obstetricians had to act on what they knew.[67]

Hodge's treatise considered disproportion of the pelvis and fetal skull to be the central calculation for understanding the progression of a given labor. Hodge, DeWees, Cock and Meigs all referred to disproportion, Cock to the greatest degree. Reflecting his practice and his times, Hodge's concern as an educator focused not so much on anticipation of a coming birth so much as how to deal with the one at hand. He assumed that a physician referencing his book would be attending a birth that seemed stymied or to be going on too long, suggesting that investigating the bony physiology of the laboring woman would help to determine the next step. Disproportion was a heady matter. Hodge maintained that no statistical measure of the pelvis could provide an absolute figure denoting pelvic proportion to the rest of the skeleton. Just as a narrowed pelvis might stop the process of birth, Hodge urged, "a similar disturbance of the progress of labor will be induced if the head of the child be enlarged above its 'standard' dimensions; in other words, the labor may be disturbed, rendered tedious, difficult or impractical, from a disproportion existing between the size of the head and the passages of the pelvis."[68] For Hodge, pelvic contraction was the determinant of obstetrical procedure and the forecast of outcome.[69]

Hodge was a thoroughgoing mechanic. His concerns for birth included presentation or the position of the fetus as labor began in earnest. Fetal presentation at the onset of labor projected the path the fetus was to take during birth unless the attendant intervened. Was the fetus head down and facing backwards, or was it one of the several variations on this "standard" presentation? Obstetricians clarified and categorized presentation in the development of medical education in obstetrics. In Hodge's view, presentation provided a foundation for the choices the obstetrician had to make. In his framework there were several possibilities, including surgical intervention.[70]

The text formulated three degrees of contraction. The first was a three inch measure of the anterior posterior diameter of the superior strait, the *conjugata diagonalis* (sacrum). The second was a three and a half inches of the lateral diameter with a 2–3 inch *conjugata diagonalis*. The third degree was less than 2 inches between the pubis and the *conjugata diagonalis*. Hodge was describing degrees of deformity in flattened and narrowed pelves.[71]

The first degree "irregularly contracted" pelvis might cause fetal death by putting pressure on the fetal head. The dangers were also great for the mother.[72] Here Hodge urged his students to let the labor go ahead without intervention. There was little hope for the infant with the threat of damage done to its cranium.[73] He chronicled the likely result of tears: vesico-vaginal fistulas for the mother. Prolonged pressure of the fetal head on the pelvic floor deoxyfied vaginal tissues, causing death to those tissues. In the most simple and probably most frequent kind of vesico-vaginal fistula, a tear occurred in the vaginal wall, causing urinary incontinence which began some days after birth had occurred.[74]

In cases of second degree deformity Hodge saw a few choices, none of them easy nor likely to produce a positive outcome. If the infant had died, he suggested perforation, which involved bringing the infant out by craniotomy, draining the inside of the head first. If the child lived yet, the alternative was symphysiotomy, the severing of the bony conjunction at the pubic symphysis of the mother, opening up the maternal pelvis to allow the birth of a live baby. This was risky and the aftermath did not promise recovery for the mother, not to mention that she might not regain the ability to walk.[75]

The third-degree distortion of the pelvis offered dire choices as well. Gatrostrohysterotomy, essentially sterilization plus Caesarean section, Hodge saw as preferable to craniotomy. Once again this abdominal procedure (with a very high rate of mortality for the mother) was a chance to save both mother and infant, which Hodge saw as most desirable. He wisely urged obstetrical surgery before labor had gone too far. The lack of antiseptic procedure rendered this an unlikely choice, despite Hodge's enthusiasm, for the intervention.[76]

Hodge built his approach on the conceptualization of distorted pelves as defining of complicated labors. His obstetrical instructions involved procedures well ahead of his time—most physicians were unlikely to proceed with these operative obstetrics. Hodge's text represents historical evidence for obstetrical understanding and possible but not essential direction. Few American physicians acknowledged contracted pelves among their patients. If American physicians acknowledged the condition at all, they believed it a largely European problem. Still, the problem remained relevant to their practice.

* * *

In 1883, Boston physician H.R. Storer published a "Report from the American Medical Association's Committee on Obstetrics" abstracting case reports from twenty-four U.S. journals over the preceding year. From sources ranging from Philadelphia Dispensary Reports to various individual institutions, the committee counted 16,493 obstetrical cases between 1839 and 1883, finding only two contracted pelves, two deformed pelves and 3 pelvic measurements. There was also one case of a Caesarean section done on a woman with a contracted pelvis. The committee added that the only justifiable use of such radical surgery was for a woman in labor with a contracted pelvis.[77]

* * *

Contracted pelves. Much ado about very little? Perhaps, though physicians in Europe and America apparently confronted obstructed birth often enough to consider the problem at length. Obstetrics developed and grew as a science in consequence, in the process redefining both the perception and the culture of childbirth. The veneer of empirical study established a new authority, a regime dedicated to scientific inquiry. The distorted pelvis recognized as a danger, one obvious step was to identify the cause. Attention focused on rickets.

Two

The Riddle of Rickets

By the middle of the nineteenth century, obstetricians in Europe and America were fully conscious of the dangers posed by a distorted pelvis. Vexing questions arose from an awareness developed over more than three centuries. Physicians sought to define the contracted pelvis in exacting terms, invoking ever more precise statistical measures, only to debate the indications identified. How large a pelvis was deemed adequate? More importantly, what was to be done to ameliorate the perils of a pelvis too narrow? If a seemingly healthy woman did possess a contracted pelvis, a birth canal far too small, how had such a condition come to be? Most commonly, doctors pondering the issue offered the same essential answer: rickets. A childhood disease had stunted proper skeletal development. That answer raised the most troublesome issues of all. What was rickets exactly? The cause, the cure? Despite ongoing and historical investigation, the disease proved enigmatic throughout the remainder of the century. Rickets was baffling, and to some extent remains so today.

* * *

The disease is complicated, apt to arise from a variety of conditions tied to both environment and nutrition. How long rickets has plagued humanity is a question impossible to answer; certainly it predates modern times. In the last twenty-five years archaeologists have consciously begun to look for evidence of rickets in the context of industrialization and urban growth. Many writers in the seventeenth, eighteenth and nineteenth centuries concluded that widespread rickets, especially in England and continental Europe, resulted from pollution and other side-effects of industrial development. Recent archaeological studies have sought to verify the perception, only to discover conclusive evidence of rickets—and contracted pelves—at pre-industrial sites both in Europe and America. Armed with a new-found interest in rachitic bone lesions and contracted pelves, archaeologists have made several discoveries of the disease, permitting comparison of its incidence through time.[1]

Newly discovered evidence indicates a considerable incidence of rickets in the days of the Roman Empire. Recognizing that the disease in later times accompanied urban growth, archaeologists at Historic England and McMaster University of Canada investigated eighteen graveyards dated to the Roman era, when urbanization first spread across Europe. The sites, ranging from northern England to southern Spain, yielded 2,787 skeletons for examination. Of the children uncovered, more than 5 percent exhibited the telltale signs of rickets. Shockingly, many of the victims were very young infants. "Some were suffering even in the first few months of life," archaeologist Simon Mays noted. "The inescapable conclusion was that people were keeping their infants indoors too much." English cemeteries saw the highest frequency of the disease, a discovery unsurprising given the subsequent history of rickets.[2]

In 1998, British archaeologists Donald Ortner and Samuel Mays completed examination of a medieval collection of bones found in northern England near York, studied for the express purpose of discovering the presence of rickets. From the remains of adults, young children and infants ranging from AD 950 to 1500 at the Wharram Percy cemetery, the authors found the marked presence of rickets in 8 of 687 skeletons (adults and children), using these cases to develop and demonstrate a paleoarchaeological methodology to research rickets.[3] In the Middle Ages, children were dying with the disease.

The archaeological description of rickets reflects current understanding:

> Essentially [rickets] is a failure to mineralize the protein precursor of bone known as osteoid, complicated by disruption of development at the growth plates. This may result from a deficiency of vitamin D in the diet, failure to absorb vitamin D during digestion, failure by the kidneys to convert vitamin D precursors to vitamin D, inadequate exposure of the skin to ultraviolet light necessary for the conversion of vitamin D precursor to vitamin D, and the failure of the kidneys to retain phosphate, one of the components of bone mineral. Inadequate exposure of the skin to sunlight is the most common factor causing rickets.[4]

Particularly of note is the expression of certitude that underlying malnutrition is significant in the incidence of rickets, a position true in many cases true but ultimately misleading.[5]

Comparing the Wharram Percy site with other graveyards from before and after the beginning of industrialization strongly suggests that industrialization did result in higher infant and child mortality and a notably stronger incidence of severe rickets.[6] In 2002, archaeologist Mary Lewis studied four English graveyards to compare urban conditions in the medieval period with the effects of early industrialization.[7] The focus of Lewis's study was child health as a measure of the impact of the two social historical processes. Based on remains in a London graveyard dating from 1729 to 1859, the study concluded that children's health deteriorated markedly only well after urbanization was underway, and only with the coming of industrialization.[8] The culprit? Rickets. Fifty-four percent of those excavated in the cemetery showed signs of rickets and/or scurvy.[9] Although conclusions regarding the social status of the children found cannot be absolute, for the most part evidence suggests these children came from well-to-do families. Rickets was not simply a disease of the poor and undernourished. Nor was the disease necessarily a product of urban industrialization and accompanying environmental degradation. Archaeological discovery has both confirmed and expanded the historical puzzle of rickets.[10]

* * *

Early writings on the subject came from England. Oxford physician Daniel Whistler (1619–1684) labeled the disease "the rickets" in 1645. The name's folk origins derived from a Saxon word originally used in Dorset, the word *ruckets*, meaning "to breath with difficulty," suggesting the English people actually named the disease before medicine did.[11] Rachitis, the scientific name established in 1650, traces back to a Greek word for spinal disease. The French referred to the condition as "Rachitisme."[12]

Facing what must have been a sizeable outbreak of rickets, Francis Glisson (1597–1677) produced the first examination of the disease in the modern context, publishing *De Rachitude* in 1650. Glisson, physician and professor at Cambridge, thought rickets a new disease, although there was written evidence that it went back at least to the time of Soranus of Ephesus.[13] Glisson also used the name rickets, maintaining that the condition came primarily among the well-nourished children of the well-to-do. (One historian posits that the epidemic was blamed on wet nurses, as wealthy women of the period sent their children out to nurse.[14]) Glisson and hundreds of doctors since have identified the disease by similar appearance and symptoms. With some exceptions, infants and young children were the most common victims. Indigestion and stomach ailments were common. A crooked stance with bowed legs or knock knees, a bent spine probably derived from contracted pelves, swelled joints especially at the extreme end of the long bones, the wrists and the ankles, characterized rickets. Children between one and two years old looked stunted in growth, sometimes uneven in their legs and arms and thorax. The head shape was often noted as peculiar to the disease; it could be long or square but seemed to be larger than the rest of the body—the Olympian forehead. This may have been an illusion, as rickets arrested growth in the child, creating disproportion between the body and the head. Many argued that hydrocephalus, or water on the brain, was very common among rickets victims and caused enlarged skulls. Some saw these children as precocious, others saw them as slow. They had a stillness about them, uncharacteristic of a very young child usually eager to move. Glisson described the affected child as being somewhat listless.[15]

By 1650 many knew rickets as "the English disease." The first to use coal in manufacturing and the heating of homes, the English people endured dark sun-starved days and physical damage from the blackening fuel.[16] The use of coal and atmospheric toxicity continued for centuries. Subsequent ready access to the rachitic skeletal remains of children testified to the extent of the disease's presence. From the 1600s well into the twentieth century, knowledge of rickets came from dissection and autopsies—morbid anatomy. Doctors referred to studies based on skeletons held in medical research laboratories or museums, exemplifying specific variations in the effects of rickets.[17]

Ambiguities, especially by our standards, in the definitions both of rickets and contracted pelves fog the landscape of these years, limiting our ability to know much about women's bodies in labor in the eighteenth century. Probably the innovation and application of forceps involved cases of rickets, just as did Baudeloque's pelvimetry. Glisson identified symptoms of the pediatric condition and named it "rachitis" at nearly the same time that the Chamberlins introduced the forceps to assist childbirth. Ramifications from each remained mostly within separate medical arenas but were relevant to each other. Intermittently, physicians brought understanding of rickets to bear on complications of childbirth as they determined whether the use of forceps might apply. Assumptions made concerning the origins of contracted pelves as rachitic were usually unspoken yet offered one of the strongest explanations for the "deformed" pelvis, even in van Deventer's time.

Over three centuries, practitioners came to perceive a significant threat to childbirth from a deformed or contracted pelvis—a threat increasingly perceived to originate in rickets. That perception transformed the practice of obstetrics. As clinical medicine gained strength, case records began to refer to contracted pelves. Despite the essentially certain connection, specialized physicians rarely elaborated on the connection of contracted pelves in adults to the rickets of children, although that relationship was assumed. Investigators considered the contracted pelvis only in the context of labor and childbirth, seeking effective methods of intervention in difficult delivery. By the end of the nineteenth century, in the midst of a pandemic of rickets, many physicians argued that the disease threatened the lives of women giving birth. First European doctors, then

Americans, reaffirmed the determination of rickets as the source of contracted pelves. Rickets became an international context for growing medical intervention in birth.[18]

* * *

Attention to rickets became especially prominent in the nineteenth century, when physicians and scientists elaborated on early studies of the disease. Practicing in London, Sir William Jenner (1815–1898) provided a profile of patients and a portrait of the progression of the disease. Many of his contemporaries heralded the details of his lectures to medical students of 1859 and 1860; so much so that they were printed in 1895. Jenner drew upon the experiences of Charles West (1816–1898), a contemporary English children's doctor, to emphasize the pervasiveness of rickets among children in Great Britain and urge physicians and parents to watch for early symptoms. These included signs that medical scientists witnessed repeatedly. Failure to walk at the usual age suggested the beginnings of the disease. Indigestion indicated possible rickets. Slow dentition, infant teeth erupting after the first year or later and early loss of teeth and decrepitude of teeth warned of the presence of rickets. Jenner emphasized that rickets was a general disease, not simply in the bones but in the whole body. As the condition progressed the child became emaciated with a swelled and hardened belly; the spleen swelled and the liver hardened. In his lectures Jenner discussed the pain the child felt in response to touch. Young children lay still with their arms outstretched so as not to arouse pain. They avoided physical contact with parents and other children. As the disease progressed, some children could no longer hold their heads up. Jenner shared Glisson's understanding that rickets was a disease associated with seemingly healthy, fat babies as well as children visibly failing to thrive. Later in the disease, about the age of a toddler, children's bodies became crooked and misshapen from the pliability of bones, especially long bones, as they stood erect. When rachitic bones weakened, sitting up caused pressure on the pelvis and resulted in narrowing. Walking caused bowing of the leg bones. At the same time bones thickened. Jenner and other physicians of the second half of the nineteenth century, throughout Europe, the British Isles and the United States, saw pelvic deformity originating in a child between one and two years old. First the long bones lost their shape, then the joints swelled. Not only should children not sit up too early, but they should also not put weight on their legs for fear of bowing them.[19]

In very young children, Jenner and many others observed the infant's cranial bone sutures. The fontanelle, or the infant's soft spot, closed much more slowly for a patient with rickets, providing an early symptom of the presence of the disease. The sutures bringing skull bones together gapped in some cases or failed to meet completely, especially around the occipital bone at the back of the head, creating soft spots known as craniotabes. Jenner carefully detailed all these symptoms, with a warning (no doubt influenced by Polish pathologist Rudolf Virchow [1821–1902]) that rickets was systemic and not localized in any one bone alone but in all bones, arguing that "rickets, then, is essentially and purely a disease of nutrition, not of one part only, but of the whole body."[20] Abraham Jacobi (1830–1919), a New York physician and premier early pediatrician, concurred with Jenner's interpretation regarding craniotabes, urging practitioners to look for them to catch the disease early and begin treatments.[21]

Practicing in Germany, Rudolf Virchow offered an unusual point of view. An accomplished anatomist, Virchow employed cadaveric dissection to study bone cells, establishing a new understanding of cellular activity: "all cells from cells."[22] Rather than resulting from spontaneous generation, life was entirely cell-based.[23] Lecturing at his Physiological Institute in 1847, Virchow used the study of rickets to demonstrate his cell theory. The disease was becoming increasingly significant in the 1840s and 1850s, both in Germany and internationally. Employing microscopic images of cells from tumorous tissues in a goat's jaw, Virchow exhibited the chaos in bone growth resulting from disease.[24] The jawbone exemplified normal bone growth at the cellular level and also cartilage calcification and a variety of interruptions in bone growth. His slides, subsequently published and translated, showed the "normal processes of bone formation" and the visible irregularities in calcification from rickets.[25] Through this example Virchow established that rickets was not about bones softening or exudation (oozing) at the epiphyses as previously understood, but about pathological growth of bone. The example of rachitic bone cells provided Virchow with pathological cells for comparison with layers of bone growth in normal cells. His lecture showed students and fellow medical professionals how bone tissue developed as cartilage and explained the early formation of marrow spaces. Analyzing rachitic tissue, Virchow demonstrated a new way to look at sickness at the cellular level. The disease appeared in the bone but involved more than a locus in the bone.[26]

Not all were convinced. American obstetrician Hugh Hodge, viewing rickets as the origin of "irregularly contracted pelves,"[27] focused on early formation of skeletal and especially pelvic distortion as the infant sat up and learned to walk. Ever the mechanic, Hodge looked at the human body as a machine, contending that the weight of the anatomy on developing bones brought distortion. Hodge noted the contention of other writers that young children should stay still to avoid bowed legs and other skeletal strains. The simple act of sitting could put pressure on the pelvis, causing deformity. In many practitioners' minds, rickets seemed to predispose the individual to varieties of pelvic irregularity. Medical scientists in the 1920s labeled this a "mechanical theory," an alternative to Virchow's cellular concept.[28]

* * *

An ongoing problem in the identification and comprehension of rickets was misidentification with seemingly related diseases. In his lectures from 1860, William Jenner set about to distinguish rickets from tuberculosis, syphilis, and scrofula, these being the four key diatheses—particular constitutional susceptibilities or vulnerability to given diseases—he perceived among children. According to Jenner, rickets occurred more often than the other three. He identified the symptoms of each disease and showed how each was distinct yet connected. Scrofula is a specific form of tuberculosis affecting the throat, which Jenner dismissed. The diatheses thus become a triad: syphilis, tuberculosis and rachitis—a pervasive threesome of disease persisting through the mid–1930s.[29]

Based on the concept of diathesis, a rachitic child probably also had syphilis or tuberculosis, or was likely to come down with one or the other in the future. A physician often encountered a child carrying two or more of the diseases. Tuberculosis and syphilis were life-threatening illnesses not easily treated. Rickets had the potential to heal in the early years of life if caught early enough and turned around, but was also liable to recur. Advanced rickets had the potential to kill when the thorax became misshapen; when another disease developed breathing became difficult. Measles, scarlet fever, whooping cough, diphtheria and other childhood diseases increased the likelihood of such a child's death.[30]

Weak rickety children with tuberculosis or syphilis faced an uncertain future. Jenner and Jacobi understood a diagnosis of rickets to mean a child was likely to have tuberculosis or syphilis or scrofula and easily might die from the combination. In such cases, death certificates rarely revealed rickets as an underlying condition. In one case Jenner described a six-year-old girl who suffered from extreme rickets. For years she could not walk. She finally learned to walk, only to fall down the stairs to die from weakness in the aftermath. She suffered from tuberculosis, which for the record was the cause of death.[31] With the diatheses of so many seemingly related diseases, nineteenth-century physicians often saw rickets as secondary to some other affliction resulting in the death of a child. If a fatality did occur, the cause was generally attributed to a different condition.[32] Much the same proved true for women in childbirth. If a woman with a pelvis warped by rickets died while giving birth, the record rarely reported her death as caused by rickets.[33]

Doctors in the past often variously categorized as rickets what are several diseases in today's medicine. Hunchbacks and other spinal ailments for instance came under the category of rachitic.[34] Many confused scurvy with rickets since scurvy involved bones and teeth. In the late nineteenth century Thomas Barlow, an English children's physician, urged some distinction between scurvy and rickets, arguing strongly that what many called acute rickets was in fact scurvy. Hemorrhage (which typified scurvy) beneath the skin caused swelling and epidermal pain much like but different from rickets. Barlow clarified the distinction between the two but ignored the fact that they so often occurred together.[35]

Other disorders resembled rickets. Tetany, a muscular syndrome, shared many symptoms. Rarely did a patient have tetany without first having rickets. In the nineteenth-century physicians treated them more or less as the same disease. *Laryngysmus stridulus*, spasms in the throat, including a crowing cough, were attributed to both tetany and rickets. Convulsions and a contraction of the wrists and hands in spasms also characterize tetany. Eventually separating the diseases, doctors diagnosed tetany by identifying elevated phosphorus and low levels of calcium in the blood in the 1910s.[36]

Osteomalacia, a disease afflicting mature women, found a separate definition from rickets. Extreme softening of the bones made adult women so fragile they could barely sit up. Physicians recognized such cases almost exclusively among parturient women and treated them as anomalies. Only recently have scientists declared osteomalacia as essentially an adult form of rickets, derived from the same causation. Osteomalacia is increasingly common in the United States among older women today.[37]

As Jenner noted, concurrent affliction of diseases in an individual child contributed to confusing diagnosis, syphilis serving as an example. Presence of the disease tainted the treatment of rickets patients, as society at large and medical practitioners specifically often considered syphilis patients to be morally compromised.[38] Race, class and sex juxtaposed, making it much easier to blame the disease on those with little power—particularly women and children of other races and classes. Inheritance of syphilis indicated "predisposition to a host of other disorders including … general underdevelopment and idiocy."[39] The disease itself was complicated. Unlike rickets, doctors understood syphilis to come from contagion of an unknown origin. While newborns frequently showed immediate symptoms of syphilis, they debated whether babies were ever born with an established case of rickets. Illustrating the confusion, the French doctor Antoine Portal (1742–1832) early in the nineteenth century recommended treating a rickets patient with anti-syphilitic and anti-scrofular medicines.[40]

* * *

How prevalent a disease was rickets? Where was the condition most likely to be found, among what manner of people? By the middle of the nineteenth century, awareness of rickets had grown to a point where determined efforts to answer such questions began.

Situating sickness in the environment came out of an earlier medical tradition which stressed human health as tied to nature. Balance in that relationship created good health: imbalance, sickness. Climate and geography dominated medicine as interpretive tools and as significant factors before laboratory science uncovered and declared the potency of microorganisms.[41] The nineteenth-century industrializing environment—or human habitat—experienced multiple changes, especially in the soil, air and atmosphere, biomass and water. Toxicities including sulfur dioxide permeated the atmosphere. Often times social and political leaders were unaware of the adverse effects of industrialization on the human habitat.[42] Though leaders were unaware of industrialization's effects on human health, rickets must be studied in a framework emphasizing the connections to environmental history.[43]

An outstanding example derives from the work of August Hirsch (1817–1894), who taught medicine in Berlin, Germany, where both rickets and industrialization made their mark. Berlin was growing at a rapid rate in the 1870s and 1880s; immigrants flocked to the city, only to live in poorly-built and crowded tenement houses. Smog darkened the sky; the sun rarely broke through the atmospheric layers. Children found few places to play outdoors.[44] Holding a professorship awarded largely as recognition of his two volume *Handbook of Geographical and Historical Pathology,* Hirsch recognized the growing incidence of rickets in a second edition published in 1886. Perceiving geography as central, Hirsch linked the epidemiology of various diseases to geographical region. While not fully understanding the details of environmental change, he drew attention to the lack of knowledge concerning the global historical geography of disease.[45]

Although Hirsch acknowledged an agreement among physicians internationally that many more very poor children suffered from rickets and suffered the worst cases, he felt that the disease—occurring also among children of wealthy parents—showed the secondary importance of diet in the disease's origin. He called the dietary factor, including the weak diet of poor children and the issue of breast milk versus artificial feeding of infants—"errors of hygiene in the child's upbringing."[46] Artificial or "bad food" was partly to blame for rickets, but was secondary to geography in terms of climate, the lack of fresh air, and the absence of outdoor activity. He maintained, "the air is saturated with moisture and tainted with the products of organic decomposition."[47] Hirsch forcefully argued that the environment could cause rickets and that medical scientists ought first to carefully gather data on the incidence of rickets around the world before pronouncing the origin of rickets. The statistics at hand had little value.

Geography seemed basic to understanding of disease etiology, Hirsch thought, though he declared the evidence for rickets meager. Hirsch's work built on the already extensive international publication on rickets. In his presentation, latitude clearly showed climatic affinities for the occurrence of rickets. Common knowledge and observations over time demonstrated that the tropical zones had virtually no cases, while the temperate zone, including Europe and North America, had many. Higher and lower latitudes showed very few cases. Hirsch and other scientists were puzzled that Greenland, Denmark, and Sweden experienced no rickets. "Its principal seats are Germany, England, Holland, Belgium, France, and Northern Italy."[48] Greece, Turkey, Southern Italy had virtually no rickets, but rickets occurred in Beirut. In North America, Hirsch's research in medical journals and institutional records found cases in several large central cities—Cincinnati, Baltimore, New York, Philadelphia. His geographical emphasis stirred further investigations.[49]

Recognizing connection between place and disease, many living in England knew the British Isles to have the most cases and the deepest history of rickets. Following Hirsch's lead, the British Medical Association established a committee to investigate the geographical distribution of rickets, as well as rheumatism, chorea, cancer, and urinary calculus. Directed by Sir Isambard Owen (1850–1927), the report found differences in the environmental impact on the various diseases. Rickets had a decided presence in urban and industrialized areas, and rural locales such as mines and coalfields, along with seaports. Accompanying maps illustrated the presence of each disease, color coded to show the most disease-ridden areas.[50] The maps clarified the boundaries of rickets in the population and its clear association with identifiable geographical areas; blue areas represented solid rickets while red and purple sectors were rickets-free or mostly free. The landscape of rickets varied somewhat. Major industrial centers such as Lancashire, Manchester, Cheshire, Yorkshire and some rural areas—the coal fields between Birmingham and Wilverton for instance—presented almost solid blue. In northern Scotland, Glasgow was another center of nearly "universal" rickets, as the author put it. Coal-related areas of South Wales contained a strong presence of rickets while in Ireland, Dublin and Belfast had the worst outbreaks of the disease.[51] English men and women wondered why they should have rickets—the English disease—while other peoples deemed inferior had little or none.

There was rickets in the industrializing United States as well. Archaeological studies demonstrate a clear connection between African American populations and the disease. Recent digs at African American graveyards provide data establishing and clarifying the presence of rickets in skeletons and the relationship to historical contexts, including slavery, industrialization and other factors influencing social status. In a seventeenth- and eighteenth-century African Burial Ground in Manhattan uncovered in 1992, archaeologists found abundant evidence of weakened bones and high infant and female mortality rates. Women too suffered from poor diet—: "skeletal evidence of rickets, stress from malnutrition, and teeth worn down to stubs from chewing whole grains."[52] Of 419 men, women, and children's bodies excavated, almost half were children under twelve. Most of those buried were born in Africa. Bowed limbs were the surest sign of rachitic disease in the cadavers. For bones to become bowed or misshapen the afflicted had to be mobile—not a newborn infant. The disturbing evidence showed slavery was particularly brutal in New York City; the demographics of the dead implicate rickets and slavery in the inability of children to live to adulthood and for the slaves to reproduce.

Archaeologists have also studied skeletal remains from an antebellum free African American community in Philadelphia dating from 1823 to 1848.[53] The churchyard of the Philadelphia First African Baptist Church revealed signs of rickets in the remains of 108 individuals. Buried at the site were thirty-six men, thirty-nine women, thirty-three infants under one year of age and twenty-seven older children. Historical records indicate most members of this church were free Blacks, never enslaved. Thirty percent of the adults had signs of healed rickets and ten percent of the children had active rickets at the time of death. Archaeologists observed bowed leg bones in both children's skeletons and those of the adults—certain to be the effects of rickets. Thirty-five percent of male bones and twenty percent of female leg bones showed bowing. The average adult female pelvic brim index was small, meaning the bony true pelvis—the top half—was unusually narrowed and flattened in all the females, indicating the presence of a contracted pelvis, a hallmark of rickets. There were also marks of malnutrition which exacerbated the effects of the disease.[54] Judging by the skeletons, the study concluded that the average age of death for women was 38.9 years, men, 44.9. Warped female pelves and further evidence of diseases of growth, along with evidence of difficult childbirth, marked several remains. The findings provide rare evidence regarding the health of African Americans engaged in the labor force of early American industrialization.[55]

This study compared the ill health apparent in the skeletons of the

Philadelphia individuals to that of a group from the same time period, made up of industrial slaves in Maryland, concluding that similarity between the two groups predominated. Industrialization figured in the context for both groups and helped to explain the individual's health status at death. While the archaeological evidence cannot answer quantitatively how much rickets occurred overall and does not answer definitively where it came from—such material evidence reminds us that there were pockets of life—communities—where rickets commonly affected man, woman, and child alike.[56]

Statistical evidence for the extent of rickets and associated ethnicity in nineteenth-century America appears in the *Mortality Statistics of the 7th Census of the United States, 1850*, administered by J.D.B. DeBow. The census, though sparse in terms of numerical significance, shows respect for the potency of the disease and outlines a mortality from rickets across region and race—evidence contrary to the common assumption among historians that rickets went unrecorded because no one considered the condition a cause of death. The census provides a glimpse of mortality from rickets, one of sixty-one listed conditions reported by census marshals and enumerated state by state.[57] Edward Jarvis, Massachusetts's consulting physician to the census, suggested changes to the organizing language and statistics but did not question "rickets" as a mortal disease.[58] At Jarvis's behest, a final statement of all the names of disease categories used in the census appeared at the end of the report. Each enumerated death was counted under a single category, including "rickets," with twenty-one states reporting mortalities. Pennsylvania and Tennessee had the most deaths, ten mortalities in each. Fourteen states listed one or two such deaths. The remaining seven states reported between two and ten.[59]

Enumerated with mortal rickets were northern, southern, central, and midwestern states, mostly among infants and young children, whose deaths were reported as sixty-three out of seventy-three cases—86 percent.[60] Admittedly there is ambiguity about what rickets meant to the census takers, as eight different seemingly minor conditions were subsumed under rickets, including ringworm. DeBow's report was not lacking for statistical anomalies. Still, the census offers significant insight into perceptions of the disease in 1850. Judging from the report, both whites and African Americans suffered from severe rickets, but the latter suffered in greater proportion to their presence in the population.[61]

* * *

In the second half of the nineteenth century, investigations into rickets turned more and more to the multiple facets of its environmental setting. The troubling recognition of large concentrations of rickets in industrializing nations fostered two closely inter-related quests. The more pressing was the search for a cure—the obvious goal of the health profession. But finding a cure rested to a large extent on comprehending the cause of the disease, and that was a mystery. Ongoing research did suggest nutritional deficiencies lay at the root of rachitic suffering, a possibility contradicted by the maddening existence of rickets in well-fed children. The widespread presence of the disease in definable geographic settings suggested a latitudinal, climatic, or environmental factor, though such hypotheses raised far more questions than answers. Other researchers sought underlying causation in differences of human physiology, offering suppositions based on heredity and race. Failing to establish a definitive cause, finding a cure proved exceedingly elusive.

Since the "English Disease" first appeared and came to be understood as a disease of growth, medical practitioners naturally turned their attention to questions of diet. Nurture is culturally and historically constructed, altering through time. Ever since Glisson's *De Rachitide,* students had puzzled over the interrelationship of rickets, poverty and poor nutrition. Glisson considered the disease as originating primarily in overfeeding. Yet in the nineteenth century, the predominance of poor patients led many to consider inadequacies of nutrition as a key to the disease.[62]

Long before much was known about rickets, chemists began to experiment with the elements of phosphorus and calcium in relation to human metabolism. Using cadaveric bones, researchers ascertained that calcium phosphate formed the hard cover of bones and teeth. With that knowledge they began to explore the mineralization of bone during growth, using various salt compounds. As early as 1801, Swedish chemist Jons Jacob Berzelius isolated the ratio of calcium to phosphate in the body—eventually an essential clue to evaluating the degree of rickets in a given patient. By the middle of the century, scientists had discovered the importance of lime salts in bone for supplying phosphorus, and further identified the increased excretion of lime salts in urine as symptomatic of rickets. The chemistry of bone mineralization came to inform medical understanding of the disease. Lime salts became a popular compound at apothecaries.[63]

Justus von Liebig (1803–1873), a German chemist with a wide following among English physicians in the 1840s and '50s, expanded the reach of chemistry into nutrition.[64] Liebig established a new area in physiological chemistry, closely tied to his laboratory teaching and study of the "energy-producing function of food through techniques of controlled measurement."[65] Categorizing food into carbohydrates, fat and protein, Liebig's studies investigated respiration and oxidation as part of digestion—exploring food as fuel for animal and human bodies.[66] American author Henry David Thoreau took considerable interest in his work, noting, "According to Liebig, man's body is a stove, and the food the fuel which keeps up the internal combustion in the lungs."[67] Relying on laboratory experimentation with animals, Liebig sought to "lay bare the chemical relationships between the inorganic world and plant and animal life."[68] Though parts of his science were later disproved, Liebig and others who had similar interests contributed to a new scientific interest in nutrition, metabolism and food, laying a necessary foundation for the rise of agricultural science and biochemistry by the end of the century.[69]

Liebig's research helped generate celebrated English physician John Snow's (1813–1858) study of rickets in relation to variations in breadmaking. Renowned for his successful investigation into cholera in London, Snow's venture into rickets came toward the end of his career. Snow compared certain nutritional aspects of poor communities in London, where rickets was common, to smaller rural villages in Northern England where poverty existed but not rickets. After eliminating milk as a factor, Snow considered differences in the types of bread consumed between the city and the smaller villages. In London, for lack of cheap fuel for baking, most bought bread from bakers, while in the small villages nearly all made their own bread at home. Commercial bakers used alum, sometimes in illegally high quantities, most likely to whiten the bread. Snow recognized that the alum blocked the body's absorption of calcium and phosphate (found in lime salts), causing rickets.[70]

Sir William Jenner wove nutrition into his theoretic framework for the diathesis of rickets in 1895. Jenner understood rickets to be a disease of nutrition in which there were four agents: "the nerves, the cells, the blood, and the blood-vessels."[71]

> In rickets ... there is necessarily no pathological exudation or new formation [of bone]; there is, so far as we know, merely a change in quantity and arrangement of normal structures and secretions. This is true not only of the bones and muscles, but of the secretions of the skin and kidney. Rickets, then is essentially and purely a disease of nutrition, not of one part only, but of the whole body.[72]

The question of how nutrition and rickets intersected persisted. Physicians more steadily involved in the treatment of rickets patients began to use lime phosphate and calcium phosphate in treating patients.[73] Many saw a link between the imbalance in the diet of the working class and the onset of rickets, though no specific evidence emerged. Others worried about the food newborns and infants received, debating the question of milk in the infant diet, along with breastfeeding and weaning issues. Most, like Jenner, argued that the mother rather than a wetnurse should breastfeed the child, and not for too prolonged a time period. Some doctors dabbled in

Two. The Riddle of Rickets 45

the growing practice of physician-prescribed supplemental infant feedings as a therapy and prophylactic. Inconsistencies arose as physicians observed specifically-identified populations and found no certain correlation between breastfeeding practices and a child's coming down with the disease. Treating the disease confused practitioners because of its inconsistency of incidence. Rickets predominated among poorer working class people but existed across lines of economic status.[74]

Nutrition was a vague word in the nineteenth century, ambiguous and new to the parlance. August Hirsch saw nutrition as important, but in a different sense: "All the authorities are agreed that the morbid process [of rickets] is fundamentally a disorder of nutrition, having its root either in something wrong with the upbringing of the child itself, that is to say an acquired condition, or in a morbid diathesis born with it."[75] His language reveals the polar possibilities—rickets, both hereditary and environmentally caused. The inconsistency in incidence of rickets came from ambiguous data regarding the presence of the disease among the very poor and the very rich. Just as importantly, geographical inquiry had uncovered that malnutrition offered an insufficient explanation as the origin of the disease. In one way or another, environment looked to be involved. That realization opened the door to a considerable range of possibilities.

* * *

The nineteenth-century industrial environment—a new form of human habitat—brought multiple changes, especially in the soil, air and atmosphere, biomass and water.[76] Toxicities permeated the landscape. Even the urban household could become an important a source of disease. A strong belief in science and technology as progress blinded many to the possibilities of dangerous repercussions for humans. Often times social and political leaders were unaware of the adverse effects of industrialization on human health, or denied the likelihood of adverse effect.[77]

Seeing that many white children in Northern Europe suffered rickets, yet many other children of various skin colors from different cultures and nations around the world did not, European and American researchers (anthropologists and medical scientists alike) began to look around the globe for answers to the riddle of rickets. Europeans were impressed by the lack of rickets in poor tropical regions. Colonization of countries in the southern hemisphere brought experience of diverse ethnicities and cultures; rickets did occur in some settings, but minimally. Rickets was the "English disease," mainly afflicting those of European descent. Adolfo Murillo, a Chilean obstetrician, offered some perspective at an 1894 pan–American medical conference, obviating the false dichotomy claiming European superiority. Chileans experienced well-managed and uncomplicated births; the industrialized northern hemisphere suffered widespread rachitic disease.[78] By the late 1800s, many observers found an explanation for international rickets in the rapidly growing industrial environment.

Changing the environment seemed the solution to rickets. Urban crowding, polluted air, "the want of free air" and exercise all contributed to the high prevalence of the disease among children.[79] Most geographic studies noted a seasonal shift in the incidence of rickets, "coming into sudden prominence in the spring, only to disappear in the early summer," suggesting that climatic patterns, the amount of sunlight seasonably available in temperate latitudes, might play a role. Children born in the late summer and autumn had a much greater chance of suffering from the disease the following spring.[80] Abundant sunlight served perhaps as preventative or possibly even a cure for rickets—some less severe cases healed with the coming of summer. William Buchan (1729–1805), a Scottish doctor of the late eighteenth century, had described rickets as a disease treatable by outdoor exercise—better known fifty years later as the necessity of play in childhood. He maintained the importance of open air. "It is a common notion, that if children are set upon their feet too soon, their legs will become crooked." Not so, he protested. "The limbs of children are weak indeed, but their bodies are proportionably light; and had they skill to direct themselves, they would soon be able to support themselves."[81] Popular Scottish writer Andrew Combe (1797–1847) pleaded much the same case in the mid- and late-nineteenth century.[82] In the 1820s, Polish physician Jedrzej Sniadecki (1768–1838) transported sickly children from industrial Warsaw to open spaces in the countryside, providing an opportunity to play in the sunshine. His efforts were ignored.[83]

Seasonal change may have influenced the presence of rickets, but little was done to systematically study the influence of the seasons until after World War I. Most cautious physicians accepted the observation of seasonal impact only by qualifying it with the importance of other factors.[84]

* * *

An enduring piece of folk wisdom involved treatment of rickets with cod liver oil. Those who fished the Atlantic in Northern Europe, including Northern Scotland, used the fat laden oil as a powerfully effective remedy for hundreds of years—keeping people in a Northern sun-reduced and prolonged winter context free of rickets. At one time cod liver oil had gourmet status. Use began with treatment of rheumatism and developed quickly to treat other conditions, including rickets. By the early 1820s Dutch scientists urged further exploration of the remedy's chemical properties, offering a prize for the best essay. Communicating to a Berlin medical journal in 1824, the German physician D. Schütte reported the effective use of cod liver oil in treatment of rickets.[85]

While there was a long successful tradition of using this treatment, most physicians throughout Europe caught on to its beneficial properties quite late, never understood why the oil worked, and by the end of the 1800s relied on it less and less. Unlike English and German practitioners, the French did adhere to its medicinal value, declaring the substance delectable. Armond Trousseau (1801–1867), Parisian professor of clinical medicine and rickets expert, repeatedly recommended the use of cod liver oil in the 1870s, only to abandon the practice toward the end of his career.[86] Trousseau first learned about the potential cure cod liver oil represented from his teacher, who in turn had heard of the oil's success via a patient from Holland whose parents swore by it.[87] Interest continued. Famed physician Antoine Marfan (1858–1942) was an advocate of cod liver oil well into the twentieth century, though he looked past the oil for the disease etiology and held to the idea that some yet-unidentified infection or toxicity served as the basis of the disease. Marfan suspected the root cause was syphilis.[88]

Ironically, the perception of rickets as a nutritional disease helped to supplant use of cod liver oil. Reasons for the falling-off in therapeutic use of the substance varied. Cod liver oil had drawbacks in its indigestibility and strong taste.[89] By the second half of the nineteenth century, physicians were trying a variety of remedies and struggling to isolate them. In 1882, Max Kassowitz (1842–1913), a leading Viennese expert on rickets and its treatment, began advocating the importance of phosphorus in treating the disease. Phosphorus did help patients, but in experiments, doctors, especially Kassowitz, often put phosphorus in a base of cod liver oil. Kassowitz convinced others that it was the phosphorus and not the cod liver oil that remedied the disease.[90]

By the close of the century, those who advocated cod liver oil were few.[91] Though geographic studies showed that in temperate climates where residents used cod liver oil—the fishing countries of the far northern hemisphere—there was no incidence of rickets, the logic of the oil as a prophylactic or remedy lost hold. According to pharmacology historian Aaron Ihde, this was the period of "Dreckapotheke"—distrust of the use of an apothecary treatment from the past. Germ theory had gained such a strong following by 1900 that medical practitioners and researchers expected a sudden, specific and presumably microscopic disclosure of the origin of rickets.[92] Folk remedies found few advocates.

* * *

To some nineteenth-century practitioners, nutritional considerations and environmental influence seemed at best partial answers. Treatments involving diet or fresh air may have helped to some degree, but did little to explain the rampant presence of rickets. That the disease was so endemic in such widespread quarters of defined populations suggested a pre-disposition, a natural susceptibility to contraction of the condition. Inheritance *versus* environment posed a different question for medicine concerning the origins of diseases and sometimes the nature of therapy. Questions about the heredity of syphilis, rickets and other diseases persisted throughout the nineteenth and into the twentieth century.

The concept of diathesis—constitutional susceptibility to specific diseases—provided an explanation combining inheritance and environmental influence into one. Doctors understood that a rickety child was vulnerable to other life-threatening diseases and more likely to die. William Jenner insisted that physical, mental, familial and environmental factors contributed to the diathesis of rickets, meaning certain babies and very young children were more likely to fall victim, depending on circumstance. A diathesis denoted a permanent vulnerability to one disease and a secondary vulnerability to other diseases—"pathological tendencies" which "we do not call disease." Rickets was systemic, not a disease limited to the bone, but instead "a general disease."[93]

Calling rickets a diathesis masked uncertainties. Despite his insistence on diathesis, William Jenner wavered between environment and heredity as the ultimate cause, much as Hirsch waffled. Their contentions confound our present day dichotomy of nature *versus* nurture. Jenner admitted, "I know of no facts to prove that rickets is hereditary. The health of the mother, however, has a decided influence on the development of rickets in the child. Whatever renders her delicate, whatever depresses her powers of forming good blood, *that* tends to induce rickets in the offspring."[94]

Neither delicacy nor anemia was passed down, Jenner added, rather rickets came from too little iron. Mothers made a strong impression on the health of the child—including "forming good blood," or not. Jenner took the argument further to maintain that poverty might make the parents "worse fed, worse clothed, and worse lodged," their health problems exacerbated by bearing too many children.[95] Yet wealthy parents with too many children also resulted in a weakened mother with rickety children. The more Jenner focused on motherhood the more he saw the need for proper knowledge of when and how and with what to feed the child—including the emphasis many shared on breastfeeding's pivotal role. In addition to the hygiene of the mother, the target for his blame became largely but not exclusively, the lifestyle of the poor.[96]

Consideration of motherhood was central to the ongoing analyses of rachitic disease. Although most doctors and medical researchers thought babies were never born with rickets, Jenner and many of the succeeding generation of physicians argued the existence of inherent weakness as a setting for the onset of the disease. Simply look at the health of the mother, they said, to find the propensity of a child to suffer rickets. This point of view mediated the polarity of nature and nurture. Mothers were part of the fetal environment but were also united as one with the fetus before birth, passing on inherited characteristics. Victorian culture placed mothers at the center of society, though in reality the culturally ascribed meaning of motherhood shifted according to class and race.[97]

Nineteenth century ideas of heredity varied greatly from the gene-based, essentially biological definition found in genetics today. Nature *versus* nurture, or heredity *versus* environment, posed a different question. Scholars and scientists thought climate and the environment shaped the individual on many levels, having a more direct role in the individual's health and heredity than we grant today. Try as they might to separate explanations, physicians and scientists brought both the environment and heredity together to explain the disease, struggling to clarify the context. Heredity and environment offered opposing poles of explanation. Although many recognized industrialization as linked to rickets, most assigned filth, dirt, and poverty as the real cause. Such conditions could be blamed on congenital habits.[98]

* * *

Underlying the suspicions regarding a hereditary component to rickets was a far more insidious assumption. If a pre-disposition to the contraction of rickets was passed through the bloodlines, which bloodlines were at issue? Researchers had at hand a ready answer, steeped in western tradition stretching back through the millennia, fully supported by more recent "scientific" investigation. To the minds of far too many practitioners, no biological characteristic was more heritable than race. In Europe, and even more so in America, steadfast adherence to racial stereotype did more to cloud the investigation of rickets than any other factor.

Three

The Impediment of Race

A great many ironies cloud the legacy of the Scientific Revolution. The history of science regards Francis Bacon as the first to emphasize empirical methodology in the investigation of nature, often overlooking the Englishman's stated purpose in developing the scientific method: human domination and control of the natural world. The intent, constructed on the assumption that "man, if we look to final causes, may be regarded as the center of the world,"[1] inspired anthropocentric constructions founded on no empirical evidence at all. Chief among these was an artifice known to respected savants throughout the western world as the "Great Chain of Being." The Chain was nothing more than a reflection of European self-centered identity, an expression of faith in their own sacredness, cloaked in the façade of science. More to the point, the construction was a vehicle employed to promote and sustain both racism and sexism in European thought.[2]

A chain is a series of links joined together to form a single fiber. The image of linkage was essential—the Great Chain of Being was a hierarchical strand embodying all life, with God at the upper end, those newly-discovered little one-celled creatures the last link. The concept had been around since ancient times, but found new credence with the advent of science. "Man" was generally thought to be in the middle, the highest among the animate forms found on earth, linked to the lowest form of myriad angelic spirits. Each animate form connected to the next lower, down through the whole of creation. Defining the order of beings grew to be the great challenge of natural science—which creature ranked higher than which? Comparing cadaveric bones of many species, scientists were busy at work by the late 1700s, constructing the chain.[3]

A reasonably obvious assumption (note: these were all assumptions) was a link between humans and some form of the great apes. The orangutan, maybe. But certainly not all kinds of humans were linked to apes directly. By the late eighteenth century, racial classification had entered the picture, European investigators defining their own type as the highest link. Just how many human types existed was much debated; Swedish taxonomist Carl Linneaus listed four, based on continental location and skin color. No matter who did the counting, African Blacks—"Hottentots"—ranked lowest. Race had become a biological determination.[4]

Anthropology in eighteenth and nineteenth centuries led the way in establishing race as a social, political and economic organizing principle—the fundamental classification of human beings.[5] Physical anthropology, the study of bones and fossils, had a particularly central role in defining race, based on skeletal measurement. In its early history, even before the field's specialization was in place, physical anthropologists were "concerned with recording and analyzing the nature and sources of hereditary human variation, a topic customarily reduced to the label of race." Boundaries between disciplines were fluid, not separating medicine from anthropology. The human study of humanity helps to unfold the story of race, rickets and obstetrics.[6]

By the nineteenth century, European anthropologists had established a widely accepted system of classification, creating a hierarchical ranking of five races, despite the lack of empirical evidence. Typology provided the basis for race science. Studies of skull and pelvic differentiation perpetuated a long-standing belief that the differences among racial groups provided a foundation for a hierarchy of peoples, with white Northern Europeans at the top and Black Africans on the bottom, the "link" to non-human primates. Race designations would vary from era to era, but belief in the superiority of Caucasians would endure. Medical researchers in Europe and American readily adopted such hierarchies, with whites (and males) afforded the highest rank.[7]

The pseudo-science of racial classification took shape amidst far older perceptions of race persisting throughout Europe. From at the very least the time of the Greek philosophers, various cultures recognized differences in appearance and behavior, generally attributing the disparities to location and environment. Expanding the frontiers of empire in western Europe, the Romans encountered what they saw as three types of barbarians: Gauls, Germans, and Celts. With the passage of time, these came to be seen as races of people—biologically, culturally, archaeologically—each with their own identifiable peculiarities. Subdivided by history and geography, they became the Irish race, the Scottish and so forth.[8] The distinctions influenced medical researchers. Writing in 1865, J.M. Guardia, a Frenchman, published a history of medicine including a chapter on anthropological theories, arguing that racial characteristics influenced susceptibility to disease.[9]

Looking at a small piece of the Irish experience offers a glimpse of how assumptions of racial superiority blocked objective understanding of rickets. The British identified the Irish as different—a separate race. Overtaking Ireland beginning in the early 1600s (at the very time rickets was spreading rapidly in England) the British put the Irish on reservations and proceeded to populate the island with English and Scots colonists. Famines resulted; over hundreds of years the Irish suffered from intermittent malnutrition and starvation. British overlords made little effort to maintain records of health among the Irish natives, largely failing to track even mortality.[10]

Despite the widespread certitude that rickets was an English disease prevalent in urban settings, there was some association of the rural Irish with rickets. A story comes out of the famine years, bringing to light one of the more important signs of rickets—the contracted pelvis. Among Irish women, deformed pelves were common to the point of universality. A seventeenth-century physician recorded a story related to him, intimating that at the birth of a female child the midwife immediately broke the infant's pelvis. "The wild Irish women do break the ossa Pubis [pubic bone] of the female infant." The doctor was especially impressed that the women kept the pubic bone from closing until the woman reached the age of childbearing, to ensure an easy delivery. As a result Irish women purportedly waddled for a time after giving birth. The image of "the wild women" breaking the infant pelvis characterizes the experience of the contracted pelvis as one familiar to a poor rural population, even as researchers in England and Germany connected rickets to urban environments.[11]

* * *

The female pelvis occupies an important place in the history of both rickets and race.[12] In the late nineteenth century, several anatomists' beliefs that the female body was markedly different from the male resulted in unrealistic drawings of female skeletons as smaller and childlike, especially in the size of their skulls. Redemption for a woman came "in respect to her *pelvis* [where] she set a standard of excellence."[13] In this area race came to bear as anthropologists eventually argued that white European women had the biggest and hence the best hips.

An episode unfolded early in the nineteenth century demonstrates the profound differences in perception, understanding, and approach regarding pelvic size. In 1815, highly esteemed French comparative anatomist Georges Cuvier (1769–1831) in 1815 became involved in the study of the body of a young Khoi-San woman, Saartjie Baartman (1789–1815). A slave, Baartman performed in England and France as an exhibit and curiosity for white audiences under the name "Hottentot Venus." The man who held her in servitude displayed her in sexually provocative clothing, making her appear to be naked. She performed with song and musical instruments unique to her ethnic origin that likely entranced her audience—the *ramkie* (a forerunner of the tincan guitar) and the *mamokhorong* (a one string violin).[14] Unfortunately some onlookers pursued her as a curiosity and a freak. Rumors spread about her reputed labial apron, her *sinus pudoris*—a physiological trait attributed to women of the Hottentots. Unable to see the richness of her ethnicity and the confines of her context, Europeans mistook her sexuality for animality.[15] Georges Cuvier became obsessed with curiosity about her sexual anatomy.

Cuvier contributed heavily to the shaping of race hierarchies with his strong emphasis on a biological or hereditary concept of race, basing his classification for species, "on precise measurement of skeletal and especially cranial structures [for men]."[16] Cuvier's comparative anatomy added to an argument lasting into the twentieth century over whether there were multiple human kinds or only one. According to Cuvier, Saartjie Baartman's people not only rested on the line as a different type, but were closely linked with apes and monkeys. He thought little of the "Bush people" purported to be her kin, pronouncing them "the most degraded of human races, whose form approaches that of the beast and whose intelligence is nowhere great enough to arrive at regular government."[17] The Bush people no longer existed in Saartjie Baartman's time. Who exactly her people were remains unclear, as she had migrated south in Africa.[18]

At the age of twenty-six in 1815 Saartjie Baartman died of a prolonged sickness, probably pneumonia, in Paris. Her story is largely one of exploitation and abuse. Throughout her illness she fought the mental and physical probings of Cuvier and other anthropologists, struggling to cover her body and remain free of the autopsy knife. Cuvier performed the autopsy. Curiosity appeased, he preserved her bones and prized body parts, especially her genital apron, in the French National Museum of Natural History (now known as the Musée de l'Homme).[19] Cuvier published his autopsy report in 1817, describing what he deemed to be Saartjie Baartman's sexual and reproductive anatomical anomalies.[20] Her pelvis, compared to other female pelves in various racial groupings, was the smallest and according to Cuvier's estimation the least endowed to reproduce. Expecting evidence supporting his definition of the Hottentot race, Cuvier found it. Baartman's captive exhibition betrayed the deep misrepresentation of South African women as animal-like freaks-of-nature. Relying on the specious construction of a linear chain of all earthly beings, anthropologists such as Cuvier determined that the peoples of southern Africa stood at or near the missing link.[21] Race groupings inevitably typified these people as subhuman yet endowed with elements of human physiology and culture.

Soon after Cuvier's report on Saartjie Baartman, Dutch anatomist

Gerardus Vrolik (1777–1859) wrote an essay presenting, "Observations upon the Differences of Pelves of Various Races." His work, published in 1820, expressed the early idea that pelves were analogous to skulls for identifying specific racial types. "The difference between the pelvis of the male negro, which could not be of firmer mass or have stronger bones, if taken from some wild animal, and that of the negress which unites delicacy and lightness with roundness ... recalls to the memory the pelvis of the ape."[22] Though there was an element of femininity in the female pelvis, the race of the bones overrode their sexual/gender qualities. Applying the concepts developed by comparative anatomists, Vrolik argued that the shape of a black female pelvis was specific to the shape of a black cranium, enabling birth.[23] In 1830, German professor Moritz Ignaz Weber (1795–1875) published on the same topic in 1830, elaborating on the placement of female pelves lower or higher in the human hierarchy. He sorted pelves into four types—European, American, Mongolian, and African, describing these as oval, round, four-sided, and wedge-shaped. "Females in general were considered a sexual subset of their race; unique female traits only served to confirm their racial standing."[24]

Ever refining the concept of the Great Chain of Being, scientists and philosophers had developed a linear scheme of sexual differentiation. At each link of the chain (from the angels downward), the female was declared the inferior of the male, essentially existing for the reproductive role. Women's place in the human hierarchy fell with each race, subordinated to a perceived superior male intelligence measured by craniometrics. Women in the theoretically subordinate race categories suffered the double stigma of representing a lesser race and being female.[25]

The pelves of African and African American women became an expression of assumed duality—the savage versus the civilized. The more civilized the woman, the more difficult birth, especially for male babies, as their brains were bigger. Comparing a "white" fetal skull with a "Negro" fetal skull, English obstetrician William Tyler Smith (1815–1873) in 1849 observed "they are good types of the cranial development, the one of ignorance and partial barbarism, and the other of an enlightened Christian civilization."[26] Drawings by Smith demonstrated the "facial angle" of the two skulls, explaining how the specific shape of each called for the accompanying shape of the female pelvis.[27] The reasoning suggests a Lamarckian argument, popular at the time, contending that traits were inherited as a result of successful adaptation in terms of function. Complementary fetal head and maternal pelvis permitted an easy birth. As obstetrics taught the birth process, emphasis on the cephalo-pelvic proportion and the fetal journey turned to issues of race, ease of birth, and race mixing.[28]

By the 1870s several authors presented quantified data from skulls and pelves from various museum collections, using individual items to represent different races and sexes. At the Paris Museum of Natural History, anthropologist Paul Broca (1824–1880) employed his forty instruments to undertake countless anthropometric measurements. Many doctors and anthropologists commonly used such tools for the assessment of skulls in terms of various race traits or characters, including the cephalic index, which became a measure of intelligence. Certain that intelligence was related to brain size, and that the size of the skull indicated the size of the brain, Broca employed some highly deceptive mathematics to verify the predetermined hierarchy of races. Venturing further, he concluded that the males of each race indeed possessed the superior intelligence, never pausing to consider that skull size was related to body size. Quantification also dominated the search for what many thought of as scientific meaning of the pelvis. Pelvimetry may have proven useful to determine whether an expectant mother could safely birth a child, but the larger goal was to identify characteristics defining race.[29]

To some, the obsession with numbers did little to address the essential issues. Scotsman J.G. Gaison (1854–1932) complained about the proliferation of measurement techniques for the pelvis, pointing to the work of medical doctor and anthropologist Renée Verneau (1852–1938) as an example. Verneau provided guidelines for making fifty-five different pelvic and sacral measurements to distinguish forty-two categories he called races. Gaison complained that Verneau gave no sense of "relative importance" of these measurements in his book, *Le Bassin dans les Sexes and dans les Races*. The implication was that each measure was significant in and of itself. Gaison added, "Great differences exist among anthropologists also regarding the mode in which measurements are to be made, measurement being often taken in different ways or from different points."[30] What purported to be a science proved difficult to apply consistently. Meanwhile, anthropometrics increasingly strengthened an already-constructed ideology of race.

Paul Broca invited Verneau to the Museum of Natural History in Paris to study 140 adult pelves.[31] Like Cuvier, Verneau placed priority on establishing Baartman's pelvis as the smallest in the collection. Verneau added the subjective observation that the "Venus Hottentot's" pelvis came close to replicating that of the Negress and a little of a female monkey. "In general, the Negro pelvis was characterized as animal-like or bestial; the Bosjemane pelves incomparably smaller in dimension than the European pelves."[32] Bigger meant higher quality.

The illustrations featured in Verneau's eventual book, published in 1875, exemplify the meaning of race in the nineteenth century. Carefully rendered lithographs highlighted the bones of Saartjie Baartman's pelvis—incorrectly identified as "bosjesmane"—along with a French "francais" pelvis, and that of a "negress." Other plates presented Hindu, Australian, Tasmanian, Chinese, Egyptian and Turkish specimens. "Francais" referred to a nation, not an ethnicity or a race; presumably Verneau was promoting his reputedly "Gallic" ancestors. "Nègress" was a thoroughly familiar race designation, but in description unworkably vague and impossible to substantiate. Of the sixteen lithographs, Saartjie Baartman's only was identified by name.[33]

Like so many anthropologists in his time, Verneau insisted that one or two pelvic samples could represent a whole population designated as a race, despite the fact that the evidence offered no generalizable meaning beyond the individual traits. Race categories were unavoidably inconsistent, as Verneau's designations exemplify. The pelvis itself was no longer the issue—politics and society were. Ideologies based on a multitude of racial categories swept the globe, seeking to justify colonization and human exploitation.[34]

Seeking to distinguish pelvic types mathematically, University of Edinburgh Professor and anatomist William Turner in 1886 developed a system of pelvic classification based on Paul Broca's skull classifications. Despite recognizing variance by individual and by sex within Broca's categories, Turner sought to classify pelves morphologically—by structure and shape. Utilizing the work of Vrolik, Broca, Verneau, Weber and others, Turner established a sacral index—"the ratio of the anteroposterior to the transverse diameter of the inlet × 100."[35] This index allowed him to use the ratio of length to width of the pelvic brim to compare pelves and compute racial categories. He knew the numbers were arbitrary; the sample very small.

Turner named the European pelvis platypellic—the designated highest form, the widest, oval and associated with white European women. At the other end of the spectrum was the doliochopellic—again thought to be found among so-called Bushmen or Hottentots—the longest and the closest to chimpanzees and other primates. Australian Aborigines, Polynesians, and Malays also fell into this category. A mesatipellic classification designated a round female pelvis, deemed to characterize Tasmanians and Melanesians generally. Africans proved to be ambiguous in pelvic shape, mesatipellic, but closer to platypellic—European white—than any other race. Turner emphasized the point, concluding his essay by stating "In the Negro, again, the pelvis ... approximates more closely to the European than to other black-skinned races."[36]

* * *

While European analysts did their best to perfect the "science" of pelvic classification, cultural descendants on the far side of the Atlantic

Three. The Impediment of Race

Ocean endeavored to contribute their perspective to the discussion. Social forces rising from the inescapable impacts of immigration and slavery played a large part in the development of America. From the inception of Europe's American empires, race was a determinant in social and cultural hierarchy. Radical ideologies came to challenge evolving racial notions, especially during peaks in waves of immigration. The centuries-long conflict over American slavery intensified the debates. Race permeated American self-identity. An embrace of Anglo-Saxon heritage came to define American thought.[37]

That Anglo-Saxon heritage of course derived from America's colonial origins. Real Americans were thought to be white and Anglo-Saxon, conveniently ignoring the Dutch, French, German, Celtic and other European origins of so many among their number. To say nothing of the considerable populations of Native and Black Americans. Americans had a lot to consider when the discussion turned to racial considerations. The bald contradictions between the ideals expressed in America's Revolution, the grim fact of American slavery and the repeated oppressions of Native Americans made race an extremely sensitive issue in the United States.[38]

In the 1830s and '40s some radical abolitionists posited that the mixing of the races was the only way to end social disharmony.[39] The idea of racial amalgamation proved unconscionable in the South and in most of the North as well. Where slavery was illegal, segregation and other racial practices pervaded society. Many saw the mixture of races as the death knell of civilization. In the South, no one could easily talk about masters' sexual aggressions against slave women, but this was a common phenomenon during the slave centuries, and the offspring of these unions lived marked lives.[40] Physicians such as Hugh Hodge and Charles Meigs pondered the future of a world facing what they thought of as racial degeneration. Their prejudices and their fears shaped their approach to a supposedly empirical science more than they ever realized. Because his writing focused on the physiology of birth in language denuded of emotional connection, Hodge's description of the disproportion of infant skull to female pelvis never appeared in a racial context. The mingling of races stood as a taboo topic rarely made explicit nor pursued.[41] Still, the implicit meaning was there. The ramifications of this racially-defined approach to childbirth would permeate medical practice as time went on. Subsequently, the study of pelves became the study of racial differences and their meanings.

* * *

In the early nineteenth century, Americans as well as Europeans argued whether all humans had a single origin, as portrayed in the Old

Testament and the story of Adam and Eve—monogenesis. Polygenists argued that perceived races actually represented separate species, meaning specifically separate origins for each race and an inability of any one race to breed across racial lines.[42] Nineteenth-century American history reveals an ever-increasing obsession with racial differences emanating from anthropological studies of bones from human skeletons and other animals. In the antebellum years scientists and medical men came together to create the pro-slavery American School of Anthropology. Strengthened by a guise of Baconian empiricism, biologist Louis Agassiz and physicians Samuel Cartwright, Josiah Nott, Samuel Morton and George Gliddon put forth tracts arguing African Americans had a unique physiology. Their polygenism maintained blacks were "physically inferior ... liars, malingerers, hypersexual, and indolent."[43] They presented these so-called race traits as biological truth. Other forms of ethnic stereotyping pervaded American research. The pseudo-science of phrenology appeared at about the same time as the American School, helping to establish a sort of geography of the brain detailing indelible human racial traits.

In 1820, Philadelphia physician Samuel George Morton (1799–1851) began collecting human skulls from across the world. By his death in 1851 he had accumulated more than a thousand, a putatively representative sample of the various peoples inhabiting the planet. (Morton's vast collection of mostly male skulls still lines the walls at the Academy of Natural Sciences of the College of Physicians and Surgeons in Philadelphia.) Morton studied and measured these skulls, delving into what he erroneously thought were the separate origins of multiple races of humans.[44] Following the work of European anthropologists, he postulated a hypothesis that the size of the cranium would vary in a hierarchy defined by race and sex, believing (like Broca later on) that cranial capacity indicated brain size—the larger the skull, the greater the intelligence. This conviction reified the idea that the abilities and strengths of humans varied in a fixed linear hierarchy of races, white European males at the top, white European females superior to all other female types.

Mistaken in his self-assessment as objective and scientific, Morton's untested premises, based on belief in the superiority of white men, led to subjective errors in his measurement of the cavities in his skulls. Those measurements provided the evidence allowing him to argue he had proved the lesser intelligence of the so-called lesser races.[45] One hundred-fifty years later, Steven Jay Gould revealed the unconscious subjectivity Morton wove into his study. Though he had followed the scientific method, Morton failed to consider the question of skull proportion to skeleton in the individual. Worse, his pre-assumptions that the Caucasian race was biologically separate from other races, and that bigger skulls meant greater intelligence, were egregiously false. Methodologically, his unquestioned premise of the innate superiority of white men led to errors of bias. Samuel Morton mismeasured his skulls.[46]

The damage was done. Establishing a hierarchy of human intelligence based on skull size, Morton "proved" the lesser intelligence of what he perceived to be the lesser races and the lesser sex.[47] His skull studies confirmed what many researchers wanted to believe. Race mattered. The bones provided the evidence men such as Aggasiz, Hodge, and Meigs had anticipated. Meigs called Morton "my friend, Samuel George Morton, distinguished author of the *Crania Americana*," citing a key publication used to promote the American School's perspective.[48]

Morton and Meigs were contemporaries in Philadelphia. Meigs took profound interest in a second measure of human skeletal structure: the female pelvis. Morton was attentive to bony pelves—to put it mildly. He presented his friend Meigs with "a pelvis of an Egyptian lady of rank from the tombs of Thebes, which specimen … [was] one of the most perfect specimens of the female pelvis I have ever seen."[49] Part of the fascination with female pelves came from an interest in comparing male and female anatomy as the basis for gender difference. Morton, Meigs, and many others ranked female pelves according to race types to situate them on a hierarchical ladder from ape to civilized man. Morton and Meigs saw this "perfect" pelvis from Egypt as a product of the first civilization, the forerunner of all that was now understood as Caucasian or Western. Female pelves that deviated from this standard were "Other"—other in the sense of less—of a different race and/or sex.

Meigs was professionally interested in pelvimetric study. He and other obstetricians understood contracted pelvis as a broad designation, including a majority of the examples of pelvic malformation. Using the Egyptian pelvis as a figure in his obstetrics text, Meigs compared the illustration with examples exhibiting what most medical practitioners called a "deformed" pelvis.[50] Grouping bones by loosely defined race categories also became a standard clarifying healthy from pathological.

Samuel Morton died in 1851. His work and his connections with several likeminded renowned scientists made him a celebrated participant in the American School of Anthropology. Morton provided the veneer of numbers that empowered the less scientific observational thinking of his contemporaries. Especially important was his hand in the promotion of polygeny—the idea of humans as multiple races with multiple origins.[51] Unsurprisingly, the American School's findings provided the South with a defense of slavery during the decade before the Civil War.[52] Of greatest consequence was the American School's articulation of the idea that African Americans benefited from the institution because their race made them dependent and childlike—"a separate and unequal species."

As Linda Schiebinger put it, these scientists were sure their biological concepts of race distinctions were unbiased because they believed, "the body spoke for itself."[53] The individual's identity came from stereotyped physical traits. Sickness among African Americans simply resulted from their race. Whites were at the top of a hierarchy based on race types in categories. Benefiting from power in government and the economy, they dominated society through the juxtaposition of races. Subjectively influenced by this point of view, white physicians commonly saw the white body in an entirely different light from the African American, both in the North and the South.

* * *

In the United States, slavery and its aftermath demonstrated the power of perceived racial differences. Interpretations of phenotypical traits often portrayed young fertile African American women as highly sexualized creatures with little to no mental abilities—a particularly enduring and demeaning stereotype. Historian Jennifer Morgan argues that because the African woman in bondage in the United States defined slavery—the condition of the mother determined that of the child—"the African woman embodied the behavioral and physical characteristics that degraded an entire race of people."[54]

Varying regional constructions of race influenced African American social status, as exemplified by slavery, but affecting free men and women as well. Medical perceptions of health rested on white identification of African Americans as other. Given the dominance of white perspective in record keeping, the chances for invisibility of African American deaths are high—especially for children. Yet, evidence shows mortality from rickets in the North as well as the South. Eighteenth-century Philadelphia mortality rates indicate African Americans died earlier and at a significantly greater rate than whites following the hard cold winters of the Northern temperate zone, presumably in part because they were unable to absorb sufficient sunlight, inducing rickets. Their physiology had been conditioned by thousands of years of life in a tropical climate with an abundance of sunshine.[55]

Records of slaves, kept by owners for the most part, served as part of the political economy of Southern slave plantations, but did not address with any accuracy overall mortality rates, let alone the slaves' general well-being or ability to thrive. Known records kept outside the institution of slavery failed in the same regard. Preceding the Civil War, statistics gathered in the South were fodder for the pro–Southern, pro-slavery point of view—intended to show the well-being of the slave under the system. After the war, Southern whites delighted in statistics that demonstrated African Americans' illnesses as proof they were better off as slaves. Although some questions are left unanswered, evidence from skeletons offers stark witness to rickets, a disease which makes its mark on bones.[56]

Historical and anthropological insights help to fill a gap in evidence for the pre–Civil War African Americans. Cliometrician Richard Steckel compiled statistics of American slavery to compare heights in children of various ages and adults. Steckel found "slave children were among the smallest ever measured," concluding that "the study of human growth and development makes clear that diet, disease, and work cannot be evaluated in isolation."[57] Though merely implicit in his study, without a doubt rickets was part of the "diet, disease, and work" Steckel cited as foundation for the poor record of growth. Biology and social conditions merge in the history of all three factors. Rickets generally appeared in the young child during bone growth of infancy and early childhood, but could persist in an older child's stunted growth. Or, a child might suffer rickets as a one year old but outgrow and heal virtually all signs of the disease. Although we do not know exactly how much rickets occurred among slaves, Steckel's evidence suggests that rickets may have effectively impeded the growth of many slave children. His images are stark: African American children living in freedom had greater chances to live past five years of age.[58] Rickets may have been so commonplace among slaves that physicians overlooked the signs and dismissed its importance.[59]

* * *

After the Civil War ended slavery, American awareness of rickets strengthened as medical students increasingly learned medicine in Great Britain and Europe, where rickets was commonplace among the white population and where the study of bones and cadavers helped to promote clinical study of the disease. In the United States, medical students and physicians came to rely heavily on morbid anatomy as well, winning more ready legal access to the cadavers of African Americans and the poor.[60]

An association developed linking the incidence of rickets to African Americans and slavery. As African Americans began their life on the North American continent as migrants from tropical latitudes, they may well have been susceptible. Factors such as diet probably enhanced their susceptibility. Race prejudice, a significant social historical factor affecting health in many ways, grew throughout the nineteenth century and took new shape as the country industrialized. Despite the Union's victory in the Civil War and the end of slavery, segregation, black codes, lynchings, and other forms of discrimination tell a story of regression.

Rickets in the United States had fewer victims—who were counted—than did several European countries, yet by the 1890s many American physicians wrote about rachitic disease and various sources document its presence. Initially these analyses identified African Americans as those most commonly affected by rickets. This came about at least in part as the result of the cultural stereotyping that labeled these people in negative ways. Medical science for the most part accepted the intuitive use of skin color as the basis for hierarchical human categories of race, in fact helped to establish them as reflective of significant variability in basic human characteristics. Consequently, subjectively influenced practitioners misinterpreted rickets, tending to conclude that the disease was a product of the perceived degeneracy of the black race. Many Americans came to assume race was the dominant factor in the history of rickets. Most American (and European) doctors unabashedly saw race as hereditary, signifying for African Americans an inherent susceptibility to ignorance, sickness and early death. Jenner could adduce no evidence to suggest rickets was a hereditary disease, but he did contend that a diathesis—a constitutional weakness increasing susceptibility to certain diseases—was a factor. In the minds of too many American practitioners, that diathesis was being born African American.[61]

* * *

Social forces rising from the inescapable impacts of immigration and slavery played a large part in the history of rachitic disease in America. From the inception of Europe's American empires, race was a determinant in social and cultural hierarchy. The centuries-long conflict over American slavery intensified the debates. Social status became a profound influence on both the incidence of the disease and its definition.

Childbirth in America was no different. Issues of sex equality and gender role pushed the politics of reproduction to the foreground. Gender, like race, became a means to separate and discriminate, to privilege certain socially defined categories at the expense of others. The American investigation of rickets was woven into a fabric of racial and sexual inequity.

Four

Science Reloads

Science is a process, a never-ending examination and re-examination of evidence theoretically gathered solely through the human senses, without bias. Being human, scientists are not unbiased practitioners; assumptions conscious and unconscious creep into research method and analysis, necessitating the continuous re-investigation that sometimes overturns previously accepted scientific "fact." Alternative methods throw fresh light on old problems; newly emergent perspectives cast doubt on previously cherished conclusions. Occasionally the insight is profound enough to overturn a system of human belief and understanding—what is labeled a scientific "revolution." Even a revolution is laden with holdovers from the past; unsupported suppositions persist. So it was in the second half of the nineteenth century, when Charles Darwin published *The Origin of Species* in 1859, overturning the long-accepted belief that the world's species were fixed and immutable, a product of creation.[1]

The theory of natural selection wrought profound changes in scientific thinking regarding the origins of life, breaking through blinding limitations to establish the concept of evolution. Darwin made the environment a crucial factor in the emergence of humanity. The idea depended on a better understanding of human anatomy, the function of the body in nature. Cephalo-pelvic proportion, so critical in the human birth process and part of its evolution, was already an essential concept in obstetrical science. Evolutionary theory wrought a new awareness of bipedalism and the development of pelvic structure, providing new perspective on human physiology.

Sad to say, the embrace of evolutionary theory fed rather than discouraged racial constructions of humanity. European and American scholars absorbed evolutionary concepts through a lens focused on the racial typology advanced in the eighteenth century, enshrined in Linnean taxonomy.[2] Carl Linnaeus (1707–1778) had decreed that "human races were, somehow, fixed."[3] Believing in a common origin of all humans, Linnaeus held to a hierarchy of human races while recognizing the human species as a larger category through its ability to interbreed. Early studies of skull and pelvic differentiation had resulted in racial classifications derived largely from appearance. Perceived racial differences in morphology, skull and pelvic shape and size, skin color, jaw shape, nose and other features often over-rode objective scientific investigation. Once established, the classifications perpetuated a belief that such superficial differences among racial groups confirmed a hierarchy of peoples, white Northern Europeans at the top and Black Africans on the bottom, the link to nonhuman primates.

One of the more controversial aspects of early race science was the question of origins—monogeny, as depicted in the Bible, or polygeny, belief that humans were multiple races of different origins, the various perceived races actually representing separate species. Darwin tacitly adhered to a theory of one origin for all humans, but his concept of natural selection did not contradict the theory of polygenesis. Darwin himself differentiated among the human races by citing differences in the color of skin and hair. His writings brought human evolution to bear upon the international scientific and anthropological ideas of race already in place. Images of a chain of being gave way to visions of evolutionary progress ultimately producing white European peoples.[4]

"Survival of the fittest" (a terminology Darwin adopted very reluctantly) implied a hierarchy designating degrees of fitness. Race classifications and typology remained locked in place. By the late nineteenth century many white European and American scholars, researchers, physicians and scientists (Americans especially), believed that African Americans descended from a degenerating race, that their inability to reproduce a growing population signified the coming end of their very existence. With this concept came the idea of African Americans as pathological, representing disease and as such threatening the well-being of the white race. As historian Laura Briggs explains: "Cultural evolutionism—the idea that human groups differed in the stage of evolution which they had obtained … was the reigning paradigm in science, government, and popular discourse."[5] Linking race to evolution strengthened the hold of race on the study of female pelves as part of culture and society. A sea change in natural philosophy rippled through the western world, convincing scientists in some quarters to view race as biological: nature, in the debate of nature *versus* nurture. Evolution became an alternative way to think about race. How these ideas affected society varied from nation to nation.[6]

Darwin did not discuss the difficult and complex topic of human hierarchies at length until 1871, in *The Descent of Man and Selection in Relation to Sex*. In a presentation of his theory of sexual selection, he sustained the use of racial categories, holding to a belief in the hierarchy of life which put the Teutonic—meaning German or Nordic—race on top, men over women.[7] Sexual selection represented one path to evolution, a slippery idea acknowledging the role of male or female preference for particular characteristics, as exhibited in various species. To his credit, Darwin was willing to admit the possibility of random or stochastic change while clinging to racial and sexual hierarchies; he did not think of race or sex as fixed human characteristics. He argued that lower uncivilized people, as he saw them, could evolve according to context. Relying on what became a familiar dichotomy of civilization *versus* savagery, Darwin fell back on the language at hand, a language of racial typology and human racial hierarchies.[8]

Like every scientist who has ever breathed air, Darwin's perceptions were shaped by the prevailing culture of his times—he was a Victorian male, with all that implies. In *The Descent of Man*, he firmly maintained that sexual selection among human beings was largely the province of the male, more so than in most animal species. Men were seen to be the stronger sex by far, "man attaining to a higher eminence, in whatever he takes up, than can women—whether requiring deep thought, reason, or imagination, or merely the use of the senses and hands."[9] A few pages on, Darwin concluded that "man has ultimately become superior to woman."[10] The most radical of scientific revolutions unavoidably retains much of the conventional.

* * *

The triumph of evolution gave new impetus to anthropological research; scientists and medical practitioners turned to skeletal remains to reconstruct the human past, as well as to study disease. Darwin's ideas concerning human origins reoriented a long standing question: how were various groups, perceived as races, humanly and historically related? Determining the history of human evolution quickly became central to anthropologists around the world. In 1873 Ernst Haeckel wrote, "as a consequence of the Theory of Descent or Transmutation, we are now in a position to establish scientifically the groundwork of a non-miraculous history of the development of the human race."[11] For medical and scientific thought, interest in finding a connection between humans and apes became a secular task, presumably outside the realm of religion. Stubborn and deeply rooted, the image of a Great Chain of Being persisted—the search for ancestral remains focused on "missing links." Did humans really have an evolutionary relationship with apes? For years to come, many questioned the Darwinian theory of human descent, and sought to establish an alternative history of human evolution.[12] In 1872, Rudolf Virchow took time from his studies of cellular anatomy in Germany to enter into the anthropological discussion of human prehistory. Fifteen years earlier, German construction workers in the Neander Valley had chanced upon apparently human skeletal remains of disturbing shape. Studies suggested the skeleton, featuring a very large skull with prominent eye ridges, was representative of some extinct form of humanity. Undertaking his own examination, Virchow firmly disagreed, maintaining the bones were those of a recent pathological specimen, a victim of severe rickets and arthritis.[13] The episode was the first but not the last time anthropologists used rickets as a means to interpret human fossils and to engage in discussion of human evolution. Virchow was wrong, as became evident when more and more Neanderthal remains came to light. The controversy magnified in importance as evolutionary theory gained credence. What part did these Neanderthals with their huge skulls play in human evolution? The controversies raged on. When Dutch paleoanthropologist Eugène Dubois (1858–1940) published his discovery of Pithecanthropus *erectus* (upright man) in 1891, critics maintained the fossils were remains of an "arthritic gibbon." Europeans looked upon the growing evidence of human evolution with a mix of awe and horror; the awe derived from the determined belief their own race was far removed from a discomfiting past.[14]

* * *

The changes that accompanied medical and anthropological preoccupation with evolution and race shared a basis in the concept of heredity. Belief that race was biologically fixed intimated that phenotypical traits had to be inherited. As scientists incorporated newer biological definitions of race, they also began to think about and explore the nature of heredity. The precise mechanics of natural selection, or how it came about, remained vague. Assumptions about the nature of heredity, including Jenner's ideas about diathesis, held steadfast until there was more clarity about the problem.[15]

Physicians thought that along with physical, mental, and familial traits, social and cultural factors—what are now considered to be habits—contributed to diathesis. Such features would belong to the essentialist category of "nature" in the nature/nurture dichotomy. At a loss to explain the inheritance of biological traits, researchers confused the issue by suggesting that heredity and environment were somehow woven together into a single entity. Inheritance *versus* environment posed a difficult question for medicine when it came to pinpointing the origins of diseases and sometimes the nature of therapy.[16]

Ideas of natural selection and heredity conditioned concepts of sickness grounded in culture and social status. Many physicians considered rickets a product of environment, yet influenced by individual physiology.

What kind of disease was it? Here was an important connection with a philosophical issue touching on research into the etiology of rickets—a duality of nature and nurture. Social factors inevitably intertwined with biological explanations as doctors sought to understand the disease. As thinking about rickets became deeply entangled in concepts of race, researchers looked both to heredity and society, examining social factors in the search for possible explanations. Darwin's approach to heredity dodged the question, opening the door to eugenics.[17]

* * *

The term "survival of the fittest" was coined by English political philosopher Herbert Spencer in 1864. Reluctantly accepted by Darwin, the concept was intended to epitomize human social interactions, rather than biological competition among plant and animal species. Spencer contended that natural selection occurred within human societies, with the more able surviving the ongoing contest for success, thereby promoting progress. The philosophy, eventually known as "Social Darwinism," justified unregulated exploitation of the powerless, defined by class and race. Spencer contended that such unhindered selection would eliminate the inferior.[18]

Among those grasping the idea of survival of the fittest, the fit *versus* the unfit as a mechanism of evolution, was Charles Darwin's own cousin, Francis Galton (1822–1911), a statistician and anthropometrist. Setting out to explore the implications of natural selection, a new concept and quite vague, Galton in 1865 began to consider what he saw as degeneration in nonwhite races. Branching off from Darwin, Galton emphasized nature as the determinant in the individual and in the evolution of the human race, through heredity. Galton drew most of his evidence from the breeding of animals, an old art, but he added a crucial extension: the qualities of human character were inherited, the same as physical characteristics. Darwin was not happy with this idea.[19]

Employing mathematics and measurements to study genealogy and heredity, Galton identified phenotypes or characteristics ascribed to specific racial groups, some "unfit," others "fit." Unsurprisingly, Galton's own northern European race was declared fit above all others. Data in hand, Francis Galton propagated a school of thought devoted to the controlled use of reproduction to improve the human race. In 1883, with his cousin safely dead, Galton introduced the concept of eugenics, a word he invented to define a program of selective breeding to ensure the purification of the race (Teutonic or Aryan). With the rise of eugenics, race came to be seen still more as an inherited identity. Racial constructions not only survived the introduction of Darwinian thinking, but gained strength through the application of social science and the emergence of Galtonian eugenics.[20]

* * *

Darwinian selection overturned centuries of assumption and thought, ushering in a new era of biological research. A quieter but no less significant transformation was taking place in the field of medicine. Writers and practitioners recast disease and the origins of disease into a new framework. Considerable time would elapse between what is now recognized as a seminal moment in medical history and the subsequent implementation of the findings.[21]

The European acceptance of germ theory and the rise of laboratory science typified the enormous change taking place. The premise that disease could be the work of organisms invisible to the human eye was put forward by the Islamic world as far back as the twelfth century. The concept attracted little attention in Europe, where medical authorities generally contended disease was a product of breathing in "miasma"—foul air. French microbiologist Louis Pasteur (1822–1895) was the first to produce hard evidence promoting germ theory, isolating the bacterium to blame for puerperal fever in research undertaken between 1850 and 1864. English physician John Snow cast severe doubt on miasma theory, famously controlling an epidemic of cholera in London's Soho district by blocking public access to a neighborhood water pump. German researcher Robert Koch (1843–1910) identified the bacterial sources causing anthrax, tuberculosis, and cholera. In 1890, Koch established a set of postulates crafted to govern further research into micro-organisms and disease.[22]

Thomas McKeown has provocatively argued that history wrongly celebrates the super powers of scientific medicine at the turn of the century—that in fact rising standards of living, including hygiene and sanitation, and particularly betterment in nutrition, rendered greater health and prolonged lives in industrialized countries much more effectively than did medical science. The case of rickets stands contrary to this proposition. Rickets grew in magnitude with the coming of industrialization. The burgeoning presence of the disease demonstrates that living conditions were not conducive to health, that improved nutrition was neither universal nor well understood.[23]

While rickets and contracted pelves influenced maternal and infant mortality in a less visible way, the high incidence of rachitic disease fueled attention. Driven by a sense of the new frontiers shaped by germ theory, scientists naturally began searching for the etiology of rickets in bacterial infection. Windows into infectious disease riveted the attention of medical scientists and filtered the lens through which medical professionals saw the world. Everything looked different. Unable to locate any microbial infection, determined researchers turned to the possibility of toxic disorder, some sort of weakening poison either produced within the body or imported from the outside environment. Focused on such theories, analysts showed little inclination to look further to the chemistry of nutrition or the role of the atmosphere and sunlight, where parts of the puzzle of rickets lay hidden. Geographical and national variations in approach further obscured understanding of rickets, contracted pelves, and birth. Small wonder physicians no longer trusted cod liver oil.[24]

The array of heralded developments in the province of medicine engendered some difficult choices for working physicians. Faced with the high rates of maternal and infant mortality stemming from contracted pelves, the promise of antisepsis provided obstetrical science a window for more invasive surgical intervention. Experimental research in the use of anesthesia had made the procedure safer and more routine, opening the door to greater use of Caesarian section. Surgeons remained hesitant, and rightly so—patient death had been reduced, but far from eliminated. Nonetheless, anesthesia would become an essential means to advance the ongoing quest for greater obstetrical control of birth.[25]

In 1847, Scottish obstetrician Sir James Y. Simpson (1811–1870) became the first to use chloroform to deaden pain during birth; the child was nicknamed "Anesthesia." The intervention was controversial on grounds moral and medical. Clerics argued the procedure violated the will of God, citing the Biblical injunction that woman was born to suffer. Physicians were aware of the dangers of chloroform—an overdose could kill. Simpson was able to win public approval for the practice when Queen Victoria asked for anesthesia for the delivery of her eighth child in 1853, under its influence giving birth successfully. Simpson was also responsible for the invention of an improved form of forceps, known to this day as the Simpson forceps. In America, Walter Channing of Boston, one of a growing number of obstetricians displacing midwives in home deliveries, became the first to employ anesthesia during labor.[26] Channing published a *Treatise on Etherization in Childbirth* (1848), collating statistics showing the successful use of ether by forty-five physicians in 581 childbirth cases.[27]

* * *

Pain-killing drugs were not necessary for childbirth in either Europe or America, but the practice grew. An expectant mother desiring such treatment would consult an obstetrician, almost certainly male. Should she suffer serious injury giving birth, she might then consult a gynecologist.

The term "gynecology" entered the English language in 1847, derived from the French word—coined from Greek roots—denoting "the department of medical science which treats of the functions and diseases peculiar to women." The word originated in response to the nineteenth century rise in surgical intervention to address severe problems resulting from childbirth. The practice was originally regarded as a surgical specialty, limited to repair of injuries to the reproductive organs. With time, the increasing medicalization of childbirth generated jurisdictional disputes; the boundaries separating gynecology from obstetrics proved difficult to define.[28]

Modern gynecology grew out of surgical experiments undertaken by American Southern physician J. Marion Sims (1813–1883). Between 1846 and 1849, Sims performed repeated surgeries on African American slave women's bodies, seeking a technique to heal the "accidents of childbirth" known as vesico-vaginal fistula. Such vaginal tears resulted from prolonged childbirth. Women with the condition had suffered through unbelievably, extremely long labors—days sometimes, with the infant's head visible—before finally giving birth, almost always subjected to a physician's violent intervention with ropes, hooks, knives or other crude tools. Too often, rough techniques proved the only viable choice in cases of obstructed labor. The result was the pathology of vesico-vaginal fistula—constant urinary (and sometimes rectal) drainage. Encountering several cases among enslaved women in his Alabama practice, Sims established an experimental hospital in Montgomery, where he performed as many as thirty surgeries on individual Black subjects. He used no anesthetic, only opium before and after surgery.[29]

Achieving success, Sims moved to New York City, where he enlisted the support of several wealthy women to open The Woman's Hospital of the State of New York in 1856, the first of its kind in the United States. Devoted both to the cure of female maladies and continued research in the developing field of gynecology, the hospital attracted a skilled and determined staff of surgeons, beginning with Thomas Addis Emmet (1828–1919).[30]

Emmet published often, generally basing his work on clinical records documenting surgical treatment of patients. His written work began with a book-length publication detailing seventy-three cases of vesico-vaginal fistula operations at the Woman's Hospital. Later he published articles in various professional medical journals concerning specific gynecological surgeries. In 1877 he included the abstracts of one hundred-sixty vesico-vaginal fistula patient records in his text, *Principles and Practice of Gynecology*. The two sets of patient records provide rich material regarding the births that preceded the vaginal tears. Though Emmet did not employ a lens of contracted pelves in his records, he treated the aftermath of what were undoubtedly examples of such cases, thereby providing an image of the childbirth experiences resulting from complicated deliveries.[31]

His purpose was to chronicle the kinds of cases that resulted from the "accidents of childbirth." In *Vesico-Vaginal Fistula* (1868), Emmet detailed patients' obstetrical pasts, presenting material including the year of the patient's entry into the Woman's Hospital for treatment of the vaginal tears, her age at the time of the birth resulting in the tears, the parity of the woman (how many children she had had), where she was born (ethnicity or national origin), how long her labor, the nature of the intervention, the child's condition upon birth, what anesthetic or how much ergot (a rust fungus parasitic on rye, long known to induce labor contractions) was used, how many surgeries physicians attempted to try to repair the vesico-vaginal fistulas, and the result of the surgery. Women experienced aggressive interventions—from forceps to craniotomy, blunt hooks, ropes and traction—in forty-five out of seventy-three births.[32]

Women in these clinically-described cases endured long hours of labor, in half the cases giving birth to a no longer living child. The women whose babies were either stillborn or died at birth labored an average of fifty-nine hours (two and a half days). Women giving birth for the first time labored for an average greater than sixty-six hours. One hundred-forty hours (four and a half days) was the longest labor in the recorded cases. This was especially long considering that Emmet counted only hours of hard labor, beginning when the membranes ruptured. Much of the infant death resulted from obstetrical intervention, when doctors were forced to destroy the fetus in order to save the life of the mother. Instruments used included hooks, crochets, and perforators. Blunt hooks could result in a living child, but not often.[33]

Emmet understood his cases to have originated in prolonged labors. His meticulous records and clinical descriptions provide a better understanding of what a troubled childbirth was like. The cases especially show the unusually difficult nature of some births, the extremity of complications at mid-century. He avoided discussion of contracted pelves, focusing narrowly on the high incidence of vesico-vaginal fistulas, emphasizing the innovations in surgical gynecology. Many physicians practicing in America resembled Emmet in their avoidance of the European-originated framework concluding that contracted pelves resulted from rickets. Many were now in a prolonged war with midwives over control of obstetrical practice, arguing that gynecological extremes warranted the medicalization of childbirth.[34]

Emmet provided a context for some of the women he treated, who were likely poor immigrants. Of the seventy-three cases presented in 1868, twenty-one, a little less than one-third, were Irish. Most likely these were women forced to emigrate during the famine years 1846 to 1851, when more than a million people left Ireland. The women were born before the potato failure, indicating the probable presence of rickets more than twenty years before the famine struck. As infants, these women were victims of the worsening social conditions exacerbated by the famine. Formerly, the standard diet among the hundreds of thousands of Irish tenants had been a nearly perpetual round of buttermilk blended with potatoes, a nutritious if bland fare. By the 1820s, market conditions dictated that landlords (largely absentee English) export more and more of the milk produced on farms, leaving tenants without. Deprived of virtually the sole source of needed calcium in the diet (even a constant diet of potatoes provided just 4 percent of requirements), childhood rickets was the consequence. The disaster in Ireland began long before the crop failures.[35]

Of Irish descent, Emmet treated his Irish patients with a sense of nationalism and self-identification.[36] The fact remains that these women were experimental subjects undergoing surgery in a research hospital. Emmet published several articles in various medical journals, detailing variations in surgical approach. While European scientists such as Rudolf Virchow and Carl Litzmann had made Germany the international locus of obstetrical research, gynecology was largely developed in America. Simply put, the reason was the presence of large populations of defenseless women. J. Marion Sims perfected his surgical technique through repeated experiments on slaves. In New York, Sims and Thomas A. Emmet attracted cases from the indigent Irish immigrant population to continue their research. Their European counterparts had few such subjects.[37]

In his second set of records, Emmet encapsulated one hundred-sixty similar cases of vesico-vaginal fistula from an overlapping but mostly later period, 1862–1877, with most cases from 1867. These records did not indicate nationality or ethnicity. 55.6 percent of these women (eighty-four) had labors longer than forty-eight hours; fifty-four survived labors of seventy-two hours or more (35.8 percent). In twelve of these cases women retained urine during labor. Emmet argued strongly that the lesson from these cases was the need to use forceps more often and more quickly. Many women lost the base of their bladders through the use of forceps, but Emmet thought that was because physicians failed to help women empty their bladders before using the instrument.[38]

Neither Sims nor Emmet mentioned rickets or the contracted pelvis in their numerous cases, though later physicians reflected that rickets and contracted pelves must have been the origin of the gynecological surgeons' renowned problematic births.[39] Writing on the subject in the 1870s, William Thompson Lusk suggested that T.A. Emmet's vesico vaginal fistula cases came from contracted pelves—quite possibly reflecting the influence of rickets across the population. In spite of this insight, Lusk, like many others, denied a significant incidence of contracted pelves in the Unites States.[40]

Statistics alone do not tell the story. Contrary to England, where rickets was recognized as a common disease, the United States reported rickets and contracted pelves inconsistently, varying by time and place. Such reports as do exist indicate that after the Civil War, cases steadily increased. Though case records at times referred to a contracted pelvis, the origin was generally left uninvestigated. Unfortunately for the chronicling of rachitic disease, if a woman with a deformed pelvis died in childbirth, the cause was seldom attributed to rickets.[41]

* * *

Although Thomas A. Emmet wrote as a gynecologist, not as an obstetrician, he did speculate on the causes of extremely severe and difficult births. Of course, he had his suggestions for the reform of medical practice, but he also held a kind of philosophy about the state of the human race. Like others of his time, he understood human health to be in part a product of the environment. The first chapter of his *Principles and Practice of Gynecology* was titled "The Relations of Climate, Education, and Social Conditions to Development." As a second generation Irish immigrant Emmet thought about the new world in a unique way, contemplating what he saw as a succession of original races of people and animals immigrating and replacing one another in populating the North American continent. He was concerned about the degeneration of humanity due to the intermingling of superior and inferior races, especially in the early republic. In the handwritten first draft of his chapter, he wrote and then crossed out the words:

> The cause of this tendency to deteriorate is yet obscure, but it is not impossible that the peculiar nature of our climate has a share in it. When immigration to the United States shall have ceased, and the population shall have become more homogeneous, the problem will be somewhat simplified.[42]

Struggling with how to best articulate his ideas on such a political topic, Emmet replaced them with:

> A thinking man who has had opportunities for observation, cannot divert himself of the conviction that the physical development of the women of our land is becoming deteriorated. Unless the causes of this be quickly sought out and removed we must eventually become enfeebled, after the human stream, which has given us vigor, ceases to flow into our country from other lands.[43]

Emmet's views of the health of women and the American people grew out of his work as a gynecologist. He saw immigration and issues of race and ethnicity as profoundly intertwined in reproduction and sexuality. He believed human degeneration to be the explanation for the surgical cases he encountered, the reason behind the obstructed births. The far more likely cause—the growing incidence of rickets—he never discussed.

Emmet was far from alone in his speculations. The need for gynecological surgery wanted explanation. Seeking an answer, American obstetrician George Engelmann (1847–1903) published his book *Labor among Primitive Peoples* in 1884. Practicing at lying-in institutions in St. Louis while teaching at the Post Graduate School of Missouri Medical College, Engelmann found time to write an anthropologically-based comparison of what he called the "civilized and savage." His format mirrored the well-worn anthropological approach, a comparison of his own experiences with medical writings from other cultures. He based his research on correspondence and surveys of practitioners—mostly missionaries—in the field. He found rickets to be uncommon in tropical zones.[44]

Engelmann devoted much attention to cultural variation in birthing positions, describing birth among distant peoples as admirable and well-done. The real lives of women of "other" ethnicities were in many ways invisible to him; he was unable to see the childbirth experience of other cultures as painful. Judging by his elected standards, the further the distance from civilization, the easier, more straightforward and instinctive their labors seemed to be. Engelmann emphasized a familiar theme: "intermarriage, weakened organization, and the languid neurasthenic condition of subjects in civilized communities" created problems in childbirth. Modern women were simply too sensitive to give birth without pain medicine from doctors.[45]

Among the people Englemann studied were Native Americans living in the United States. Many American writers, including physician Alice Stockham (1833–1912) in her book *Tokology*, spoke of easy births for Indians as a kind of role model for the mainstream American woman. Such representations portrayed the nature of Native American births mistakenly.[46]

Industrialization and a sense of the accompanying advantages and disadvantages of what most perceived as a higher civilization motivated many medical writers. Engelmann was heavily influenced by the work of Armand Corre (1841–1908), a French practitioner in marine medicine. Possessing a closer affinity for anthropology *per se* than Englemann or Emmet, Corre published a text for an audience of young doctors in 1882. The work provided elementary lessons in obstetrics, female sickness in childbirth, and the health of newborns. Corre's essential framework was race, grounded in a bowdlerized version of natural selection. Claiming a scientific background, he juxtaposed the most deformed black female pelvis to those of monkeys and again to what he described as a magnificent gorilla skeleton at l'École de Brest. All were situated in the hierarchy of the

Great Chain of Being.[47] Comparing childbirth across cultures, Corre provided details of various ethnic expectations for female behavior, indicating that birth differed with race. In some remote indigenous cultures, fathers performed the role of accoucheur, a sharp contrast to western European practice. Corre acknowledged that childbirth itself did go equally long (for as many trying hours) among the various human groups he considered.[48] He too argued that rickets did not frequently occur in tropical zones.

Thematically, the work of Argentinian researcher Juan Samuel Gache Solvera (1859–1907) resembled that of Corre and Englemann, his writings examining the experience of childbirth in what he defined as different cultures. Gache was curious to discover why some South American countries experienced numerous cases of contracted pelves, leading to difficult births, and some did not.[49] His interest was comparative, to try to understand his own perception, and that of many American physicians, that the United States had so few cases of rickets. Writing in 1903, he applied his assumptions of a typology of multiple races to the incidence of pelvic deformity in the Americas. For instance he argued that in Paraguay, where there seemed to be many cases of contracted pelves, there was a high incidence of interracial sexual exchange. Gache noted that the indigenous people had no difficulty in childbirth while "a generation of decrepit and corrupted people worsened by poverty" suffered difficult births. In Gache's estimation rickets and contracted pelves plagued interracial unions.[50]

Such interpretations reveal the way in which "scientific" presentations used subjective racial categories to weave speculations of a racially-fixed human hierarchy, explaining obstructed birth. There was essentially nothing of objective science in the conjectures of Gache, Englemann, or Corre, or of Thomas Addis Emmet for that matter. No method, no data, no proof. Nothing more than guesswork constructed on superficial research and a tiny number of personal observations, a grasping for some alternative to explain the apparently growing incidence of obstructed childbirth.

* * *

To the eyes of medical science, human reproduction had become a highly complicated process, demanding ever greater specialization. Even as the surgical practice of gynecology arose to meet the problems stemming from obstructed childbirth, doctors came to more carefully consider the physical welfare of the child successfully born. The word "pediatrics" entered the English language in 1849, constructed from a combination of Greek words denoting a healer of diseases (children). Throughout history, healers had recognized the problems of health endemic to the growing child, but the development of modern pediatrics began with *The Diseases of Children and Their Remedies*, a text published by Swedish physician

Nils Rosén von Rosenstein (1706–1773) in 1764. Care centers for children, established in France beginning in 1802, had appeared in several European countries by the middle of the nineteenth century.[51]

Pediatricians focused on two central arenas—infectious disease and nutritional disorders. Sickness often caused the death of children, especially before the age of five. Diseases such as diphtheria, whooping cough, hepatitis, measles, meningitis and scarlet fever swept through homes in cities and in the country, often carrying away several children in one family.[52] Tuberculosis and syphilis spread easily and deeply in an industrializing world.[53]

By encouraging women to bear numerous children, society had long accommodated the high incidence of child sickness and the associated mortality. Historian William MacNeill observes that "even high rates of infant mortality were relatively easily born."[54] A large family was a hedge, practical and emotional, against the likely death of one or more children. As birth rates began to fall in the latter half of the nineteenth century, the western world turned increasingly to medical science to save the fewer offspring born to most families.

With the recognition of germ theory, doctors treating infants and children began to see them as especially susceptible to contagious infection. Epidemics came every year at least; childhood diseases became an especially fertile ground for bacteriologists. Though diseases with the power to make history knew no boundaries defined by race, class or sex, social factors shaped both the childhood experience of sickness and the societal response to the problem. Domestic environment to a great degree reflected social status; culture and class often defined health and medical treatment. To be effective, pediatric practice had to be oriented to social context as well as public health. Children remained almost invisible, acted upon at the bottom of the ladder of social hierarchy. Few laws protected them from exploitation and few hospitals existed for their treatment. Especially vulnerable were the large numbers of foundlings and orphaned infants institutionalized in major urban areas. These children beckoned to some practitioners, presenting an opportunity to develop and innovate medical therapies. To this day, the ethics of medical treatment of children are poorly defined legally.[55]

* * *

So matters stood as the nineteenth century drew to a close. Once the nearly exclusive province of midwives, scientific exploration had redefined human birth, delineating a process so fraught as to demand not one but three medical specialties. The obstetrician was prepared to exercise authority in the birth itself; the gynecologist stood by to repair any resultant injuries; the pediatrician could supervise the newcomer's proper care. Science has a way of both clarifying and complicating at once. More ominously, scientific definition could create authoritarian walls, making the experience of childbirth a cold, rigid, and institutional procedure.

Five

American Research Impaired

Issues of race blind us. Because race is a powerful controlling signifier of social relations, economics and politics, application of the concept obfuscates meaning, obscures understanding. Historian Evelyn Brooks Higginbotham argues that race permeates the language of American history.[1] The social and cultural construction of race transcends other meanings, making categories of class and gender invisible despite their inordinate presence in the past—everything is understood and represented in terms of race. As race changes meaning from era to era, the power and impact of such a culturally-derived concept becomes illusive.

The metalanguage of race was thoroughly in place throughout the United States by the close of the nineteenth century. Though the Civil War had ended slavery, culture and law reasserted racial barriers to the nth degree. Violence against African American men accompanied fiercely enforced segregation in the South and the North. Primary to national purpose, race distinctions expanded along lines drawn around various ethnicities perceived as different and lesser beings than the governing white, theoretically Anglo-Saxon majority shaping the development of the nation. Prejudice and exclusion governed national foreign policy.[2]

By the 1890s, hope for racial equality had faded throughout the nation. Ruling whites collectively reestablished a social order forcibly subordinating African Americans, punishing them ostensibly for the color of their skin. In 1905, the U.S. Supreme Court's decision in *Plessy v. Ferguson* made segregation the law of the land, thereby strengthening and recodifying separation of Blacks and whites.[3] As W.E.B. DuBois articulated, "the problem of the twentieth century is the problem of the color line."[4] By the 1920s miscegenation laws outlawed racial intermarriage in many states. Several would enact sterilization laws for selected "unfit" types. Lynchings were frequent from the 1870s through the 1930s—justified most often by false charges of African American male sexual aggression against white women. The law of the land was shaped to protect white supremacy in the name of so-called white purity.[5]

Five. American Research Impaired 79

* * *

From the early days of abolition, Philadelphia had been home to the greatest number of free African Americans. In the nineteenth century, New York and Baltimore began to overtake Philadelphia, exhibiting a higher rate of growth for the African American population. The Civil War era and its aftermath brought a small but steady movement of people out of slavery and into northeastern cities. In 1860 Pennsylvania had 56,949 free Blacks living in the state; Maryland had 83,942; New York had a free Black population of 49, 005.[6] In 1870, Pennsylvania's population included 65,294 African Americans; Maryland's was 175,391; New York state's free Black population grew to 52,081. The increasing use of race as a framework and then an explanation for the incidence of rickets paralleled the migration of African Americans.[7]

Maryland's African American population had multiplied at the greatest rate. Baltimore was the biggest nucleus, home to 25,000 free men and women in 1850. Forty years later, the city's Black population had risen to nearly 67,000. Baltimore would become a center for treatment of rachitic contracted pelves. Philadelphia continued to house a large population of free Black women and men, living in outlying areas as well as within city boundaries. The "City of Brotherly Love" was another center of growing interest in rickets and the contracted pelvis. Medical ties to New York City, Washington, D.C., and Boston were strong, the exchange of views, information, hypotheses regular.[8]

By 1916, the trickle of African Americans moving northward had become a strong and persistent flow moving from the rural South to Northern cities, a vast movement of people known as the Great Migration. Besides Eastern cities—Baltimore, Philadelphia, New York, and Boston especially, newer western cities became home, including St. Louis, Chicago and Cleveland. The movement consisted of African Americans in many different circumstances, some in families, most leaving children and the elderly behind, moving to Northern cities in great numbers—1.6 million by 1940. They migrated to find work. Often their lives endured poverty, poor sanitation and meager living conditions in large industrializing urban centers. Much of their health care likely came from Black midwives, thoroughly marginalized by mainstream medicine. There was limited access to Black hospitals and few Black practitioners or nurses.[9]

Accompanying this Great Black Migration was a so-called "New Immigration" providing labor for the great burst of American industrialization in the latter half of the nineteenth century, to continue until the end of the Great War. Prior to 1860, migrations had largely emanated from western Europe, the reasonably familiar peoples of France, Germany, Scandinavia and the British Isles. On the Pacific coast, an immigration of Chinese laborers, mostly male, began in 1849, continuing until the Chinese Exclusion Act brought the migration to an abrupt end in 1882. Diverse ethnic groups began to emigrate from Southern and Eastern Europe in large numbers after 1870; by 1920, 4.1 million Italians and 7.8 million eastern Europeans (encompassing a bewildering array of ethnic identities) reached the shores of America, settling mostly in larger cities. Native born whites, forgetting their own status as the descendants of immigrants, readily classified these newer European immigrants as inferior human beings, worthy of little more than prejudice and mistreatment. This unfamiliar presence further complicated issues of race and poverty in traditional eyes.[10]

* * *

In Europe, analysts, researchers and writers built their studies on the idea that rickets was most often an affliction of the poor in their countries, while elsewhere in the world poverty did not generate the disease. In the latter half of the nineteenth century, population shifts resulting from migration occurred in many places across the globe, redefining the geography of rickets. This was especially true in the United States.[11] Studies of health, latitude and race—resting on "the regional human geography of race"—found that the Black mortality rate was higher in the Northern cities (typified in their latitude in degrees north) than the white mortality rate, but only slightly higher than whites in the rural antebellum South. Such scholarship suggests the importance of seasons and sunlight—governed by latitude—in morbidity and mortality, making the seasonality of rickets a likely component. The study also discovered that during the post–Civil War years, when Black migration out of the South began, African American mortality rates were consistently higher than whites in urban areas above the fortieth parallel.[12]

By the end of the nineteenth century, the neglect of African American health, especially among those whose families were left with nothing after the war's end, was extreme. As Christian Warren contends, "freedom from slavery ... brought a crisis of health."[13] The difficulty African Americans endured maintaining survival increased the denigration mouthed by many whites, who blamed their biological heritage for their poverty and ill health. Many believed the so-called race was degenerating.[14]

While discussions of environmental factors versus inherited or congenital factors in the etiology of rickets continued, a steady medical exchange regarding the incidence of the disease hummed in the background. In the United States of the 1870s, only a few physicians reported cases of rickets. Their voices came mostly from New York, Philadelphia, Washington, Baltimore and Boston, cities where August Hirsch had recognized a notable presence of the disease in his geography of 1886. Though American physicians differed regarding the incidence and effects of rickets, they shared in the growing international attention devoted to the difficulties experienced in a small but intriguing number of childbirths, difficulties often attributed to contracted pelves. The science of obstetrics was gaining strength.[15]

* * *

Examining obstetrical experience through the peculiar lens of race led American researchers in contradictory directions, obscuring comprehension of the critical issues. While some researchers identified what they believed to be a marked biological tendency toward rickets among dark-skinned people, others interpreted their evidence to reach an entirely different conclusion. Certainly childbirth differed with race, they argued, but rickets was not the distinguishing factor.

During the Civil War and after, many African Americans sought refuge in Washington, D. C., believing freedom and equality would be theirs. There they met the endemic assumptions of racial typology at every turn. Though Washington's Freedmen's Hospital mission was established to care for people newly freed from slavery, one doctor practicing there, Joseph Taber Johnson (1846–1921)—a white physician—brought his pre-conceived notions of ethnology to bear on a study of childbirth among the African American patients he treated. Visualizing race as a biological absolute, Johnson expounded upon the anatomy of Black women and babies—the newborn cranium and the maternal pelvis—in its relation to gorillas. Having established race as the critical component, he took the argument further, demonstrating the role of class in childbirth. The more educated and civilized the individual, the more difficult the birth.[16]

Johnson, who practiced at the Freedman's Hospital in its first years, published an essay in 1875 regarding the "Apparent Peculiarities of Parturition in the Negro Race." He drew from five hundred of his own cases, eight hundred attended by two young Black doctors associated with the hospital, and seven hundred cases passed on by "granny midwives."[17] Johnson argued that, in his experience, freed African American women had few deformed pelves and that overall, their birth experiences were uneventful. Externally their pelves seemed narrow, but internal measurements were normal. He described the comparatively easy births of these patients. Not only did he belittle the intelligence of the birthing African American women as being of the "lower race," he belittled the practitioners from whom he gathered case records—the granny midwives, a category identifying Black midwives from the South, and his African American associates at the hospital, "two busy colored physicians."[18]

Contradictions in his comments derived from the racial blinders he wore—he saw African American women as uncivilized in comparison to over-cultivated white women. Misperceived animality, according to such observers, gave Black women the ability to give birth without pain, while "overcivilized" white women suffered terribly.[19] Unafraid to express his sexual attraction to his phenotypical representation of African American women, the grace of their walk as opposed to the waddle of white women, he portrayed them as the opposite of white women with difficult births and highly nervous civilized ways. Although he did connect rickets to a kidney shaped contracted pelvis, Johnson found little other evidence of contracted pelves in these patients and deliberated extensively over the influence of race. In the end he had no doubt. Johnson's stereotypes of race shaped the world of his practice.[20]

Following in the footsteps left by Samuel Morton and Charles Meigs, Johnson put the pelves of the African and the African American low in the evolutionary hierarchy, an expression of the persistent duality—savage versus civilized. The more civilized the woman, the more difficult the birth—especially for male babies, as their brains were bigger. Johnson argued that cases of cephalo-pelvic disproportion always involved white or sometimes mixed-race male babies.[21] Class, for Johnson and others like him, served as a distinction among whites only. Mixed-race was a category of its own.[22]

Johnson's essay developed a picture of birth as varying according to race. Adopting Dutch anatomist Gerardus Vrolick's idea that the female pelvis and the fetal head shared a complementary race-based shape, he reproduced drawings comparing "facial angle" of the "Negro" fetal skull to the "White" fetal skull. The size of the Negro head was supposedly smaller, hence the birth was easier—a Lamarckian argument, popular at this time, arguing traits were inherited as a result of successful adaptation in terms of function. (The doctor did admit that some educated African Americans showed intelligence—specifically the Black physicians whose data he used.) Complementarity of fetal head and maternal pelvis facilitated birth—cases of miscegenation, from this point of view, brought trouble. As obstetrics had established the birth process with an emphasis on cephalo-pelvic proportion, now the fetal journey involved issues of race and race mixing.[23]

* * *

Joseph Taber Johnson's contentions regarding the relationship of race and the ease of birth notwithstanding, two American physicians, Robert Harris and John Parry, both from Philadelphia, professionally recorded experience with rickets and race relatively early. Each had attended obstructed births and founded their studies of rickets on difficult labors wrought by contracted pelves.

Parry's work began with a review of the statistical incidence of rickets coming from Europe. Though the exchange was international, a great proportion of the studies of rickets from 1870 to 1914 came from Germany, Austria, England and Scotland. Somewhat rough, the cited numbers showed that rickets affected children in Europe at a significant rate, varying there from twenty to more than thirty percent. Such reports were standard in medical articles, evidence of prevalent rickets in countries similar to the United States politically, economically and socially.[24]

In the United States, quite the opposite was true—few talked about the presence of rickets among infants and young children. Parry was an exception, reporting in 1872 that twenty-eight percent of the sick children between one month and five years old in the Philadelphia Hospital children's departments suffered from rickets.[25] African American patients were an important component of his patients. Well-steeped in the current medical literature, Parry considered the association of race distinctions with cadaveric evidence of the disease. Performing numerous post-mortems to study the skulls and brains of infants and young children who died of rickets, he commented on the skull shape and the deterioration of the brain tissue—"the pale, watery brain, the substance of which often has the appearance of cornstarch."[26] Most common he said were the "rachitic long heads ... among negro children ... [and] very rarely among the whites."[27] Parry identified this specific long head shape, known as doliocephalic, as a trait of African American infants with rickets. He suggested the square head, possibly meaning white, was more common, but did not clearly identify its racial base, if indeed there was one.[28] In a footnote, Parry explored the meaning of "dolichocephal," clarifying that the skull shape was not an inherited race trait but rather the consequence of an "effusion of serum" around the child's brain.[29]

Race was not a purposeful conceptual basis guiding Parry's observations. Despite this lack of intent, his statistics pointed to a predominant racial factor in his cases of contracted pelves.[30] (A text on childhood sickness by American authors J. Forsyth Meigs and William Pepper followed a similar path. *A Practical Treatise on the Diseases of Children* devoted several pages to rickets without invoking race as a factor.)[31] Parry's treatise on the nature of rickets was lengthy and educating, the implication being that physicians did not know the subtle early characteristics of infantile rachitic disease so carefully delineated by Jenner. Parry considered his own clinical experiences in the light of Jenner's observations, and wisely noted Trousseau's emphatic embrace of cod liver oil, urging its use in the treatment of the disease.[32]

In Philadelphia lived one woman whose birth histories were so extremely severe as to excite publication and reference among several doctors, including John Parry. An adult somewhere in her twenties, she lived in a different world from them—a world of urban poverty and deprivation. In the late winter of 1874, W.H. Parrish, a physician at the dispensary service of the Philadelphia Hospital, attended her final birth in a "garret, a most dismal forbidding den, so low that by persons of ordinary stature the erect posture could not be assumed. The leaky roof let in the wind and rain, and there was no fire or means of counteracting the chilling effects of the weather. Such was the setting for the third craniotomy." A Black little person "living alone, the woman suffered severe skeletal disfigurement resulting from childhood rickets—her femurs were 'bent forward' ... and the tibiae are moderately crooked—leaving her barely four feet tall." At the time of Parrish's visit, other occupants of the house constituted "a mongrel crowd of whites and negroes in various stages of drunkenness, and exhibiting all the evidences of abject poverty, wretchedness, and degradation."[33] No words from the woman survive except those quoted by physicians. Certainly she did not see her neighbors in the same terms as the doctors who wrote up the case. We know she experienced sexual intimacy that left her pregnant four times and that she died of puerperal fever in her garret four weeks after her third craniotomy. Though she had visits from medical personnel in the postpartum days, for the most part she was unattended.[34]

In the clinical records doctors called her Josephine Scott, but we do not know if this was the name she herself used. During her final pregnancy she protected herself as best she could, hiding from the staff of the Philadelphia hospital dispensary. Though she had sought their assistance repeatedly in years past, by the last pregnancy she feared their treatment and tried to escape another craniotomy by going to the Bedford Street Mission Hospital. A woman physician there fetched Doctor Parrish after forty hours of labor without progress. When Parrish came to help her, she denied her history of craniotomies, pretended "stupidity," and would give no information about herself. Whether she willfully withheld information remains unknown. Parrish's language shows he felt alienated from the patient's way of life.[35]

In spite of Parrish's harsh assessment, he admitted that Josephine Scott's extreme exhaustion caused him to etherize her, merely to examine her. Such a pain killing therapy was becoming routine for white women, but not African Americans. Parrish calculated a pelvic diameter of one and seven-eighths inches, indicating this birth was dangerous. No hope existed to save the life of the infant, whose head still floated above the pelvic inlet. The doctor and his associates struggled to hold the fetal head still to effect perforation and to empty the brains to permit passage. At the time, Parrish felt he would be lucky to save Scott's life, as her contracted pelvis thoroughly blocked the progression of the birth. Without alternative choices, a craniotomy risked everything—a path this patient had already followed twice.[36]

After the delivery of the destroyed fetus was finally accomplished, Parrish reported that she now "confessed" to memories of the two previous craniotomies done at the Philadelphia Hospital, and, Parrish said, "we then recognized her as Josephine Scott."[37] What the doctors knew about her was actually very little. Her second craniotomy had been performed by John Parry, who recorded that "she could give no definite account of herself."[38] Parry reported she did not really feel any pain, quoting her words after the second gruesome craniotomy, "[I] did not mind having a baby, that it did not hurt [me] any."[39] Echoing Joseph Taber Johnson, white doctors commonly argued that African American women had an easier time given birth and did not feel pain.[40]

Perceived race and social status difference created barriers in perception and communication. Though this patient was heavily sedated during these operations, she clearly had undrugged moments and plenty of time to consider the procedures she experienced—enough to hope for a different outcome with each pregnancy. She depended on the doctors to help her through dire labors but feared and mistrusted them at the same time.

When "Josephine Scott" died of puerperal fever, doctors objectified her extremely contracted pelvis as a prized rare case. Her conjugate pelvic diameter was a centerpiece for Parry, who judged her pelvic inlet anterior/posterior diameter to measure one and one half inches, an eighth of an inch less than Parrish measured. This was considerably below the three and one/half inch limit proclaimed by German researcher Carl Litzmann and American physician Hugh Hodge to be the bottom of the normal range. Like the rare European cases Parry had read about, this patient's traumatic birth meant for him the publication of a lengthy article in which he argued for abandoning craniotomy.[41]

In the article, Parry described himself sitting at "the bedside of a suffering woman in the most trying moment of her existence."[42] As he described the woman's delivery over several pages, the language shifted to detail an ever more violent yet tedious piece by piece destruction of the head of the patient's fetus. Parry first seemed to suggest this patient was a "lady," but when talking more specifically he succinctly made the woman's lesser social status clear, if tactfully and without judging her further. Because she was "colored," she was a "girl"—more a child than an adult. Parry said she was twenty-four; the next year Parrish posited she was twenty-eight years of age. Overall, Parry's concern was not so much for her well-being as for how her case could provide an example to protect women of greater affluence and more secure social standing—white women—from pain and trauma giving birth. For Parry, the lesson was to heed Robert Harris's advocacy of Caesarean section.[43]

In the last decades of the nineteenth century and the first decades of the twentieth, numerous extreme obstetrical surgeries moved in and out of favor, often in the name of the contracted pelvis. Joining Harris, Parry sought to establish a medical protocol using Caesarean Section instead of craniotomy in any birth where the mother's pelvic conjugate diameter measured two and a half inches or less. Writing in 1879, Parry hoped to see the day when seventy-five percent of women who underwent Caesarean section lived.[44] In 1871, Harris had published the first in his series of four articles chronicling births exemplifying extremely difficult yet purportedly successful experiences—Caesarian Sections without antisepsis, often without anesthetic. He found that 60 percent of the women in cases surveyed recovered from the surgery; the year following he wrote of improvement, with a recovery rate of 70.1 percent.[45] The chief obstacle was infection; hospital precautions developing in Europe had yet to reach across the sea. Harris included descriptions of the shape of the pelvis in his abstracted records, referring to specific conjugate diameters of contracted pelves, measured internally. Nineteen of the patients (32.2 percent) measured a conjugate diameter of two inches or less. Of his fifty-nine cases, twenty-six, or 44 percent, were labeled as quadroon, slave, mulatto, French-creole, or Negress, a number far out of proportion to the general population. (Rather than an indication that non-whites were more likely to suffer contracted pelvis, the fact was that minority patients were far more often the subjects of such experimental surgery.)[46]

Across lines of race, twenty-four of the women Harris described died within a few weeks of giving birth, while twenty-six recovered fully. Some women survived the Caesarian birth only to bear another child or two and then meet their demise from a second such experience. Several of the birthing women exhibited contracted pelves and may have had rickets. Five cases explicitly reported deformity from rickets. Two were white women and three were African American. Harris used one doctor's drawing of a pelvis to declare the patient's deformity rachitic. All but one of the mothers with such a deformity died. Harris proudly announced that the five children had lived.[47]

* * *

As American doctors continued to consider the symptoms and incidence of rickets, they more willingly discussed the significance of race for the victims. By the latter years of the nineteenth century, doctors had intensified the professional exchange about the presence of rickets and urgently warned one another of an ongoing epidemic. Studies from the period frequently refer to multiple cases of rickets among former slaves, and possibly those free men and women who never knew slavery directly. Published medical reports increasingly categorized dark-skinned people as the population most affected by the disease in the United States, despite the undeniable fact that Americans first learned about rickets from European physicians whose patients were white English, German, French, and Dutch children. Plainly white people contracted the disease just as readily as any other ethnic group, yet most American researchers continued to insist rickets was a product of racial disposition, an inherent constitutional weakness specific to biology.

Nineteen years after Joseph Taber Johnson published his findings, another Washington D.C. physician, George Acker, published "Rickets in Negroes," an 1894 work intended to inform other practitioners of the great extent of the disease among his African American hospital patients. The article was one of the first to discuss rickets employing an explicitly racial framework. Acker associated the disease with the diatheses of tuberculosis and syphilis—"the scrofulous diseases"[48]—having seen patients who suffered both before displaying symptoms of rickets. He traced the ill health of these patients to the end of slavery and the loss of paternalistic care from the slave master, though he admitted slaves probably had rickets too. His language degraded African Americans even as he fully described the dimensions of poverty in which they lived:

> Anyone who has been brought in contact with them knows of their shiftless, improvident ways. Being placed on their own resources and without any restraining influences they suffer from intemperance, impure air from overcrowding and want of ventilation, and insufficient clothing.... The race is undergoing serious physical decay.... [This] is due to inherent weakness or physical degeneration, and not to any special fault in the environment.[49]

Acker found "Negroes are almost without exception rachitic."[50] He thought these patients carried a proclivity to the disease, in fact inherited it. Acker discounted the importance of climate, stating that African Americans were susceptible to rickets in any climate. The symptoms of the disease paralleled the standard symptoms of rickets Jenner had identified. As race defined the incidence, Acker's tone and words denigrated the very people who suffered. In his estimation, these people were simply degenerating, weak in many ways. His stereotyped point of viewed mirrored the eugenicist concept of fit and unfit human beings, which in turn meshed neatly with ideas of traits peculiar to specific races.[51]

Statistics for African Americans are such that accuracy in numbers of births and child deaths is virtually impossible. Historians Edward Shorter and Phillip Cutright considered the effect of rickets on Black health and fertility. Their so-called "health hypothesis" argues that rickets, venereal disease and infection in childbirth led to infertility, precipitating a decline by deforming the pelvis.[52] As demographer Richard H. Steckel noted, the mortality rate for Black children fell with the end of slavery. For African American adults, the rate of mortality stayed nearly the same until 1920.[53] Cliometrician Stanley Engermann concluded that African Americans experienced a steady decline in population from 1890 to 1940.[54] Engermann addressed the decline in terms of fertility, suggesting that African Americans experienced a demographic transition similar to whites, though different because of their historical experiences. The Great Migration from rural life to urban industrial settings was accompanied by a lessened rate of reproduction, apparently through the use of birth control.[55]

White physicians commonly saw the white body in an entirely different light from the African American, even in the North. In the late nineteenth century, many highly-educated professionals maintained that African Americans as a race were declining due to failure to reproduce successfully, because of high infant mortality and morbidity, and through general enfeeblement. Rickets was to be expected. As John Haller described physicians' views, "the post-war Negro was succumbing to disease in far greater numbers than the antebellum generation, and that the Negro seemed precariously close to extinction."[56]

George Acker looked at the situation with a jaundiced eye. "This is a serious subject for consideration, and should engage the attention of the health authorities, for we now have a prolific race of unhealthy, degenerated beings who will prove a menace to the interests of the country."[57] Falsely reporting higher rates of African American reproduction, Acker pushed the medical approach to rickets around a corner, locating an abundance of the disease in the large population of African Americans living in the United States capital. In a contradictory and camouflaged way, the argument fed the idea of race suicide—that the survival of the white race was endangered by the presence of a diseased and degraded yet "prolific" African American population. Arguing at once that Blacks were unhealthy, degenerating, and poised to overwhelm the country was American racism at its most heinous. George Acker's pronouncements regrettably reflected American sentiment at large. Across the nation, extreme racial discrimination characterized law and behavior.[58]

African American physicians practicing in Washington possessed little power or opportunity to publicly rebut Acker's tone and interpretation. Few in number and fiercely determined, they focused on the overwhelming task of bringing health and well-being to sick African Americans.[59]

Five. American Research Impaired

* * *

The growth of pernicious racial thought and behavior was not without answer. Separate health care seemed one solution to the adversity. Black leaders abhorred the thought of accepting segregated institutions, but saw no alternative. Many feared the eventual end of their race, as the high rates of death and disease outweighed the birth rate—the "degeneration" advanced by Acker. Discounting such interpretations, Daniel Hale Williams (1856–1931), a physician and Black leader, argued for the importance of accessible medical care for Black people and for the presence of Black physicians and Black hospitals. In 1891, he founded the Provident Hospital in Chicago, which became a biracial training center for medical students.[60] African American physician Francis Mossell (1856–1946) trained at the University of Pennsylvania and opened the important and successful Frederick Douglass Memorial Hospital in Philadelphia in 1895.[61] Despite such attainment, the harsh realities of segregation continually challenged the well-being of patients and the quality of health care. Money was a problem; white hospitals attracted much more funding.

The traditions defining Black culture in America made issues of health care especially challenging. Even as some Black physicians applied themselves to creating their own hospitals, problems remained and in fact grew. Migrating to cities from rural areas, some African Americans people brought with them a folk culture of medical practice, often grounded in herbal remedies. Doctors represented a ghostly threat. Many believed there were night-riders wearing white sheets, night doctors who kidnapped Blacks for experimentation and sold their cadavers for autopsies—stories perhaps perpetuated by slave masters.[62] Daniel Williams offered insights to the challenges of caring for Black women, describing with contempt the heritage of folk medicine to which many ascribed. He warned, "they have a natural dislike and horror of hospitals."[63] Still, Williams was empathetic to their fears. In his experience the women consulted once they came to expect appropriate ameliorating treatment. How many, he asked, have these women been misdiagnosed?[64]

Health issues, as framed in a culture of race distinction generated by whites, became a significant concern of African Americans. Fully aware of the developments in medical research, community leaders sought to improve the standards of medical care available to the Black population. Beginning in 1895, W.E.B. DuBois (1868–1963) headed an annual conference in Atlanta, devoted to "the Study of the Negro Problems." The eleventh such conference, attended by an elite biracial group including DuBois and anthropologist Franz Boas (1858–1942), considered "the Health and Physique of the American Negro." Though much of the discussion centered on efforts toward improving health care, participants took time to consider the impact of segregation. DuBois and his colleagues questioned assumptions underpinning the racial categories established by whites, challenging their validity. Speakers demonstrated the fallacies of racial typology, addressing the scientific ideas afoot equating brain size and differences in head shape with race. Their conclusions challenged the validity of mainstream scientific assumptions degrading African American intelligence and blaming them for the origin and spread of disease. Urging the separation of medical research from the idea of race, the conference emphasized that prejudice and stereotyping blinded white scientists in their work. Accompanying the rise of modern medicine, the concept of race had become a metalanguage in the medical system, impacting and influencing every aspect of its practice, resulting in racialized medicine (conscious or unconscious). DuBois published the edited reports of the meeting the year following, providing a wealth of information about the lives of African Americans, the availability of health care, the exceedingly limited opportunities for Black education in the field of medicine.[65]

Opposed to pressuring whites for legal and political rights, Booker T. Washington (1856–1915) took a different tack. Research conducted at his Tuskegee Institute in 1914 fully established the health crisis among Blacks—45 percent of Black deaths were preventable; the economic costs of early mortality ran to one hundred million dollars. Washington responded by launching a National Health Improvement Week in April 1915, subsequently observed as National Negro Health Week. A climax to his self-help movement, Washington spoke to three thousand people, mostly Black, at the Bethel A.M.E. Church in Baltimore, where he contended that whites needed to help better the health of Blacks for the good of society as a whole.[66] Voicing a premise that germs did not honor racial lines, he condemned segregation, urging reform of living conditions to address the high rate of sickness and disease among Black people. Negro Health Week was highly successful in terms of Black participation (and some white), but in the final analysis did little to better the serious problems of health care.[67]

Despite the efforts of Washington, DuBois, Williams, and countless others, racism in all its forms remained far too entrenched in American medical thinking to effect meaningful change in research or health care. Continued insistence on racial construction would persist, obscuring the science devoted to untangling the etiology of disease—rickets especially.

* * *

The question of race in the etiology of rickets only grew more complicated. In an 1895 study of Italian immigrants, medical practitioner Irving M. Snow chose a different framework to associate the origins of rachitic disease with race.[68] Snow, a physician in Buffalo, New York, presented his paper, "An Explanation of the Great Frequency of Rickets Among Neapolitan Children in American Cities," at the American Pediatric Society's sixth annual meeting.[69] Among the first in the United States to devote himself to pediatrics, Snow's study heightened the impression of race and ethnicity as key factors in American rickets. Snow predicted that in the future, three fourths of the sick Italian children who came to his clinic at the Buffalo Fresh Air Mission Hospital would have rickets. Most of his Italian patients came from southern Italy—Naples and environs. This was amazing, Snow contended, citing August Hirsch's geography of disease. Heretofore, rickets was known only in northern Italy. Snow set up a research study comparing ethnicities of immigrants in Buffalo. He looked at two hundred immigrant children—one hundred-eight Italians and ninety-two of other nationalities. Among the Italian patients, seventy-six were rachitic; among the others, only eleven had the disease. Most of the Italians exhibited advanced symptoms such as the appearance of rachitic rosary lining the rib cage, craniotabes, narrowing and deformity of the chest, or muscular weakness. Surprisingly, most were overweight.[70]

Determining that southern Italy was not a locus for rickets, Snow researched conditions in the region. He concluded the residents of "the Italian colony in Buffalo" were better off than they had in Naples (except for rickets), and possibly better off than other immigrants of different ethnic origin elsewhere. Comparing races (without mentioning African Americans), he stated, "Concerning the hygiene of the skin, the Italian babies were never as clean or as well cared for as the average American Irish, or German. However, to say that they were, as a class, filthy would be untrue." An awkward complement at best, but kinder than George Acker.[71] Snow thought the parenting and provision of clothing and food was good. He had a positive assessment of the appearance of the parents, "strong, healthy, young people. The women are well-shaped and have easy labors."[72] Although Snow defended the goodness of his Italian patients, his double-entendre reference to the shape of the women patients or mothers of patients, kept explicit the idea of an ethnic, other racial group and the subjective state of women, especially women immigrants.

Snow was puzzled by the incidence of rickets among his patients. His work included a systematic comparison of the climates of Naples and Buffalo. He found an answer that looked to explain the prevalence of rickets among Neapolitans and African Americans alike—though he never made the connection. Drawing from Hirsch, Snow attributed the cause to exposure to a climate of cold, damp weather. "The intrusion of a southern race into a northern climate is an occurrence that has few parallels in history."[73] Migrating north made people sick with rickets, necessitating changes in lifestyle. For Snow, this included lessons in hygiene, nutrition, and ventilation, as well as infant care. Keep your children in open fresh air with as much sunshine as possible, he cautioned. In the final pages he brought the lesson back to the Teutonic or Nordic races, warning that migration to a different climate impeded reproduction and threatened health. Unlike Acker, Irving Snow did not blame race for the presence of the disease so much as he found the environment—the home environment—responsible.[74]

After Snow read his paper, attending members of the American Pediatric Society participated in a lively exchange of views, sharing experiences and putting forth individual interpretations of the etiology of rickets, noting the great variety of possible explanations. Race and rickets opened up discussion among notable members of the audience, including L. Emmett Holt (1855–1924), a well-known New York City pediatrician, J. Henry Fruitnight (1851–1900), also of New York City, and George Acker.

J.P. Crozer Griffith (1856–1941) of Philadelphia reacted with bewilderment to the idea that migration to a damp colder climate might cause rickets, as he considered the many generations of Black Philadelphia residents who "ought to have become acclimatized by this time."[75] He saw no difference between his white and the Black cases. He suggested that an inherent affinity, a propensity, for rickets was associated with African Americans. Griffith argued that there were different classes of African Americans, that Philadelphia had a unique history affecting the epidemiology of the disease. His later publication, a handbook on the care of children, does not mention variation of rickets by race, though the work makes numerous references to signs of rickets and details how to treat them.[76]

L. Emmett Holt, a young man rapidly becoming a nationally recognized leader in the new specialty of pediatrics, agreed that Italian and African American children suffered the most severe rickets. If an Italian or "colored" child came to the hospital with a serious disease, the child likely had rickets in "a marked form."[77] In other words, a child with rickets was not likely to get treated for the disease—or even diagnosed as such—unless he or she contracted a severe illness, such as tuberculosis or pneumonia, whooping cough, or measles. This meant that rickets cases were undercounted, and that such children, African Americans especially, were more likely to die with rickets.[78]

Audience members tossed around personal beliefs about the poor, their health and diet. George Acker argued for a better environment and possibly the use of an emulsion of phosphorus and cod liver oil. Still, he concluded climate was of little import and what he saw as a peculiar physiology accounted for sickness among the African Americans. What little denial of the racial factor occurred failed to quell the overwhelmingly race-based exchange; climate and inherent traits, though posed as opposites, both led to race as the etiology of rickets.[79]

S.S. Adams, a physician from the District of Columbia, referred to Acker's essay on African American patients, stating that very few whites in Washington had rickets. Maybe, he thought, this was because there were very few poor white people, whites being considerably outnumbered by Blacks in the area. Like Snow, Adams urged education in hygiene as the key response to the high numbers of rickets patients.[80]

The emphasis on hygiene was revealing. Regardless of the types of patients they treated, many physicians in one form or another saw race as the context explaining rickets. If not biology, the culprit had to be ignorance of proper sanitation practices. To combat the problem, researchers urged the teaching of proper hygiene to immigrant ethnic groups and African Americans.

Rarely characterized precisely, the concept of hygiene was evolving in meaning in the late nineteenth century with the coming of germ theory and health reform. Middle class ideals of lifestyle and habitation combined with developing theories of proper sanitation and cleanliness to define proper behavior. Wellness was tied to proper use of newly advanced plumbing sanitation technologies; never mind the fact that hot running water and indoor toilets were not possible for many, particularly in poorer neighborhoods.[81] Nutrition was regarded as part of hygiene. Discussions among practitioners considering rickets focused on breast feeding and, as it was called, artificial feeding of infants. Though most doctors agreed breastfeeding helped keep an infant well, they often criticized mothers for their particular approach. In the end mothers were often blamed for the growing prevalence of rickets. White American doctors always identified a patient by race if (s)he was not white and often belittled the African American women's abilities as mothers—collectively or individually—unable to portray them in that fundamental social role, or to recognize the impact of poverty on their efforts. Concepts of hygiene and nutrition were habits that on the one hand could be improved by education, but on the other limited by supposedly inherited racial failings.[82]

Doctors' perceptions of the incidence of rickets came largely from the nature of their practice. J. Henry Fruitnight took a different tack in the discussion, presenting a list of ethnicities in his New York practice by frequency of the disease. He found the greatest number of rickets cases among Italians, but the second largest group was Teutonic—the English and the Scandinavian. Fruitnight went on to enumerate Slavic and Bohemian immigrants as suffering more rickets than found in the British Isles—thought by many to be the locus of the largest outbreak of the disease. "He thought this was due to the sudden transition from the environing conditions under which their ancestors had lived for centuries." A profound change in climate could leave any human being susceptible to rickets, regardless of racial classification.[83]

* * *

While the perception of rickets as a race-based disease largely defined American comprehension, that conclusion directly contradicted European experience. No one in America addressed the contradiction. Instead, physicians at their professional meetings expressed race-based opinions, debating why the African American or the Italian communities should be afflicted by the disease. Some felt the Italians case was really puzzling, but very few questioned the widespread presence of the disease among Blacks. Etiology conflated with stereotype, confounding so-called scientific efforts to understand and treat the disease. Assumptions of race made objective investigation into the origins or incidence of rickets impossible.

At various points in time, American medical writings reported that upwards of eighty percent of the nation's children suffered from rickets. Observations of such magnitude surely suggested that people of many and diverse ethnic backgrounds suffered the disease. Impressions based on race and ethnicity obscured diagnosis, making accurate statistical accounts extremely difficult. The confusion resulting makes an historically accurate rendering of how many people living in nineteenth-century America actually had rickets, and who those people were, maddeningly impossible.

Migration and immigration found a way into perceptions of sickness and health. Practitioners treated their racial interpretations as common knowledge, based on everyday observation. There were, of course, exceptions to what looks to be a cultural bias; some physicians did refuse to accept race as an element of the discussion. But not many. Particularly in the eastern United States, physicians generally assumed, insisted, or simply accepted the common understanding that African Americans were the most commonly afflicted with rickets, along with Italian immigrants. Social response grew into xenophobia among far too many members of the well-established dominant class. Southern and eastern Europeans, the Chinese and Japanese, and other newly emigrated groups suffered from a general disdain at the hands of the medical profession. Though rarely articulated baldly, habitual segregation and denigration of African Americans defined most medical research, dominated clinical procedure, and biased medical writing. The metalanguage of race so clouded perception, rickets was inevitably to remain one of the great puzzles of American medicine.

Six

Combating a Riddle Unresolved

From the 1870s through the 1910s and beyond, rickets had a particularly strong influence on Western society. Widespread recognition of the disease and the attendant contracted pelves brought awareness of a growing presence, apparently connected to the advent of industrialization and migration, transecting climates and geographies. By the latter part of the nineteenth century, physicians were enumerating and exploring myriad rachitic symptoms, searching for an explanation. Rickets most directly affected children—killing some, affecting many. Significant but far more difficult to trace, contracted pelves, a consequence of rickets suffered in childhood, significantly affected some adult women giving birth.

Laboratory discoveries transmogrified medical practice and the theoretical understanding of sickness and health, but failed to offer any satisfactory answers for the treatment of rachitic disease. The movement of peoples across the globe, accompanied by extreme alterations in the patterns of life, brought increased physical contact and nutritional exchange. Rickets seemed to spread, becoming an enigmatic reminder of the incomprehensible effects of social, political and economic metamorphosis. Migration from warmer latitudes to temperate climes seemed to create particular susceptibilities. Patterns in the United States proved especially mystifying. Industrializing rapidly, home to a large population of African descendants, attracting immigrants from Europe and Asia, rickets assumed an enigmatic presence. American practitioners maintained incidence was small and limited to darker skinned peoples, defying European evidence to the contrary. Not until the twentieth century did some assert a nearly universal prevalence of rickets in the United States.

Two hundred-fifty years of scientific investigation into the puzzle of rachitic disease had produced myriad suppositions, conjectures, hypotheses, educated guesses, and very little in the way of answers. Rickets was a nutritional disease. A product of industrialization. A consequence of poor hygiene. Hereditary. Not hereditary. A characteristic of race. Microbial. Toxic. Seasonal. Associated with other diseases—scurvy, tetany, syphilis.

There were cures, maybe. Phosphorous. Cod liver oil. Proper breastfeeding (not for too long). Fresh air. Sunlight. The floundering would continue well past the close of the nineteenth century.

* * *

The fact that free-roaming wild animals never got rickets while captives in zoos became rachitic intrigued many medical researchers.[1] In 1889, a dietary experiment by English surgeon Doctor John Bland-Sutton (1855–1936), carried out in a London zoo, sparked interest in nutrition as a cure for rickets in humans. Invited to treat lion cubs after "more than twenty litters" from the same lioness had died of severe rickets soon after birth, Bland-Sutton offered them a diet of goat flesh, bone dust, milk and cod liver oil. Stunningly, the cubs recovered. Although Bland-Sutton never published the study, word of his success spread and interest in dietary remedies for rickets ensued. Ongoing experiments in zoology, primarily looking for ways to strengthen the rachitic bones of domestic animal bones contributed further evidence, but no definitive resolution to the question of the source of rickets.[2]

Few were ready to accept cod liver oil as good therapy. Writing of Bland-Sutton's success, London pediatrician Walter Butler Cheadle (1836–1910) mistakenly attributed the cure for rickets to dietary supplementation of animal fat—triggering a years-long debate over its importance.[3] Cheadle attempted to use fat and cod liver oil to treat rickets in rats, without success.[4] Scientists sought a more appropriate research animal, but were unable to experimentally induce rickets in any species. Doubts about the science of food supplements, their impact on human physiology and health, endured.

While his nutrition experiments yielded little, Cheadle did resolve at least one of the puzzles surrounding rickets. William Jenner, John Parry and several others had debated whether tetany and rickets were one and the same disease. Cheadle recognized Jenner as the first to recognize the convulsions of tetany in association with rickets, noting that "*tetany* is a curious state of painful muscular contraction, a tonic spasm, chiefly of the hands and feet; it is also closely and especially associated with rickets. In these cases laryngismus is a constant accompaniment, and tetany often follows an attack of diarrhoea, to which rickety subjects are unusually prone."[5] Though often accompanying rickets, Cheadle was able to demonstrate that tetany was a very serious yet separate disease. His work was confirmed early in the twentieth century, when bloodwork became the modus operandi for testing potential rickets cases. Such tests identified tetany by a low level of calcium not necessarily occurring in rickets. One source of confusion eliminated. Larger questions of diet remained unanswered.[6]

Six. Combating a Riddle Unresolved

* * *

European and American researchers (anthropologists and medical scientists alike) began to look around the globe for clues to the puzzle of rickets. Common knowledge and observations confirmed that tropical zones exhibited virtually no cases of the disease, while the temperate zones had many. The nineteenth-century western outlook translated this observation, imposing a geography of nations, cultures and races. The world got smaller as people traveled more easily. Communication and contact via telegraph, expanded print, railroads, and steamboats opened the world to medical research, fostering high-powered intellectual exchange. Industrialization and urbanization were radically transforming the human habitat.[7]

Hidden in the history of these years lay another killer of children—the Great Famine in northwestern India from 1876 to 1879, a famine killing millions of people. Florence Nightingale wrote in 1877, "The more one hears about this famine, the more one feels that such a hideous record of human suffering and destruction the world has never seen before."[8] Although the story was publicized in a London newspaper with photographs as the disaster happened, the famine disappeared from public memory very quickly. Invisibility was a product of the race-based hierarchical structure of colonialism—the subjectification and subordination of native populations. The history of the famine provides context for subsequent European efforts to discover the etiology of rickets in the habits of foreign cultures.[9]

International medical researchers mulled cases of rickets and other health problems among impoverished urban populations in Germany or England, but ignored those colonized and starving to death in remote areas of India. Though many considered rickets a wasting disease marked by diarrhea, most medical writers saw this condition as the opposite of famine. But famine and diarrhea were wasting diseases, apparently the consequence of malnutrition. Perhaps rickets was a disease of malnutrition after all. Nutrition remained an ambiguous concept, often viewed as an aspect of the environment, a perspective that added to the confusion. Even the word "famine" was used variously, with ambiguity and ambivalence. Medical writers at the time of the famine—even the forward-looking German physician August Hirsch—failed to recognize the impact of political, economic and social forces on colonial populations, or the famine's significance for medicine and history.[10]

In his geographical survey of diseases published in 1886, Hirsch never mentioned the Great Famine of 1877, nor any other specific famine. He released a second edition in the 1880s, featuring a section on "Dysentery and Diarrhoea," this time including general discussions of famine, wasting disease and malnutrition. Never considering the power of government to cause or exacerbate famines, he categorized such events as a disease without social cause, either endemic or epidemic. Rickets appeared in this edition for the first time, without contrast or interconnection with famine.[11]

Unlike the sometimes tropical diseases dysentery and diarrhea categorized by Hirsch, the German physician linked rickets to a specific temperate climate and latitude. Beirut was his one exception to the rule of the "immunity of warm countries" he and many others attributed to rickets.[12] Hirsch ascribed some incidence of diarrhea and dysentery to famine and drought and reviewed endemic dysentery in India, perhaps implicitly referring to the famine of 1876–79. Discussing specific areas in the Deccan Plateau where the famine originated, he wrote: "In fact the drought was so great and exceptional in many of these [epidemics], that it appeared to those who have recorded them to be an especially notable part of the etiology."[13] Hirsch saw climate as part of pathogenesis but was reluctant to identify drought more specifically as a cause of famine, despite the growing record of climatic patterns indicating periodic drought (known today as El Niño–Southern Oscillation events).[14]

Regarding rickets, August Hirsch saw nutrition as important, but in a different sense: "All the authorities are agreed that the morbid process [of rickets] is fundamentally a disorder of nutrition, having its root either in something wrong with the upbringing of the child itself, that is to say an acquired condition, or in a morbid diathesis born with it."[15] His language encompassed the polar possibilities—rickets, either hereditary, or environmentally caused. All the authorities agreed, said Hirsch, that the inconsistency in recorded incidence of rickets came from ambiguous data regarding the presence of the disease. For August Hirsch, rachitic disease came from climate and environment mostly and diet only slightly, especially among the poor.[16]

* * *

In 1890, a radically different interpretation of rickets appeared, contending the origins of the disease lay in the environment. English physician Theobald A. Palm (1848–1929) investigated the disease from a missionary perspective, following several years of practice overseas. Palm had carefully studied Hirsch's *Handbook of Geographical Pathology*, and was thoroughly familiar with the British Medical Association's map detailing the occurrence of rickets in his native country. Palm's home in Cumberland harbored significant rachitic disease.[17] His mission took him to Japan, a uniquely industrializing Asian country where rickets was absent. Writing as a scientist, Palm corresponded with other practitioners, mostly fellow missionaries, gaining information about rickets among the poor in Asian countries, comparing geographical and international variations in incidence.[18]

The question many medical researchers asked—without mentioning race directly—was why do children of Northern European nativity suffer from rickets but not children of other races, such as the Hindu children in India, living in extreme poverty? More than a coincidence, several of Palm's correspondents wrote about India, describing conditions in the areas where the famine had occurred in the 1870s—Kashmir, Punjab, and Madras. No one asked how can we rescue so many people, including infants and children, from dying of starvation and diarrhea? Instead, they puzzled over the absence of rickets. No mention of that horrific past appeared, yet every contributor noted the extreme poverty and deprivation of his locale. In the face of horrifying conditions, physicians reported few if any symptoms in the bones of patients warranting a diagnosis of rickets. Palm wanted to know why people in China and India, living in what he considered the world's worst poverty and filth, escaped the disease.[19]

Palm found multiple examples in Asia to contrast with England, drawing from the works of others as well as his own experiences in Japan. One interesting such study came from William Huntly of Glasgow, who wrote on rickets in Rajputama, a country of great poverty, where "rickets is substantially an unknown and unrecognized disease."[20] The desert climate involved long seasons of hot dry weather. The culture of day-to-day life included close association with animals, including their excrement. Adding nutrition to climate, Huntly described an Indian diet which was mostly grain-based, mixed with pulses. There was no consumption of milk. All of which, Palm pointed out, stood in the face of those who argued a deficiency of animal fat was the root cause of rickets. He proceeded to a clear and logical argument disputing the many different suggestions offered as possible explanations of the disease. Mothers in Rajputama nursed one child until the next was born; European and American analysts urged early weaning to avoid rickets. Indian children suffered from widespread sickness, including fevers, intestinal disorders, and bronchial afflictions, but still exhibited no rickets. Palm emphasized that there was a great deal of syphilis, yet no rickets. Conjunctivitis was common; many considered eye disease to be affiliated with rickets. Not in India. Overlooking the fact that these children were sickly and needed medical attention, Palm and Huntly instead considered the question, why did they not have the rickets while children at home did?[21]

Data in hand, emulating an established basis of comparison for nations around the world, Theobald Palm put the Japanese experience of specific cities next to others of similar latitude. He fully considered environmental and cultural factors of diet, clothing and other issues of lifestyle as well. Factoring English smog and atmospheric pollution into the equation, he reached the conclusion that sunlight was a major factor in rachitic disease. Arguing that the Japanese climate had specific advantages as regarding rickets, in particular "the strength of the direct rays of the sun,"[22] Palm urged more investigation into the effects of light on the human body, touching on skin and pigmentation. Over several pages, Palm wrote about the "Chemistry of Light," drawing analogies with studies of plants, including the work of Darwin, studies of animals, and the role of sunlight.[23]

This was not a new idea. As far back as the eighteenth century, William Buchan, author of the widely read *Domestic Medicine*, had emphasized outdoor play and fresh air as essential to childhood health. Popular writer Andrew Combe pleaded the same in the mid- and late-nineteenth century.[24] Palm added scientific specificity to the commonsense notion. Echoing these writers, echoing August Hirsch, thinking more of his homeland and its plague of rickets, Palm declared, "It is in the narrow alleys, the haunts and play-grounds of the children of the poor, that this exclusion of sunlight is at its worst, and it is there that the victims of rickets are to be found in abundance."[25] Palm concluded that poverty and dietary weaknesses had nothing to do with rickets. These "[areas] which are grossly negligent of ordinary hygienic precautions, though they pay the penalty in other ways, are not scourged by rickets." The disease instead resulted from "climatic conditions"—in a word, the lack of sunshine.[26] The children of the impoverished famine ridden areas spent hours in the outdoor sunlight. Lack of sun was the cause of rickets.[27]

Looking at other societies to understand his own native land, he compared cultures and communities, with the presumption of hierarchy of human worth. Scientific interest in climate led him to objective measure of neutral factors, but subjective bias influenced subsequent interpretation. His "Chemistry of Light" made reference to skin pigmentation in a general way, yet labeled residents of the tropical zones as "other"—deeply pigmented human beings. Writing for a white audience back home, Palm noted "the changes in the skin, sun-burn and freckles, we are familiar with."[28] An indication that racial perception went hand in hand with the politics of his geography. Palm judged Asian society as implicitly lower than English society. His mind was open to alternative explanations of rickets, but division by skin color remained, a presumption he shared with most whites. Culture shaped perception. Palm understood rickets to be a disease of pale-skinned people. In America, the presumption was largely the opposite: darker-skinned human beings were thought to be the victims. In both instances, racial judgments clouded scientific investigation.[29]

Six. Combating a Riddle Unresolved 101

Despite the inherent racism, Palm's insightful approach was well ahead of his time. Consideration of the role of sunlight complemented multiple observers' emphasis on the role of industrialization. Though many Europeans (and a few Americans) saw manufacturing as a key context for rachitic disease, no one understood how or why industrial conditions were so instrumental. Palm's Chemistry of Light became one more theory, interesting but ultimately mysterious. Physicians and scientists continued the struggle to clarify the origin of rickets. More than thirty years would pass before an argument for sunlight resurfaced.[30]

* * *

In an essay on "The Etiology of Rickets," published in the *British Medical Journal* in 1908, Leonard Findlay considered the questions of diet and environmental setting in the framework for an animal experiment, a somewhat informal, yet soon to be pivotal study. Pathologist and pediatrician at the Outdoor Department for Sick Children at the Royal Hospital in Glasgow, Findlay would make a strong international impression as the founder of the "Glasgow School on the Aetiology of Rickets." Well aware of Theobald Palm's insights into the power of sunlight, Findlay addressed climatic and dietary factors in the disease.[31]

Findlay used dogs as subjects. His experiment was very simple; two border collie puppies provided the data for analysis. Both puppies became rickety, exhibiting bowed legs; one stayed tied up while the other was allowed to run. The puppy running free recovered, while the other had to be put down as a result of the disease. These pets became the enduring basis for Findlay's clinical argument that exercise combined with fresh air alone was the key to recovery from rickets. Further experiments followed.[32]

Many years later, in a presentation before the American Medical Association, Findlay underscored the importance of his home city in giving him authority on rickets:

> Though Glasgow is not considered, at least by its visitors, a pleasant place for the habitation of man, yet it is, perhaps chiefly if not entirely for that very reason, an ideal home for a school of medicine, Glasgow, as you know, is a veritable beehive of industry, and thus unfortunately possesses all the qualifications for engendering disease. Within a comparatively small area there is a population of a most heteregeneous [sic] nature of over 1,000,000 persons, who, in many quarters, are literally huddled together. Disease of the infant and child is especially rife.[33]

Industrial and domestic coal burning accounted for toxic smog in the manufacturing center, notorious as a locus of rickets. In 1909, the year following the border collie experiment, a toxic fog in Glasgow killed 1,063 people.³⁴ To Findlay, widespread rachitic disease was very much the product of an industrial environment.

The Scottish physician was careful to distinguish his findings from the work of Theobald Palm, noting that "the confinement of the children, which we find wherever rickets prevails, does, of course deprive them of some fresh air and sunlight, and thus reduce their resisting powers, but it is not entirely, or even mainly, on these grounds that it exerts its baleful influence, as my experiments prove."³⁵

Acknowledging that the underlying cause of rachitic disease remained elusive, Findlay insisted the cure was both simple and obvious:

> want of exercise is the chief etiological factor in this unfortunately too common malady. It is possible that there may be a toxin responsible for the immediate results but without lack of exercise this toxin will not produce any injurious effects.... Until this specific toxin is isolated and its nature and mode of formation understood, any such idea is mere theorizing and an easy refuge for ignorance.³⁶

Firmly wedded to the environmental perspective, Findlay's essay critiqued another theory gaining ground late in the nineteenth century. The notion of heritable rickets, encouraged by the advent of Darwinian natural selection, had grown central to international exchange debating the origin of the disease. Proponents of inheritance were momentarily sustained by the work of Austrian physician Max Kassowitz, who reported in 1882 (as part of his research on the efficacy of phosphorous) that 80 percent of newborns in Vienna were rachitic. He contended the disease was congenital.³⁷ Drawn to the idea of heritable rickets, inspired by the sensational report, physicians carried out further studies to test Kassowitz's findings. Research conducted in 1897 found rickets in just 12 percent of newborns. Six years later, there was but a single case.³⁸ Findlay traced the history of Kassowitz's decline, noting that the hereditary theory was based "on macrosopic appearances alone, and not on the finding of any characteristic histological changes in the bones." The work lost credibility with the realization that Kassowitz had misdiagnosed early rickets. Possessing fundamentally little anatomical and physiological knowledge of the newborn as substantially different from adults, Kassowitz and his followers had identified the softness and open aspects between newborns' cranial bones and sutures as craniotabes—rachitic lesions. The identification was wrong—the softness constituted instead a non-rachitic congenital disorder, possibly related to syphilis.³⁹ The problem was to separate symptoms of rickets from indications of entirely separate congenital conditions.

* * *

Six. Combating a Riddle Unresolved

Still, some physicians were convinced the disease was in some fashion an unintended consequence of modern civilization, the rise of cities, the growth of industry. In 1906, David Paul von Hansemann (1858–1920), Berlin pathologist and assistant to Rudolf Virchow, presented a paper emblematic of the international recognition of rickets as an ongoing crisis. "On Rickets as a Folk Disease," would influence many fresh practitioners of the new pediatrics. American pediatrician Edwards A. Park (1877–1969) referred to Von Hansemann's essay, as "one of the great papers on rickets, by far the greatest written on the etiology of the disease."[40]

Von Hansemann described rachitic disease at great length, cautioning his international audience that rickets was the consequence of modern civilized life and demanded serious attention. Although it did not kill children immediately, the disease carried side effects that crippled people and shortened lives. With a foreboding sense of war approaching, Hansemann envisioned a German army of weak rachitic soldiers with flat feet, bowed legs and knock-knees, similar to the rachitic lions in the London zoo, animals that had lost their strength and the ability to reproduce. Rickets presented a riddle for science to solve, with greater import as a symbol of the historical moment. Hansemann's observations, contrasting the wild and the natural, came to be understood as the theory of domestication.[41] His summary:

> Domestication does not relate merely to those things which pertain to the house ... but refers to every effort on the part of man to further the survival of the race and of the individual by artificial means and to aid in the struggle against the forces of nature. By this definition it becomes at once apparent that not alone does man domesticate animals but has domesticated himself.[42]

Domestication was a catchword encapsulating an impression of life in the early twentieth-century western world. The word "Civilization" reflected a belief that society had evolved to its highest level. Yet, there were social flaws and, obviously, diseases. In Hansemann's eyes, "Every effort to further the race" (meaning the white race) was lost. The German physician saw rickets as a metaphor for social deterioration, insisting the disease was an indictment of the well-being of society as a whole. In an effort to establish the etiology of rickets, a member of the white intellectual elite advanced a critique of modern civilization. Von Hansemann supplanted the celebration of an industrial "revolution" with an image of the domestication of human life. His observations presented a troubling corollary to the opposition of civilization to savagery.[43]

Rather than devoting attention to the growing presence of atmospheric pollution, von Hansemann considered the impact of industrialization on cultural behavior. Historians today view the rise of "domesticity" as part of the profound changes in Western economic, political and social life occurring as industrialization proceeded, beginning in some places as early as the 1500s. The words "domestic" and "home" appeared in the English vocabulary in the late 1700s and early 1800s, reflecting a new cultural awareness developing in response to an industrializing society. People were sundered from nature. The locus of family life and remunerative work, traditionally carried on under the same roof, had begun to separate. Increasingly, men and women left home to work, often in unhealthful places. The home became a kind of fortress, a barrier against the surrounding environment. Connection to the natural world, the out of doors, the seasons, grew limited. People were tamed. Human health suffered.[44]

To illustrate the connection of rickets to domestication, von Hansemann drew a parallel to the health of domestic animals, noting that caretakers often failed to recognize the rickets many exhibited. Through research in Berlin, in Tokyo and with the help of a Japanese assistant, he studied the incidence of rickets in zoos. At von Hansemann's request, a zookeeper in Tokyo captured an indigenous wild monkey (maccacus speciosis), kept the primate captive for a prescribed time and then shipped the creature to Berlin. Studying this monkey, Von Hansemann confirmed his suspicions that captivity produced signs of rickets, concluding that only domesticated animals contracted the disease. Animals free in nature escaped rickets because they lived outside the confines of domestication, an interpretation similar to the theories advanced by Leonard Findlay the previous year. The origins of rickets lay in the lack of outdoor exercise.[45]

Drawing from anthropological studies, physicians generally assumed that nations in contact with the West would inevitably witness the onset and increase of rachitic disease as manufacturing took hold. Yet, despite Japan's rapid industrialization in the last half of the nineteenth century, von Hansemann, like Palm a decade before, was struck by the lack of rickets in Japanese society. The German physician admired the nation's child-rearing, which insisted on outdoor exercise no matter what the season. Japanese cultural practice protected them from the debilitating effects of industrial civilization. The wooden airy structures of Japanese homes, with oiled paper windows, open courtyards and gardens, kept children from rickets. Such homes did not wall in the interior to the absolute exclusion of the outdoors. German stone houses, with their thick glass windows, kept children inside and harbored rickets among them. German houses and the attendant domestic culture captured children and sickened them.[46]

Though he referred to Japanese scholars as colleagues and peers, von Hansemann still believed that in order to be free of rickets Japanese society had to be less domesticated (read civilized) than Germany. Von

Hansemann's understanding of the etiology of rickets led him to conclude that full-blown industrialization produced the disease. Thus, he compared the rickety animals in the zoo to the confines of urbanization and industrialization such as experienced in America and Europe—equating animal cages to human homes. After all, zoos had appeared in the nineteenth century, part of the industrialized world.[47]

Variations on the environmental theme were many, yet von Hansemann's image of Western urbanization as a domesticating process accentuated key social factors bearing on the analysis of disease. The theory of domestication put the history of the home and its significance to health at the center of the problem. For von Hansemann, linking rickets to industrialization was a link to homes and the domestic scene, the hearth. The spread of disease and the nature of medical treatment from the early years of the century onward would depend not merely on industrial conditions, but the concomitant cultural construction of home and domesticity—an entire way of life. Domestication theory transcended the blinders that prevented people from grasping the extent of social changes in their time.[48]

* * *

True to the peculiarities of American social conditions, discussion of rickets among researchers in the United States followed an anomalous course. Long positing the disease was uncommon, physicians came to grips with the problem haphazardly, denying the growing presence, minimizing the effects, blaming the existence on racial factors. Perspective changed slowly. By the early 1900s, physicians had confronted enough cases to make the disease significant in their practices, raising questions and stimulating new scientific inquiry.

At an American Medical Association meeting in Columbus, Ohio, in 1889, John Lovett Morse (1865–1940) boldly declared race had no role in the origin of rickets. A practicing clinical pediatrician and assistant professor at Harvard Medical School, Morse was responsible for routine examinations of babies and toddlers at the Infant Hospital's out-patient department in Boston. Morse found so many rachitic rosaries in his consultations, he determined to learn just how common rickets was. Analyzing four hundred cases of children under two years of age, treated during two summer months in 1898, Morse surprisingly found three hundred-eighteen—nearly 80 percent—"showed more or less marked evidence of rickets."[49] Similar to what clinicians observed elsewhere, many of the victims were not in the hospital for treatment of that disease but when examined exhibited rachitic symptoms—especially rachitic rosaries, beaded ribs, delayed emergence of teeth, or other such signs.[50] Patient rosaries ran from mild to severe. "A large proportion of the cases were mild and would not have been recognized as rickets unless a careful examination had been made,"[51] Morse observed. Were such rosaries simply normal in Boston, or was rickets run rampant among infants there?

A rachitic rosary presented numerous small swellings of the cartilage lined up along a longitudinal line where the ribs met the sternum, creating a palpable beadlike presence under the skin. Morse concluded the rosaries were not normal. Long recognized as a sign of rickets, this particular abnormality could result in a seriously reduced ability to breathe, known as contracted ribcage.[52]

Although rosaries were the most common sign he found, the doctor altogether identified eight different "changes in the osseous skeleton ... considered as evidences of rickets."[53] These included aspects of the skull, enlarged epiphyses in the wrist or ankles, bow-leggedness or knock-knees—several commonly identified symptoms, mostly of the bony skeleton. Finding 80 percent of his patients exhibited a rachitic rosary, often in combination with one or more other symptoms, led Morse to conclude that the disease, ranging from mild to severe, had a significant presence among the poorer classes. The rosaries did not appear among more well-off patients in his private practice. Supplementary evidence, such as frequent discovery of rachitic rosary in infant postmortems, suggested the symptom was the earliest to develop.[54]

Morse was careful to stress that the Infant Hospital's out-patients were not necessarily representative of all cases in the United States, as they were children from Boston and nearby Cambridge and Somerville, plus some from more outlying and rural surroundings.[55] In terms of ethnicity, eleven classifications made up his list, ranging in number from one representative to a group of one hundred twenty-two. Arranged in order of size, "Russian and Polish Jews" accounted for thirty-eight percent; "Irish" twenty-two percent; followed by "American," "English, Scotch and Canadian," "Negro," "Italian," "German," "French," "Swede," and finally "Finn, Portuguese and Syrian."[56] Morse boldly and without qualification asserted "no race is exempt from the disease and ... the cause must be sought elsewhere."[57] Other studies had exhibited a similar distribution of place of origin, but none spoke so clearly to the point, denying any racial component to the disease.

The fact that free-roaming wild animals never got rickets, yet became rickety in zoos, intrigued Morse. Wrapping his theory of the etiology of rickets in the hygiene of sunshine and fresh air in a later publication, Morse concluded that for humans, "[rickets] is more common in the city than in the country, in the winter than in the summer, in the poor than in the well-to-do." He went on to talk about race in a general sense, referring to migration: rickets is "more common in this country in those races whose new surroundings are most different from those to which they were accustomed." Being careful to avoid specific ethnic or racial phenotypes, he went on, "the children of a pastoral race are most likely to develop it when confined to a city. This is also true of wild animals. They never have the disease when free, but often develop it when confined in zoölogical gardens."[58] Rickets seemed to be caused by modern urban civilization. "The cause of rickets in Boston and vicinity is to be found in improper hygienic surroundings rather than in race or diet."[59] He went on to say, "It is probable too, I think, that rickets is absolutely on the rise."[60]

As the number of American cases of rickets grew, the disease seemed to become more complex—in fact almost inscrutable. At the 1894 meeting of the American Medical Association, New York City pediatrician L. Emmet Holt remarked, "it [is] very singular that a disease having such a pathological condition should be so obscure in its etiology.... Rickets [is] a vice of nutrition, and one of great complexity."[61] Like Morse, the young but skillful Holt perceived that there was more to rickets than met the eye.

Following a well-worn track, Morse thought the cause of rickets involved "improper hygienic surroundings" in the poorer classes.[62] Presumably, improper hygiene would indicate lifestyle rather than diet. But for Morse and many others, hygiene included nutrition. Early pediatricians had addressed nutritional questions by vying with one another to devise the best infant artificial food. Physicians of all sorts continued to question and assess milk in the infant diet in comparison with breastfeeding, and attacked weaning issues as part of the origin of rickets. Few were ready to accept cod liver oil as good therapy, including Morse, a loyal student and assistant of Thomas Morgan Rotch (1849–1914), a president of the American Pediatric Society. Calculating the percentages of carbohydrates, proteins and fats found in human breast milk, Rotch had doctored cow's milk, providing the foundation for an infant diet supposedly bettered by science.[63] Morse advocated Rotch's approach to infant feeding. Many infants failed to thrive, but Morse remained devoted, retaining Rotch's approach long after the treatment fell into disfavor. Debates regarding the power and science of food and supplements on human physiology and health endured. Henry Fruitnight advocated the use of lime phosphate and calcium phosphate in treating rickets patients, as did others.[64]

Thomas Southworth, a physician for out-patients at New York's Babies Hospital, urged the use of "Lactophospate of Lime," finding the formula especially effective. His regime for patients, outlined at a meeting of the American Medical Association in 1908, emphasized such dietary treatment. The syrup, commonly available as a dietary supplement, was comprised of calcium phosphate (derived from bone ash) slaked with lime. The ingredients are found in cows' milk. Like Morse, Southworth was concerned to warn his fellow practitioners of the early symptoms of rickets. Unlike Morse, his work depended upon a framework of race and ethnicity, focused primarily on African Americans and immigrants from southeastern Europe.[65]

The discussion that followed Southworth's paper offered opposing opinions. Southworth and Morse argued the utility of phosphorus, Morse stating, "he had given children phosphorus until he has feared that they would light if rubbed too hard, without having seen the slightest benefit."[66] Arguments ensued over dietary details, the etiology of rickets, and craniotabes as rachitic symptoms, all of which remained points of conflict for years to come. A physician from Chicago asserted rickets was over-diagnosed, suggesting that the issue was one of hygiene above all.[67]

Hygiene figured heavily in the minds of reformers and physicians, used often as a code word for race. Joining the discussion, L.T. Royster (1874–1953), a physician practicing in Norfolk, Virginia, recalled that in the late 1890s he had been an intern in the New York Infant Asylum, where he had treated white cases of rickets almost entirely. In Virginia he attended only African American cases, perhaps revealing shifts in incidence of the disease with migration. Painting Black migration as an environmental health issue, Royster maintained, "Back of it all, there unquestionably is the standpoint of hygiene, and the nutrition of the mother. It is an inheritance of unhygienic surroundings."[68] Echoing an old refrain, Royster argued that African Americans, freed from slavery, could not take care of themselves. Maintaining an "Inheritance of unhygienic surrounding," he conflated environmental causation with individual physiology, culture, and historical context, throwing in a touch of the Lost Cause, a mourning for the lost world of slavery. Royster referred to the "inheritance of superstition" as the most deadly symptom of all. Until it was gone there would always be rickets.[69]

While it is impossible to quantify exactly, many African Americans did have rickets, constituting what appeared to be a high percentage of the sufferers. Many analysts believed skin pigmentation to be a factor; race persisted as an issue under medical scrutiny. Recognizing the power of racial interpretations in American discussion, the Scottish pediatrician Leonard Findlay agreed that rickets in the United States resided largely in the black community. In a telling statement made in 1918, Findlay asserted

> Rickets would seem to be unknown when savage races live under natural conditions, but exceedingly rife when these peoples dwell in civilised countries, *e.g.* in New York, where one hardly sees a negro child without some evidence of the disease.... I do not recall ever seeing a non-rachitic half-race negro child. It is notorious that these native races in civilized countries inhabit the worst quarters of our towns.[70]

Six. Combating a Riddle Unresolved 109

Findlay's remarks did little more than underscore the ongoing sense of confusion and frustration at the heart of the ongoing discourse. This linkage of rickets to individuals of mixed race directly contradicted "The Etiology of Rickets," his 1908 essay building a forceful case for environmental causation while denying hereditary factors. The use of "half-race" imagery ten years later simply confused matters further, amplifying the connotations of racial interpretation and implying that rickets, or the susceptibility to rickets, was heritable. The contrast of the civilized to the savage was by now very familiar, accentuating the connection to assumptions based on race. In the end, Findlay tried to escape his biased and subjective assessment, now pointing to poverty and hygiene as the root cause of rachitic disease.[71]

* * *

For American physicians, rickets was a problematic illness, in several senses. With little agreement on the rate of occurrence, much less the source of rickets, the disease presented a baffling prospect. The implications for medical science, for society as a whole, were difficult to discern. Discussion of rickets—both symptoms and treatment—evolved slowly, reflecting changes in medical therapeutics and ongoing scientific research. One thing was certain. By the close of the nineteenth century, awareness of the disease had grown enough to become a matter of public concern.

Ever willing to address (if not inflame) popular unease, weekly newspaper columns began providing space for mothers to ask questions about illness, including rickets in their children. Less often, adults with rachitic symptoms wrote in for help.

One of the first such glimpses came from *The New York Times* in January 1897. The story was based on establishing specific measurements defining the "perfect" female shape—"What a Woman Should Be." Regarded as defects were knock knees and bowed legs—well-known to be the result of childhood rickets. Marked by rickets with one of these deformities but seemingly in good health otherwise, some women lost aesthetic appeal.[72]

Changes in fashion aggravated the problem. By 1916 skirt hems had risen six inches above the ankle, much to the chagrin of fashionable but bow-legged or knock-kneed women, as reported by *The Chicago Tribune*. Some rickets' sufferers did not perceive their cases as pathological so much as embarrassing. For others, the experience was far more serious.[73]

Perspective depended in part on gender. Most of the correspondents with Doctor W.A. Evans, syndicated columnist for *The Chicago Tribune* in the 1910s, were mothers. Advice in the column was broad, but stressed oft-repeated themes. Frequently Evans suggested surgery for misshapen legs. In January of 1918, a woman described treating her son by baring his bowed leg to the sunshine and massaging the limb as a preliminary to surgery, only to find the leg straightened without further intervention. Despite the work of Theobald Palm and others, Evans cautioned readers he doubted a cure by sunshine was possible. Often he advised seeing a doctor in person to diagnose a child. According to Evans, the disease at hand could be scurvy, rickets, or tuberculosis.[74]

A different style of advice came from African American Doctor A. Wilberforce Williams, who wrote a weekly column titled "Talks On..." for *The Chicago Defender*, a newspaper targeting African Americans. Williams never referred to rickets or tuberculosis as diseases of special concern. Though joining other columnists in dismissing the clinical impact of rickets simply as the source of unsightly deformities—more a blemish than a physiological problem—Williams did consider the impact of the disease seriously. In September 1918, the doctor described what he thought to be proper pre-natal care for a pregnant woman. He mentioned rickets only in passing, but clearly considered the disease to be a threat to good prenatal health: "The reason we have so many ricketic [sic], weak bones, bow-legged and deformed children is due largely to the food given the child after it comes into the world."[75] (Note that Williams used the collective first person "we" to identify his point of view as African American.) Williams urged pregnant women to consume plenty of calcium and lime salts—supplements thought by reputable medical sources to be deficient in the maternal diet, giving rise to rickets. For both Evans and Williams, proper diet seemed the essential component.

Newspaper counsels along such lines reflected popular concern, offering an alternative point of view on the epidemic of rickets. While medical science approached the disease with a kind of tunnel vision wrought by extensive knowledge, an appreciation of the dangers, and the puzzle of etiology, lay readers responded to growing knowledge of the epidemic with practical concerns. What is rickets? How is the disease contracted; what can be done to prevent the occurrence? How do I deal with the unfortunate effects later in life? All very good questions, for which the medical profession had no real answers.

* * *

Sunlight. Fresh air and exercise. Diet. Racial heredity. Despite determined research, heated debate, fountains of ink, the medical world seemed no closer to resolving the mystery of rickets than their predecessors a half century before. Theories abounded; the situation remained unchanged. European nations continued to cope with a legion of cases; researchers in the United States had come to recognize the epidemic ongoing in their midst. Disputes over the numbers of cases, the identities of the victims did nothing to confront the essential problem; rickets was a widespread, debilitating disease, killing young children, affecting health throughout the lifespan.

What had changed, fundamentally changed, was the structure of medical response. Where once upon a time, an attending physician was likely to encounter rickets in all the manifestations—the rachitic rosaries of the afflicted child, the contracted pelvis of the pregnant woman, the horror of the obstructed birth—medical specialization now apportioned responsibility. An infant exhibiting signs of rachitic disease was the province of the pediatrician; etiology and treatment their particular task. Birth injuries resulting from bones malformed in childhood demanded the surgical skills of the gynecologist. The actual process of birth, obstructed or not, that was the obstetrician's work. Though inter-related in various and obvious ways, each medical specialty was freed to pursue the particular problems they perceived, define those problems as they saw fit, arrive at their own solutions. Science stood at the childbed, tools in hand. Rickets had come to affect childbirth, anatomically, physiologically and culturally.

Part II

Resolution

Medical Reach in a Progressive Era

The accelerated pace of change in the diversifying fields of obstetrics and pediatrics was by no means a transition taking place in a cultural vacuum. Beginning in the last years of the nineteenth century, the entirety of America was in ferment; the voices demanding change to be heard everywhere. Small wonder. In the years since the Civil War, American society had endured a vast, all-encompassing metamorphosis. Driven by industrialization, the nation's economy expanded beyond imagining. Business boomed, commerce boomed; the traditional values born of an agricultural society diminished in meaning. The expansion was horribly uneven; unparalleled economic gains were punctuated by deep periodic recession. A few became fabulously wealthy; a great many found themselves in desperate poverty. Fed by an influx of rural peoples, Black migrants from the South, and a vast wave of immigration, cities grew large, creating new and enormous problems. Rapid transformation spurred the need for still greater transformation.[1]

The period bears familiar labels: the Age of Reform, the Progressive Era. The names imply much that is ultimately misleading. Superficial interpretations leave the impression that this was a time when conscientious Americans attempted to alleviate the burdens wrought by industrialization and urbanization, bringing relief to the defenseless. To some extent true, this was by no means the ultimate intent of the reformers. What was wanted was an administrative state governed by scientific experts, men and women who would regulate not merely the abuses of big business, but every aspect of American life. The claim to scientific expertise lay in the developing fields of sociology, anthropology, economics, psychology—the social sciences where statistical analyses of human behavior became the basis for defining the proper productive life. Personal freedoms framed in the Declaration of Independence were a quaint relic of an outmoded past. As the twentieth century dawned, an administrative elite stood prepared to make all the decisions necessary to shape an American future. They would become a fourth branch of government, determining policy, ordering industrial growth, labor relations, agricultural production, transportation networks, urban affairs, immigration, charitable organizations, human health, human reproduction. A great many believed they could reserve to themselves the right to decide which Americans should have children.[2]

Obstetricians and pediatricians developed their sciences in an atmosphere redolent with self-appointed temerity grown of dubious expertise. Medical science implemented practice reflecting the values of a significant, well-educated "progressive" portion of American society. Defining the errors, the inefficiencies, the misguided practices of the human past, doctors would contribute to what they envisioned to be a safer, more ordered world. If there is a law governing history, it is that any attempt to reform human behavior can result in something infinitely worse. Perhaps Mark Twain said it best: "Nothing needs reforming so much as other people's habits."[3]

SEVEN

Johns Hopkins to the Fore

Social values, political and legal boundaries, religious beliefs and economic status—ideology—have historically created a complex texture for human childbirth. With the coming of modernity and the rise of industrialization, science and medicine fought for control of this essential rite of passage, a process many in the Progressive Era perceived to be a struggle of civilization over savagery. As the calendar turned to a new century, medical practitioners aggressively sought control of infant delivery, rationalized on the basis of rickets and contracted pelves. The culture of birth in America witnessed the beginning of profound change, driven by the increasing authority of obstetrical science. Johns Hopkins Hospital and Medical School, established in 1876, stood in the vanguard, the seat of recognized practice combining research, education and clinical experience. The institution's rapidly expanding influence did much to shape the social and political factors that eventually relocated the vast majority of births from the home to the hospital delivery room.

Four great male physicians became the guiding lights of the school's medical faculty. William H. Welch (1850–1934), the first Dean of the Medical School, was a bacteriologist brought from New York City's Bellevue Hospital. Hired in 1885, Welch in turn recruited William Osler (1849–1919) of Canada as Physician-in-Chief, director of the School's innovative residency program. Osler in 1892 published a highly popular medical text, *The Principles and Practice of Medicine*, in which he listed being a member of "the colored race" as part of the etiology of rickets. By the third edition seven years later, he insisted that "children of the Negro and Italian races" inherited the disease, a contention he maintained for decades.[1] William S. Halsted (1852–1922), also from New York, was a pioneer in anesthetics and aseptic surgery. Of particular import for this history was Howard A. Kelly (1858–1943), practitioner in obstetrics and gynecology, enlisted from the University of Pennsylvania. Intended to develop the field of obstetrics, Kelly gravitated toward gynecology as the medical school developed. These four men ascended to the heights of faculty power as the school took shape, in due time becoming honored and revered historical giants. All felt ambivalent at best about women as medical students, but tolerated them in one way or another.[2]

German medical science heavily influenced the curriculum and practice developed at Johns Hopkins. While the experience of modernization differed from one country to another, Germany and the United States were similar in the timing of an industrial surge. German medical research was regarded as the best in the world; Austrian and German facilities attracted large numbers of students from the United States, including Welch and Osler. Doctors and medical students traveled the Atlantic to learn new scientific methods and theory, studying rickets among numerous other maladies. Much of what drew them was the study of pathology—"An exciting atmosphere of the German laboratories where student and master worked side by side, where every facility needed for advanced study or research was provided, where discipline and dedication to the ideals of scientific inquiry invariably prevailed and where there was a sense of anticipation from being on the cutting edge of medical discovery."[3] "It is the master mind of [Rudolf] Virchow," declared Osler in the late months of 1873, "and the splendid Pathological Institute … that specially attract foreign students to Berlin."[4]

The Johns Hopkins Hospital, constructed in 1889 on a Baltimore city block bordered on the east by Wolfe Street, rose in a poverty-stricken neighborhood. Not far from the Chesapeake Bay Harbor, the Medical School and Hospital were separate from the remainder of the University, built north of the city.[5] Johns Hopkins, the original donor, had required in writing that the hospital and the medical school serve the poor and needy; to his credit, he insisted that the hospital be open to Blacks and that there be a "Colored Orphan Asylum" attached. Though the hospital initially had no separate facilities for Blacks, strict segregation was instituted. Wards were divided by race. Separate buildings quickly arose to maintain racial separation.[6] Despite the intentions of Johns Hopkins himself, administrators for decades refused to staff Black medical professionals or accept Black medical students. The Board did establish a Colored Orphan Asylum in 1895, something very close to a house of industry, providing a context of discipline, hygiene and white middle class regulation.[7] The Asylum emphasized social and cultural reform of the African American children, preparing them to enter the workaday world of the lower classes. Little attention was paid to actual health problems—a strikingly odd hospital approach, accomplished without question in the 1890s. Such facilities served to meet the founder's provision for medical service for those with little or nothing.[8]

* * *

Seven. Johns Hopkins to the Fore

The City of Baltimore was in many ways a metaphor for the radical changes taking place in American life after 1865. The ensuing years witnessed a rapid industrialization, sustained by a laboring force comprised of Black migrants from rural areas and new arrivals from Eastern and Southern Europe. Expanding helter-skelter, living conditions suffered; Baltimore became one more blighted industrial landscape marked by endemic poverty and disease. Rickets was to be expected.

Following the Civil War, Baltimore prospered as a city, becoming a largely working-class town. African Americans contributed heavily to the economic growth of urban Maryland.[9] The Great Migration, including a large influx of African Americans into Baltimore during the Great War, fostered a steadily rising percentage of Blacks in the city thereafter. Migrating from rural areas, these people brought with them a folk culture of medical practice carried in large part by African American midwives. Traditions included use of herbal knowledge and cures, elements of African animistic culture, and a holistic spiritual approach connecting health and sickness to cosmology.[10]

European immigration overwhelmed the city of Baltimore late in the nineteenth century. Neighborhoods housed mixed ethnicities until about 1890.[11] Immigrants from Europe found what they could in rapidly developing ghettos, many on the east side near the garment industry.[12] Too little housing, mostly in filthy crowded tenements, left many out in the cold. Immigrants and migrating African Americans alike had to make do with limited incomes and social status-defined work opportunities derived from stereotyping.[13]

Adequate health care was an ongoing concern in a city marked by determined racial segregation. Facilities open to African Americans were few. Bayview, a large Baltimore almshouse, opened in 1866, becoming a complex serving poor and indigent people ranging from widows to thieves. By 1890 nearly 80 percent of the patients were permanent, most deemed insane. Hardly an ideal setting for health treatment of the poor, but a facility open to African Americans, though segregation remained the organizing principle governing treatment.[14] In 1894, the first private hospital in the United States designated for African Americans opened on Orchard Street in Baltimore. Provident Hospital, founded by six African American doctors, served the community while affording African American medical students and physicians clinical experience in treating patients. The founders became part of an elite group of race men.[15] The hospital soon moved to West Biddle Street, establishing the foundation for what was to become a significant institution by the end of the 1920s. Provident Hospital offered unbiased medical care for Blacks in Baltimore, alternatives to the segregated wards at Johns Hopkins. Though documentation is lacking, the Provident Hospital may well have offered emergency medical care in cases of obstructed and prolonged labor.[16]

Often neglected, African American experience played a central role in the history of Baltimore and the history of the Johns Hopkins medical institutions, providing context for significant numbers of women patients served by the Hospital. Late nineteenth-century Baltimore was an industrial town with a new medical school that included white women medical students but excluded African American men and women as medical students or practitioners.

* * *

Facilities at the Johns Hopkins Hospital from the beginning included a dispensary, a separate building constructed on Monument Street behind the common wards. A free clinic available to those known as the worthy poor, dispensaries historically treated many immigrants, Blacks and working-class people in their neighborhoods. Identification of clients as "worthy poor" extended back to the early nineteenth century, requiring a reference attesting to good moral standing or circumstances deserving of broadly defined medical care. First appearing in England, such locally-centered institutions cost less to run and served more patients inclusively. Medical goodwill originally fueled neighborhood enterprises, responding to new health needs arising from industrialization and urbanization. Dispensaries proliferated in urban areas in the second half of the nineteenth century, commonly including a central building staffed by an apothecary (a pharmacist) and a doctor.[17]

As urbanization took shape, dispensaries grew in importance, even as their nature changed. The numbers of patients needing access to free care rose with the growth of city populations, including migrants and immigrants. More and more physicians, even in neighborhood settings, distanced themselves from immigrants and migrating Blacks. General practitioners often viewed such people as radically different from themselves, alien. Medical reformers saw dispensaries as essential to provide for the poor and indigent, but insisted upon efficiency of care and economy—dispensaries were to serve only the truly needy.[18] Some dispensaries included social workers and other staff to assist social relations, education and the identification of deserving patients.[19]

The Dispensary at Johns Hopkins accommodated a maximum of four hundred patients. The service did not exclude patients by race, but provided separate waiting rooms. A critical component of medical education, the building included an amphitheater seating two hundred-eighty people, a venue for lectures and classes. Combined with laboratory research, clinical experience was an early hallmark of the medical school, an integral part of the residency program developed by William Osler. Students learned medicine scientifically and practically, directly observing and treating a diversity of cases. The nature of the Dispensary placed students closer to patients and sickness, giving them a better sense of the human dimension of medical care.[20] The by-laws of 1889 for the Dispensary listed fields of treatment including "General Medicine, General Surgery, Gynecology, Ophthalmology and Otology, Laryngology, Dermatology, Neurology, Diseases of Children, Genito-urinary Surgery, and Orthopaedic Surgery," notably excluding obstetrics as a specialization, but including gynecology.[21]

In 1895, William Welch appeared before the Johns Hopkins University Board of Trustees to advocate the establishment of the OOS—the Out-Patient, Outside or Outdoor Obstetrics Service (as it was variously called)—the first provision for obstetrical service at the Johns Hopkins Hospital. Welch explained that obstetrics had been and would remain an important area of instruction, typifying a medical school curriculum including the three areas of "Medicine, Surgery and Obstetrics." Pregnancy, labor and birth comprised a gray area, neither medicine nor surgery. The OOS was to be part of the Dispensary. Welch went on to add that the Service would provide a critical proving ground for nursing students. The Board approved the plan, confirming the appointment of Doctor J. Whitridge Williams (1866–1931), member of the School's Gynecology faculty, as director.[22]

The endeavor was new and not completely thought-out. Medical students on call for the OOS in 1896 described the accommodations as less than they might have expected, characterizing them as "fifth rate hotel" rooms.[23] No plans even existed for lying-in patients in the hospital until the next year, when administrators designated a space for twenty white patients in a maternity ward squeezed into the isolation building. A separate building for African American medical care appeared on Wolfe Street, serving as such for women until the Woman's Clinic opened in 1923. Obstetrics held a somewhat lowly place in medicine to begin with— outclassed by gynecology. People in the United States expected most births to occur at home; midwives still practiced widely.[24]

Commitment to assisted childbirth stretched the Dispensary staff thin; the OOS needed the assistance nursing students could provide. Student nurses balked at the extent of time spent in the lesser tasks of attending labor during the early hours of dilation or false starts to labor, as well as required daily return visits after the birth. Nurses refused to serve in any capacity resembling midwifery. In 1898 Mary Adelaide Nutting, Superintendent of Nurses, announced that women students felt the outdoor service benefited only medical students and asked to remove her students from the OOS. William Welch and Hospital Superintendent Henry Hurd intervened in the crisis, defending the success of the OOS and securing the provision of nursing care despite the nurses' complaints.[25]

Similarly discontent, J. Whitridge Williams wanted to keep his ties with gynecology, but now practiced in a separate arena. More than anything, he dreaded being labeled a midwife. Despite the misgivings, Williams would make the most of his opportunity.

* * *

The racial conflicts burdening Maryland's history did much to shape J. Whitridge Williams's approach to the practice of medicine. Very much a product of Maryland, loyal to the region, Williams was born in Baltimore in 1866. His father, a Virginian by birth, was a practicing physician. His mother traced doctors in her family back one hundred-sixty years.[26] At an invitational lecture delivered as President of the Medical and Chirurgical Faculty of Maryland in 1916, Williams looked back on his childhood, remembering his father's Baltimore practice, including a "fine line of darky practice."[27] On the surface, the reference pertained to the treatment of those who had great need and next to no wherewithal. Deeply embedded, emboldened by cultural pride and heritage, lay a patronizing and belittling of those without. Throughout his career examples of such racialized language emerge from the record, especially from Williams's oral presentations. His language before a medical audience betrayed his condescension.[28] Williams was a Southerner who held fast to hierarchical views of African Americans, even as he treated the substantial number of Black women seeking assistance at the Johns Hopkins Hospital and Dispensary. His medical research was grounded heavily in regular access to expectant African American mothers. In the chivalric Southern tradition, despite considering them inferior to whites, Williams never failed to be overtly polite to his Black patients.[29]

Awarded his baccalaureate at Johns Hopkins in 1886, Williams achieved his medical degree from the University of Maryland two years later. Like many American students, he learned laboratory science abroad, studying in Vienna and Berlin. He read Latin, French and German as easily as he read English. Deeply ensconced in the European medical model, especially the German school of the mid- to late nineteenth century, Williams felt himself a medical scientist. He first became associated with the Johns Hopkins Medical School in 1889, volunteering as an assistant physician in the hospital's Obstetrics-Gynecology department, directed by Howard Kelly. Furthering the studies begun in Germany, he developed his laboratory research techniques under the tutelage of William Welch, learning to identify the bacteria in cases of childbed fever. Even at

Hopkins, pathology and clinical laboratory science took shape slowly. The endowment for a laboratory did not come until 1897; the facility opened the next year.[30]

Apart from puerperal fever, obstetrical practice remained outside the great rush of bacteriological and clinical discoveries of the 1880s and 1890s. For Williams, the fit with obstetrics was uneasy. Throughout his career he objected to the limitations of such a singular categorization as obstetrics, seeking to work with the whole female body and holding fast to gynecology as well. He understood the authority gynecology had won as a surgical specialization, and sought the same for obstetrics.[31] His early publications explored cases of cervical cancer and "Tuberculosis of the Female Generative Organs." In each case, the issue of race figured significantly. Black women were listed as "colored"; white women referred to as "Mrs.," reflecting their perceived superior status.[32]

Williams was talented, well-educated, and supremely ambitious. Appointed director of the Outdoor Obstetrical Service in 1895, he found himself firmly associated with the practice of obstetrics, like it or not. Making the best of his circumstance, he set about enlarging his domain, pushing for the creation of the lying-in ward at the hospital and the inclusion of obstetrics in the medical school curriculum. From 1895 until his death, Williams represented *the* authority in obstetrics, contracted pelves, and Caesarean sections at the medical school. Students and associates studied, worked, researched and wrote obstetrics under and for him.[33]

Turning his attention to the anatomy of labor and birth, Williams began the process of redefining the boundaries of the field he inherited. A medicalizing operative dynamic drove obstetrics as he launched his career: a medical impulse subjectifying women in birth. That verb—subjectifying—carries significant implications: women were viewed as subjects, underlings in need of authoritative direction, and as specimens, people available for scientific study and possible experimentation. Like many others, Williams saw the obstetrical transition mainly in terms of surgery, heavily related to awareness of contracted pelves.[34]

* * *

As obstetrics grew in the early twentieth century, obstetricians and gynecologists published reports of the incidence of contracted pelves throughout the United States and the world. Determining medicine's relationship to birth rested upon the question of incidence, developing rationales for operative procedures in case of complication. Publications presenting statistical evaluation of sometimes thousands of cases were juxtaposed against close analysis of individual cases. By the end of the century, professionalized medicine regularly incorporated numbers into peer review and assessment of therapeutic success. Contracted pelves provided impetus and framework—materials with which to analyze the mechanics of birth—but surgery was the tool of application. Williams quickly rose to national leadership, embracing the practice of pelvimetry and the identification of types of contracted pelves as the basis of modern obstetrical surgery—sculpted in terms of anatomy based on race. Williams brought the race science of pelvimetry to a central role in American obstetrics.[35]

As early as 1890, Williams understood his science of pelvic measurement as a tool to improve and facilitate the use of Caesarean section. Upon becoming departmental head, he required medical students and residents to measure every patient's pelvis. His underlings produced critically important material for Williams's obstetrical career and the institution. Publishing statistical reports in various medical journals, students, interns, and residents noted that Williams had suggested they prepare the work that followed.[36]

Absorbed with a clinical approach and determined to make obstetrics a science, Williams delivered and subsequently published an initial article on pelvimetry in 1891, contending that the history of contracted pelves established the seriousness of the condition. His study considered the work of Hendrik von Deventer and William Smellie, but embraced as models the work of Michaëlis and his student, Carl Litzmann. Williams saw their numerical standards for types of contracted pelves as a guide for American medical science.[37]

Howard Kelly listened to Williams's paper, and offered interesting comments. On the one hand, Kelly described a case he had witnessed as a caution against considering pelvic measurements as all the evidence necessary to make a decision on whether or not to use Caesarean section. This patient had delivered easily despite a measurement indicating the need for a Caesarean. Kelly then described an opposite case. Though the woman's pelvis involved even more extreme contraction and an unusually difficult fetal position *in utero* than the first case, the attending doctor scoffed at the idea of a Caesarean. He performed a podalic version, but succeeded in delivering only the fetal body without the head—apparently a breech birth. The result was the dangerous but "very old obstetrical problem ... how to deliver a loose head, bobbing about in the uterus." The mother died as well. The case exemplified the horrors of medical intervention. Kelly supported Williams's prescription of pelvimetry as a preventative measure—far less threatening to the life of the mother and child than podalic version during labor.[38]

* * *

From Williams's point of view, the assignment to direct the Outdoor Obstetrics Service seemed a prison sentence. Ambitious and aggressive,

Seven. Johns Hopkins to the Fore

he employed every maneuver he knew to increase his power and practice, urging the importance of obstetrics as an essential science whenever possible. Frustrating conflicts with the head of Gynecology ensued; Howard Kelly's seniority put Williams at a disadvantage. Kelly insisted on a firm distinction between the specialties; gynecology by far bearing the greater prestige. Students were forced to navigate the barrier between the two. Recognizing Williams's simmering anger, Kelly attempted to acknowledge Williams's growing presence without sacrificing his own authority.[39] Twice he urged the Medical Board to promote Williams to Professor of Obstetrics, each time without success.[40]

In 1899, the Board held a special meeting, called in the light of an appealing offer made to Williams by the Rush Medical School in Chicago. Acting quickly, the Board offered the director of the OOS the position of Obstetrician to the Hospital, with a seat on the Board and the promise of increased salary. A few months later Williams became full professor in a newly separated Department of Obstetrics. Kelly continued as Professor of Gynecology. The problem then was to define the boundaries between the two disciplines; lingering soreness is apparent in bylaws promulgated in 1905. Among other items, new jurisdictional rules established that in cases of contracted pelves, Caesarean sections were to be performed under the aegis of the Department of Obstetrics. Control of that issue was fundamental to the practice of J. Whitridge Williams.[41]

Even after he committed to the Johns Hopkins Medical School and firmly established his professional bailiwick, Williams continued to complain about his status. In 1916, he wrote an angry letter detailing his past grievances regarding treatment by the hospital administration and the Department of Gynecology. "After I became a member of this Board, repeated controversies with the Gynecological Department were necessary to prevent my being relegated to *the status of a mere mid-wife*.... Nor have I as yet been able to impress you with the fact that *obstetrics is essentially a surgical specialty*" (emphasis added). The Medical Board and the Superintendent hastily made repairs before his threatened letter of resignation was delivered. Unimpressed by the administration's desire to keep him at the institution, Williams made sure that a copy of his letter appeared in the public domain, on record for all to see.[42]

Williams' personality and his career as an obstetrician drew from a strong sense of masculinity and manhood. Sporting a broad mustache, he spoke with a deep, memorable voice, giving rise to his nickname, "The Bull." He steadily smoked a regimen of pipes.[43] He told bawdy, ribald stories in the classroom, enjoying the mortification of female students—he was very uncomfortable with the idea of women becoming physicians.[44] Williams generally had a coterie of male medical students in tow, creating a culture that sought to exclude women from the practice of obstetrics. Such exaggerated masculinity was a product of the time, exemplified by that symbol of Progressivism, Theodore Roosevelt. Eventually known as the Bullmoose, Teddy's idea of masculinity tied manhood to nature, physical strength and close association with the untamed west, especially as a hunter.[45] Nearly everything was bully.[46] Williams did not speak of western travels but was repeatedly tempted by Chicago, the urban connection to the West, the link between civilization and the frontier. Several of his students at Johns Hopkins came out of the West.[47]

Coupled to his staunch masculinity and determination to discourage women from obstetrics, there were the persistent expressions of racism. Repeated examples of racial stereotyping, phenotyping and use of degrading vernacular sobriquets spoke to his underlying beliefs. Williams recognized his dependence on African American patients, but interpreted this as *his* gift to *them* in their dependent, human status. Again, he was very much an exemplar of his time; racial prejudice permeated American society, making audiences receptive or at least passive in the face of his disparaging utterances. To their credit, some at Johns Hopkins resisted stereotyping as part of their practice of medical science, insisting on objectivity. But Williams was a national leader in the medical profession by the early 1900s; his voice, his image mattered. His degradation of African Americans fed the ongoing supposition that racial classification was integral to medical research and diagnosis. Medical science was shaped by racial perception.[48]

In 1915, vying for Rockefeller Foundation support to fund creation of the first School of Public Health in the country, Williams, by then Dean of the Medical School, declared "we have 100,000 darkies here with all their diseases, and their mortality twice as high as the white, and three times as much tuberculosis, and four or five times as much syphilis."[49] Letting his guard down in a somewhat protected environment, Williams divulged his approach to black patients; his desire not so much to make them well but to use them in education and research. Medical science benefited from study of their diseases, sickness and high mortalities. To his way of thinking, to treat African American women represented a progressive form of generosity.

Race and gender—the roles and status of women, interactions between men and women, relations among the defined races—are critical to the history of the OOS and the history of childbirth. J. Whitridge Williams developed a programmatic approach to obstetrics, particularly though not exclusively emphasizing surgical measures. He always insisted that in childbirth the physician should first respect "the force of nature," as he put it, to let the birth happen. Yet his formative early practice as an obstetrician and teacher emphasized the danger of contracted pelves, the consequent need for surgical intervention. The patients of course were women, emblematic of both the biological nature of reproduction and its social and cultural expression. Ethnic diversity was prominent among OOS cases; Williams reported and repeatedly emphasized that nearly 50 percent of his patients giving birth were African American. Medical students, a few of them women, none of them African American, were required to spend a term at the Dispensary, supervising at least two births. Only white women were nursing students. All were subject to the authority of the Director, the assistants he appointed. Birth emerged transformed—reconstructed on Williams's plan to create a more thoroughly medicalized event. He envisioned a hierarchy of practitioners, including obstetrical nurses, each with a specifically defined contribution. Expectant mothers would avoid midwives, seek prenatal consultation, give birth under the supervision of a specially trained medical staff (ideally headed by a dominant male physician). Basic to his perspective was a complete distrust and disdain for female midwives. Yet, his library included a number of old midwifery texts, including the work of Madame du Coudray. Williams referred to such texts, seeking obstetrical knowledge and pedagogy, even as he condemned lay practice.[50]

Williams looked to the past, drawing his sense of self as an obstetrician from history, pointing especially to Hugh Hodge, the authoritative physician at the University of Pennsylvania in the mid-nineteenth century. Hodge had seen the human body as a machine, birth as a mechanical process—Williams thought along similar lines. Childbirth was clinical, biological, dispassionate. He thought of himself as opening the future, bringing progress to an outmoded culture and practice of childbirth, delivering a superior alternative to the long practice of midwifery. After all, his was a progressive era.[51]

In 1910, Abraham Flexner's momentous *Report on Medical Education*, funded by the prestigious Carnegie Foundation, named the Johns Hopkins Medical School the model institution in the United States. The Foundation had chosen to focus their efforts on the betterment of American health care; the report established clinical science as the standard for all institutions of medical education. The designation brought enormous prestige and power to the University, magnifying the strength of J. Whitridge Williams's leadership in the field of obstetrics, the significance of practice at the Outdoor Obstetrical Service.[52]

That same report stymied African American medical education, belittling Black capabilities.[53] Accompanying the rise of modern medicine, the concept of race had become a metalanguage in the medical system, impacting and influencing every aspect of its practice and promoting racialized medicine (albeit not always explicitly).[54] Physician and historian Vanessa Gamble argues, "This racism was not limited to the prejudiced attitudes of isolated individuals. It was institutionalized in the structure of the American medical system and sadly, this institutionalized racism actually intensified as medicine became more scientific and as new standards for medical practice developed in the first decades of the twentieth century."[55] Flexner's heavy-handed criticisms offered little hope for the improvement of African American intelligence. Black medical schools languished in the report's aftermath.[56] The problem was not the lack of ability or commitment; Black medical schools suffered most simply from a lack of funds.[57]

* * *

Testimony to Williams's steadily rising influence was the publication of *Obstetrics,* a text first appearing in 1903. Though a very young and junior member of the medical faculty at Johns Hopkins, the book was exceedingly well received; a second edition appeared the following year. "The Bull" was determined to lead obstetricians toward an identification of themselves as practitioners of operative midwifery—true scientists at last. Reflecting the results of ongoing research at the OOS and the Johns Hopkins Hospital, the text was widely adopted by faculty and students throughout the nation, undergoing repeated new editions throughout the course of Williams's life, and ever after. Amended by multiple coauthors, new editions continue to appear. (The twenty-sixth edition saw publication in 2022.) Medical students read *Williams Obstetrics* still—the work remains an eponym for obstetrics, derived from experimental research and practice, molded in misogyny and racial prejudice.[58]

Eight

Intervention in Childbirth

Writing in the 1920s, physician and poet William Carlos Williams reflected on the timelessness and intimacy of home birth, describing long nights waiting, sleeping with his head on the kitchen table, dreaming a synchronized dream of the slow rhythm of waves of contractions steadily pressing on but not yet productive. By then, the dream was not entirely peaceful. The medical practitioner was beset with nagging questions: at what point should the attending doctor intervene in the birth? What was the best method to employ? The twentieth century had brought new standards to the practice of medicine.[1]

Obstetricians devoted more and more time to discussion of the techniques to use in obstructed labor. A pelvis diagnosed as contracted commonly became the warning for a potentially difficult birth, calling for surgical intervention. While the most extremely narrowed pelvic inlet clearly required extreme measures, borderline cases made the decision much more difficult. Doctors benefited from new tools in their armamentarium—anesthesia, antisepsis and asepsis, measures which improved mortality statistics (in comparison to the nineteenth century) but did not perfect them. Use of anesthesia made surgery more successful and less painful; ever-increasing attention to hygiene reduced infection and minimized the spread. New choices arose as Caesarean section became safer, bringing the possibility of saving both the mother and the child. Meanwhile, the vast majority of women (85 percent as late as 1927) experienced birth without life-threatening difficulty at home, often but not always with medical attendance.[2]

Katharine Park's *Secrets of Women* offers a cultural and gendered approach to the history of childbirth, locating a mythology and culture of violent intervention predating the rise of modern medicine. As one physician lamented in 1918, "Belly-ripping has become a mania and its maniacal ravages have invaded the realm of obstetrics."[3] Medical practitioners became sure of their surgical procedures, anxious to be in charge of childbirth, determined to be rid of midwives. Increasingly accustomed to the responsibility and the power of choosing who would survive by what operative method, childbirth in the form of medical obstetrics became increasingly masculine and surgical.[4]

In 1890, a discussion at the Obstetrical Society of New York followed a professional paper on contracted pelves, dystocia, and variation in treatment between hospital and private practice. Revealing the challenges in choice doctors faced, the palpable frustrations of the nine participating physicians surfaced as they considered the alternative suitability and success of craniotomy, forceps, and version. Most felt that craniotomy was quite safe for the mother and easily done by the surgeon. One participant argued that doing craniotomies in the home held less risk than the hospital setting. While some bemoaned the large heads of fetuses and the inability to easily judge the size before birth, others emphasized the necessity of careful pelvic measure. Proper diagnosis of a contracted pelvis could allow the physician to evaluate, prepare for a difficult birth.[5]

By the early twentieth century, diagnosis of the contracted pelvis had become a common theme in obstetrical texts. The reported incidence of obstructed pelves, the diagnostics and treatment of the condition, made rickets integral to the medicalization of childbirth in the Progressive Era. Many considered contracted pelvis to be perhaps the worst and possibly most life-threatening effect of rickets, but investigation into the causes of the disease escaped the interest of obstetrical science. Driven by the desire to supervise the process of birth, obstetricians turned instead to the problems stemming from pelvic obstruction, seeking a surgical answer. An air of desperation pervaded. Branches of medical science proceeded along separate paths; the pediatricians struggling to resolve the riddle of rickets while the obstetricians focused on the small number of nightmare births rooted in contraction. A transformation of American childbirth was the result.

* * *

Prior to the 1890s, few American physicians had even acknowledged contracted pelves among their patients. Despite the efforts of John Parry, Robert Harris and others, most practicing physicians doubted the significance of the condition, reflecting the very small number of cases reported between 1839 and 1883.[6] At a meeting of the American Gynecological Society in 1890, physician Edward Reynolds presented a paper analyzing 2,227 cases of labor occurring over roughly two years at the Boston Lying-In Hospital and the Obstetrics Department of the Boston Dispensary. He identified thirty cases of contracted pelves, little more than 1 percent. Reynolds directly addressed and quickly dismissed "the widespread incredulity of European obstetricians upon the alleged infrequency of contracted pelvis among American women, and their expressed opinion that its rarity is due to the almost universal neglect of pelvimetry by American physicians rather than any national peculiarities of our native women."[7]

Reynolds found eight further cases but discounted them, as the women were Blacks or immigrants. Separating both from his category of "Americans," Reynolds set the stage for a raging debate: Who is American? By his reckoning, African Americans were a special, seemingly irrelevant category, as were women emigrating from Europe. Eliminating them from the study, Reynolds maintained only native-born women, implicitly white, were American, and among them very few exhibited contracted pelves—far fewer than Carl Litzmann had found among German women. A nationalistic comparison of the European numbers to the American data motivated many researchers. Reynolds declared rickets and contracted pelves insignificant for American medicine, concluding that only a very small number of what he considered "Americans" had deformed pelves.[8] Skeptical of including the eight African American women who qualified for his study, Reynolds did measure their pelves and typed them accordingly. Finding just one contracted pelvis among them, he argued in a footnote against the commonly held supposition that African American women suffered a high degree of rachitic deformity.[9]

J. Whitridge Williams took note of Reynolds's work. Presenting a paper before the Maryland Medical and Chirurgical Faculty in 1896, Williams announced that he had identified fifteen cases of contracted pelves among one hundred patients at the Outdoor Obstetrical Service, nearly twice as many cases as Reynolds, in a much smaller sample. Williams counted four native-born whites, four immigrants of various ethnicities, and "eight negresses."[10] Williams objected to Reynolds's findings not in terms of the identity of Americans, but the source the physician used to compile his figures. Reynolds's numbers derived only from surgical cases. Williams had no quarrel with connecting contracted pelves to surgical intervention, but such data was not enough. Obstetricians needed to measure every patient in order to establish an accurate set of numbers showing the incidence of contraction. That determination proved an essential step toward the medicalization of childbirth.[11]

In a letter, Reynolds voiced his own objections to Williams's figures, arguing that most of his cases should not count, as they included a large number of Black women who, he insisted, just like his immigrants, were not Americans. Williams' figures for the incidence of contracted pelves in Baltimore were inflated, resulting from "his count [of the] negro race as American-born women."[12] Reynolds did agree in principle with Williams; understanding contracted pelves were essential to obstetrical practice.

Racial inheritance defined the shape of the pelvis. Williams took Reynolds's statistical evaluation as a professional challenge, continuing to pursue issues of deformity based on his own pelvimetric interpretation. Racial categories remained essential. He never addressed the issue of American identity directly, leaving that task to his assistant, Doctor George W. Dobbin (1870–1928).[13]

Dobbin was probably the most important assistant to Williams in the 1890s, appointed first resident and assistant in Obstetrics just after Williams was put in charge of the Outdoor Obstetrical Service. Dobbin wrote several articles, including two statistical analyses of patients in the OOS, mostly focused on the incidence of contracted pelves.[14] In 1897, Dobbin published a study of 350 cases, identifying contracted pelves in 11.5 percent of patients. (This number was far more in line with the 10.25 percent identified in the OOS case records for the years 1895–1898 than the 15 percent Williams claimed.) Dobbin spoke directly to Reynolds's assertion that the Black women were not American, stating "the negro, to my mind is certainly an 'American-born woman,' and we now have to consider her so in the legal sense of the term."[15] Backing off somewhat, he noted "at any rate their large number in the Southern States, not to mention the fact of their being exceedingly prolific, making it necessary and important for us to consider them in making a statistical report." Dobbin followed with a chart organized in three categories: "American," "Negro," and "foreign." A few pages later, he added one more reason to include the African Americans in medical research of the contracted pelvis: "The question of the negro race is … important … for rachitis being so common among them, they are bound to increase the percentage of contracted pelves to a marked extent, I think, in the South, we shall have to consider them as American women."[16] Slightly befuddled by the whole issue, Dobbin in his next publication devoted to case statistics referred to white patients as "so-called American patients."[17]

The debate was reflective of a society coming to grips with momentous change. Within the obstetrical profession, recognition of contracted pelves amplified a broader realization that America was becoming increasingly civilized, more like Europe. Larger questions about birth and the nature of society intertwined with the issues of race bared in the dispute defining American identity. For Williams, Reynolds and many others, discussion of the incidence of contracted pelves rested on an assumed set of distinctions between Black women and white women. Confounding medical interpretation was the fact that African American women seemed to have more abnormalities parallel to the European standards of pelvic deformities. What was the future of American birth?[18]

For Edward Reynolds and many other medical practitioners, the contracted pelvis was the fundamental breakthrough of modern obstetrics. Responding to Williams's subsequent work describing the funnel pelvis (a condition in which the anterior-posterior diameter of the pelvis is greater than the transverse diameter) at a meeting of the American Gynecological Society in 1911, Reynolds declared "Dr. Williams had had the courage and intelligence to throw the traditions of the past overboard and approach the obstetrical pelvis from the point of view of common-sense and sound mechanics, and he had revolutionized our views of the contracted pelvis."[19]

* * *

The early years of the twentieth century saw various physicians present papers offering criticisms and concerns about the use of pelvimetry. In a paper presented for the Gynecology Section of the Philadelphia College of Physicians in 1901, Edward Davis observed that "four-fifths of patients having abnormal pelves delivered themselves spontaneously."[20] While noting race as a factor in the frequency of contracted pelves, Davis did not employ racial categories in his analyses of clinical numbers. He supported the basic importance of pelvimetry, but urged recognition of factors such as poverty and malnutrition in assessing a patient. In the discussion that followed Davis's presentation, Doctor Richard C. Norris, a practitioner at the Preston Retreat, a private maternity hospital in Philadelphia, commented at great length on the inconsistencies in pelvic measure and the incidence of contracted pelvis. Turning discussion to the recommendations advanced by J. Whitridge Williams, Norris cast doubt on the necessity and the wisdom of universal internal measurement, emphasizing that the risk of infection outweighed the benefits of such a practice.[21] Not present at the meeting, Williams never answered Norris's charge in print but did change his demands for types of measure over time, sometimes arguing that his conservative use of measurement guarded against infection.

Cornell University physician and professor James Clifton Edgar (1859–1939) aired his criticisms of pelvimetry and contracted pelves in the *Transactions of the American Gynecological Society* in 1902. Questioning the very definition of the contracted pelvis, he observed, "Not only is there absence of harmony in measuring these pelves, but there is even failure to agree upon what a contracted pelvis really is."[22] Edgar complained loudly about the lack of a universally-accepted standard, arguing that "pelvimetry does not lead to mathematically accurate results."[23] For purposes of his study, Edgar closely adhered to the guidelines advanced by J. Whitridge Williams, recommendations intended to establish a universal pelvic measure of obstetrics patients. Trying for reliable figures, Edgar measured and remeasured patients, finally using anesthesia, only to throw out a thousand cases in concern for their inaccuracy. He found no way to verify the measurements once he found the cases questionable. Adhering strictly to scientific method, Edgar eventually developed an acceptable composite of records, based on twelve hundred cases of childbirth at the Mothers' and Babies' Hospital in New York City. The distribution combined eight hundred patients at the outdoor clinic, four hundred within the hospital. Edgar identified forty-four deformed pelves (3.66 percent), thirty generally contracted pelves (2.5 percent), and fourteen flat (1.16 percent)—in all, 7.32 percent (roughly one delivering mother in fourteen).[24]

His figures were much smaller than the count at Johns Hopkins. Edgar urged that disparate results of frequency came from a "want of harmony of method," but also enumerated a variety of factors ranging from social status to gender role as issues in the probability of contracted pelves. He did not deny the utility of the category of race, delineating twenty-one ethnic groups in addition to women born in America, but urged that social factors including poverty and deprivation deeply affected many immigrant women exhibiting pelvic deformity. Among Edgar's cases were thirty African American women who, as was typically the case in many such studies done in the Northeast, were listed as "no record." Challenging the assumption that deformed pelvis was the result of heredity, Edgar suggested environmental conditions of poverty and malnutrition affected American Blacks and eastern Europeans alike. Several of his patients were of the "new immigration," women of Jewish descent, victims of pogroms in Russia. In his terminology, all these groups likely experienced "misery, semistarvation, exposure."[25]

Edgar's analysis was a direct challenge to the studies undertaken at Johns Hopkins Hospital. Williams and his students did not analyze immigrant statistics, dismissing them as too limited to be significant, though there were growing numbers of such patients at the hospital and dispensary. Despite the oversight, Williams contended that eastern European women did not suffer contracted pelves, while African American women were two-and-a-half times more likely to suffer the condition as native born whites. The science of pelvimetry was a long chalk from achieving results neutral and unbiased.[26]

Doubts continued. At a meeting of the American Medical Association convened in 1905, Doctor Effa V. Davis, physician from Chicago, delivered "A Study of the Bony Pelvis in One Hundred and Fifty Cases." Roughly half the cases derived from an outdoor clinic, the remainder were home births she attended. Her motivation derived from a different source; she noted "the frequent causes of deformities in the cases handled and the not infrequent difficulty encountered in the normal pelvis," including issues of "childhood, puberty, family and general habits."[27] Davis found twenty-six of the one hundred-fifty cases (17.3 percent) presented deformed pelves. Of these, eighteen were generally contracted, and four simple flat and rachitic. Of the deformed cases, sixty-one percent gave birth easily without medical intervention; those needing assistance were most often delivered with forceps. There was just one Caesarean Section. Of the one hundred twenty-four normal pelvic cases, twelve required operative intervention (from forceps to extraction).[28]

Davis pondered some atypical variables in her discussion of the statistics. She talked about ethnicity (with no reference to African Americans) but focused more fully on the level of education among the patients. As a woman, she was undoubtedly aware of the prevalent belief arguing higher education jeopardized maternal experience. Her conclusion was that education had not harmed the bodies of these women in their adolescence, nor in the "growth and development of the bony pelvis."[29]

One of the few to directly address the issue of causation, Davis considered general contracted pelves, the most common deformity, finding them to be "a form of degeneracy." Contracted pelves thus joined inebriety, heart and kidney disease, tuberculosis and syphilis as expressions of constitutional weaknesses. Davis blamed lack of or faulty breast feeding for rachitic pelves. She felt strongly that many pregnant women remained inactive and ate too much. Babies weighing ten pounds were too big; she urged dieting for the mothers-to-be. There was skepticism in her audience; the sample size was small, the concepts challenging. But Davis presented a female perspective on the issues, and brought to bear factors largely ignored in the discussion of contracted pelves. Her tabulations supported a growing realization that the condition was becoming a concern for women of the "better classes."[30]

The complaints of Effa V. Davis, James Clifton Edgar, and Edward Reynolds were echoed by many obstetrical scientists in the early twentieth century. Numerous articles analyzing cases of contracted pelves, symphysiotomies, and Caesarean sections expressed impatience with the lack of consensus regarding the standard denoting a contracted pelvis. Wherever the standard was set, pelvic measures above that number would be considered normal. To move the designation one way or the other altered the perceived number of cases. A wide range of opinions existed, but none could transcend the arbitrariness and mistaken assumptions of race as factors in the measurement and subsequent interpretation. Many cases identified as one of four types of contracted pelves never encountered difficulty in labor; a high percentage experienced delivery without surgical intervention. This was the crux of the matter. The field of obstetrics was exhibiting a growing determination to take a firmer hand in the entire process of birth. The greater the perception of obstructed birth as a critical issue, the greater the justification for obstetrical intervention.

At a meeting of the American Gynecological Society held in 1904, Doctor Alfred Freeman Africanus King (1841–1914) of Providence Hospital, Washington, D.C., took up the long debated practice of pelvimetry. King commanded respect within the profession; he was one of the physicians who rushed to the aid of Abraham Lincoln at the moment of his assassination. King chose the topic "Uniformity in Pelvic and Cranial Measurements" to argue for the need to establish a universal definition of the "normal" pelvis. Comparing pelvimetries of the normal pelvis, he charted the numbers identified by many different physicians internationally and across time, from the work of Jean-Louis Baudeloque in the 1780s to the efforts of physician James Clifton Edgar in 1902. King contended the averages derived in competing analyses were taken from cadaveric samples with "promiscuous" pelves, compared to "selected *normal* pelves." To his way of thinking, there was no agreement on the size of the standard pelvis; the disparity of numbers defeated the point of mensuration. The purpose, King argued, was to obtain "an intelligent understanding of the physiology of parturition, in particular of that part of the process termed the mechanism of labor."[31]

King acknowledged the importance of anthropology and thereby the racial distinctions in measurement. Referring to the work of Washington physician Joseph Taber Johnson published in the 1870s, King accepted the importance of race in establishing pelvic categories, but subordinated these to the importance of establishing a "hypothetical" or "ideal" standard by which to teach. Most important was the reality of the fetal head engaged in the maternal pelvis in preparation for birth; pelvimetric numbers should serve to educate students on the parameters of the process.[32]

Several luminaries from the growing field of obstetrics were among the audience attending A.F.A. King's paper, including J. Clifton Edgar and J. Whitridge Williams. Williams allowed that King's idea of standardizing the pelvic and cranial measurements had validity, but challenged King's minimizing of the significance of racial difference, pointing to the conclusions reached in the comparative study undertaken by Theodore Riggs. After extensive discussion, the session chair declared the time had come for the American Gynecological Society to establish a standard for pelvic and cranial measure, appointing Williams, King and Edward Davis as the committee to draw up the proposal.[33]

* * *

However defined, discovery of a contracted pelvis motivated preparations for an obstructed labor. The calculus of surgical intervention

Eight. Intervention in Childbirth

changed almost yearly as doctors deliberated in journals and at meetings regarding their preferences, drawing from statistics and case studies. Questions of timing became significant. By the end of the nineteenth century, the sense of the time allotted to each stage of labor had changed for many. Doctors came to expect trouble if labor failed to move from first to second stage within twenty-four hours, judging something was so wrong that intervention was necessary. Physicians experimented with several operative choices; sometimes the procedures appeared sequentially in a single labor. Doctors competed with one another, most often through their institutional settings, to find the safest modus operandi.

Forceps were perhaps the first choice and the least harmful, depending on the instrument. High forceps were the most dangerous, indeed causing deaths, used when the fetal head was not yet engaged in the opening of the birth canal. Middle and low forceps incurred less risk. Depending on the specific case, forceps often served to bring the head out, coming foot first or head first. An alternative was to turn the baby before birth—version. Some doctors performed what was called podalic version, popular in the 1890s. During a labor which failed to progress, often breech, the attending physician turned the fetus to a footling presentation, using their hands externally on the mother's abdomen. If version or forceps failed, craniotomy was deemed necessary.[34]

The mother's life was primary. Opinion shifted slowly toward emphasis on going to greater lengths to save a living child without risking the mother's life. Given the lack of medical knowledge regarding newborn metabolism and the unavailability of alternatives for infant feeding prior to the 1890s, the odds of a child living without its mother were slim. Thinking of the infant's life before the mother's never crossed most people's minds. A living woman with a dead child might easily bear another child or more, while a newborn with a deceased mother faced an uncertain future at best.[35]

Though craniotomy remained a practice into the twentieth century, many physicians began to move away from the procedure, citing among others the writings of Adolphe Pinard (1884–1934), a well-known French obstetrician from the Baudeloque Clinique in Paris. Influenced by Catholicism and national fervor, Pinard in 1899 urged a shift to privilege both mother and child, part of a French national campaign to increase the rate of reproduction.[36] More and more, the practice of obstetrics subsumed contentious public issues such as contraception and abortion.[37] In the United States, a diminishing birth rate among the white middle class intensified the public interest in a better rate of infant mortality as well as maternal mortality. Those fears of "race suicide" grew—America needed more white middle class babies. Saving the mother's life began to lose primacy. Those motivated by religious views, especially Catholics (who maintained a strong presence and authority in Baltimore, St. Louis and a few other locales), increasingly pressured doctors to favor the child's life over the mother.[38]

In some circles in the 1890s, an early diagnosis of contracted pelvis motivated experimentation to reduce the size of the fetus—a smaller baby made an easier birth. Doctors considered denying food to very pregnant women in the last weeks of pregnancy, believing a more deliverable fetus would result. An Ohio physician, Henry Wald Bettmann, induced early labor by administering ergot. Again, the purpose was to improve the cephalo-pelvic proportion—an alternative intervention not widely supported. Most saw little to gain from early birth, observing that premature infants had little chance to live. Physicians including Adolphe Pinard and J. Whitridge Williams found the calculus of mortality more acceptable employing craniotomy rather than inducing early labors. Bettman's research did result in growing interest in the care of premature and newborn infants. Speaking in Berlin in 1892, he narrated the experience of birth as seen through the eyes of the infant, emphasizing the maintenance of life, the utility of a simple incubator (invented in France in 1878) to keep the premature baby alive.[39]

Calculating the risk of death of mother and child through statistics, doctors advocated increasing intervention. Joseph B. DeLee (1869–1942) of Chicago was among the most vehement and enthusiastic in commitment to the new order. DeLee articulated the fundamental belief that childbirth was a pathological event, rationalizing his call to empower and professionalize obstetrics. "We all know that even natural deliveries damage both mothers and babies…. If childbearing is destructive, it is pathogenic, and if it is pathogenic it is pathologic."[40] He carried this further in a later presentation, arguing that "only a small minority of women escape damage during labor." To forestall injury, DeLee advocated systematic administration of anesthetic, followed by episiotomy (incision of the perineum and vagina to prevent tearing) and forceps delivery in every primapara or complicated birth. Though DeLee did not advocate such extreme intervention in all births, the suggested regularity was disturbing. Speaking of the pressure women brought to him to end pain in childbirth, DeLee noted an increased demand for anesthesia, complicating obstetric procedure while compromising infant and maternal health. Women even begged "for Caesarean section to escape the dangers and pain of childbirth. They will tell you that Mrs. So-and-So had a Caesarean section done, has no backache, which they have."[41] J. Whitridge Williams responded in vehement opposition, espousing respect for nature and avoidance of unnecessary intrusion even as he too continued to devise operative techniques and medical procedures.[42]

Eight. Intervention in Childbirth

DeLee spoke from a wealth of experience. The son of Jewish immigrants from Poland, he grew up in Chicago, where he achieved a medical degree in 1891. After consultations with social worker Jane Addams of Hull House, DeLee in 1894 established a walk-in clinic on Maxwell Street, offering pre-natal care to largely immigrant neighborhoods. DeLee traveled to homes to attend childbirths. Five years later, he opened the Chicago Lying-In Hospital on Ashland Boulevard, a fifteen bed dispensary that quickly gained a reputation for the standards of cleanliness and success of deliveries.[43] In a text published in 1913, DeLee observed

> A distinction between hospital and home practice in obstetrics is gradually creeping into our scientific discussions. Careful study of existing conditions will convince any one that the safest place for the parturient woman is the special, well-equipped lying-in hospital. Here are all the facilities for the aseptic conduct of labor and the puerperium, here is the danger of child-bed infection properly evaluated, here only are the refinements of an operative technic possible, because the operator has the help of trained assistants.[44]

A training facility for medical students and nurses, the hospital soon attracted physicians from across the country anxious to learn the new obstetrics. DeLee's reputation spread.[45]

One characterization described J. Whitridge Williams as DeLee's "outspoken adversary."[46] Much of the sparring between the two leaders of obstetrics was theatrics, perhaps regionally based—Joseph DeLee of Chicago and the West; Williams established in Baltimore, the East and South. "Bull" Williams stood on his strong sense of Southern honor and utter confidence in his methods; DeLee was said to be a perfectionist, if generous in his associations. Certainly DeLee addressed his rebuttals to Williams's challenges in a less emotional tone.[47]

The combined influence of Williams and DeLee transcended their differences; their efforts did much to negate cultural traditions making women active participants in labor. As pregnant women—primarily white middle class and educated women whose voices were heard—demanded relief from pain and freedom from danger in childbirth, the work of Williams and DeLee, supported by their obstetrical colleagues, made childbirth a passive, very nearly an alienated experience. Educating the lay public, the next generation of medical practitioners, and the social reformers busily transforming American society, the new obstetrics constructed a birthing atmosphere built on hygiene, antisepsis, anesthesia, and instrumental intervention. The home gave way to the hospital.[48]

* * *

With the development of anesthesia, antisepsis and asepsis, Caesarean section became a more viable alternative to early labor or craniotomy.[49]

Innovative surgical techniques improved the chances of patient recovery. In 1876, Italian surgeon Eduardo Porro (1842–1902) successfully explored a new Caesarean procedure by removing the patient's uterus, thereby minimizing the chance of infection and subsequent maternal mortality. Hysterectomy seemed a small price to pay in light of the alternative; a Caesarean which sterilized the mother at least offered the possibility both baby and mother might live. By the latter years of the century the Porro Caesarean section became accepted practice but remained uncommon, thankfully left to the skilled surgeon and practitioner of antisepsis.[50] Infection remained the greatest threat.[51] If a mother was infected before or during labor, Caesarean section was not a choice, as surgery would precipitate death for the mother and child.[52]

Until 1882, physicians performing Caesarean sections almost universally operated without suturing the mother's uterus, fearing infection. Most historians credit German obstetrician and gynecologist Max Saenger (1853–1903) with developing a "conservative Caesarean section," introduced in a case of contracted pelvis in Leipzig. Saenger sutured the uterus with silver thread. The stitches still had to be removed, but the rate of recovery was much better. The practice of Caesarean section increased in consequence, though the risks were high and stayed high well into the 1930s.[53]

Modifications of Saenger's method sought to avoid infection of the peritoneal cavity; such an infection spelled certain death. Some surgeries brought the uterus outside the body before delivering the baby; an accompanying hysterectomy would leave the uterine stump permanently external. The incision beginning the Caesarean changed with time, shifting initially to a median cut into the peritoneal cavity of the abdomen, making the patient very vulnerable to infection. Joseph DeLee and fellow American physician Alfred Beck advocated a low cervical cut, vertical or transverse, developed in Scotland by J.M. Munro Kerr (1868–1960).[54] DeLee explained the incision as a way to avoid drainage from the uterus into the abdomen, limiting the danger of puerperal infection. In specific conditions the method proved safer than previous techniques.[55] J. Whitridge Williams balked at the lower cut and stuck with a median incision throughout his career.[56]

Physicians continued to explore other options in cases of extreme pelvic deformity. Symphysiotomy, an operation abandoned early in the nineteenth century, reappeared in the 1890s. The surgery simply opened the pelvis—pulling apart the bones that met to make up the pubic symphysis, breaking the cartilage so as to expand the pelvic area. In truly extreme cases, physicians fell back on pubiotomy, an operation in which the pubic bone behind the symphysis was actually sawed in half. Each procedure opened the pelvic outlet enough to allow delivery of the child—the mother's well-being was compromised indefinitely. Despite the severity of such procedures, there were several proponents. Benefits included the possibility of delivering a live child and the likelihood that, given a subsequent pregnancy, the woman could give birth vaginally without surgical interference. Barton Hirst of Philadelphia declared, "The position of this operation [symphysiotomy] in the treatment of labor obstructed by a contracted pelvis is beyond doubt the question of greatest present interest in obstetrics."[57] Adolphe Pinard and J. Whitridge Williams embraced the practice at the turn of the century; the operation gained more adherents at the Johns Hopkins Hospital in the 1910s. Choice of surgical intervention was governed by the probability of death; neither symphysiotomy nor Caesarean section was very good. Caesareans grew in popularity, symphysiotomy and pubiotomy eventually fell by the wayside, no doubt an expression of their essential destructiveness.[58]

Intervention broadened. Anesthesia—originally instrumental in Caesarean sections—became an essential tool. In 1899, German physicians developed an anesthetic combining morphine and scopoline, producing an agent that deadened pain while leaving the patient in a semi-conscious state. Not eliminated, the pain was beyond conscious recall. Soon known as twilight sleep, the combination was first employed in childbirth in 1902. The *New York Times* made note in 1915, indicating the anesthetic had no effect on the newborn infant. *McClure's Magazine* ran a feature. By the 1920s many women were demanding twilight sleep, complicating the obstetric procedure and actually compromising infant and maternal health. Anesthesia for labor left women with little ability to think consciously; mothers came to undergo birth as a completely passive experience. Historian Judith Walzer Leavitt has convincingly argued that women's pleas for twilight sleep inaugurated obstetrical domination of childbirth through the increased hospitalization for childbirth.[59]

Slowly and inexorably, medical men gained control of birth in the United States and much of Europe. Drawn to the growing array of surgical techniques, obstetrical science turned increasingly to gynecology as an accompanionate specialization, leaving child care to the pediatricians. Essential to this emerging concept of supervised childbirth was the presence of the male authority. Not every delivery demanded surgery, but growing expertise in the surgical way of birth created new and exciting capability. At the heart of this growing fascination stood the essential question: what manner of condition justified such extreme intervention? Hopefully, the science of pelvimetry held the answers.

* * *

In 1905, the Uniformity in Pelvic and Cranial Measurements Committee for the American Gynecological Society presented their recommendations. For the pelvis, King, Williams and Davis designated thirteen different numbers; some external measures, some internal. For the fetal head there were six. The committee qualified their standards by emphasizing they had avoided the exactitude and precision of fractions in order to make centimeters and inches comparable. The standards suggested were not averages, but a compromise taken from textbooks of the time. The three agreed that the purpose of measurement was to assess the proportion of the fetal head to the maternal pelvis, in particular the birth canal. There was no mention of race, only numbers.[60]

The one obvious fact to be drawn was that the science of pelvimetry had grown increasingly complicated with the passage of a century and a quarter. Jean-Louis Baudeloque, the pioneer in this endeavor, undertook four measures of his female subjects: three external, one internal. In their report, King, Williams and Davis defined standards for the normal pelvis including those four measures, and nine more besides. What is most instructive however, are the differences in the figures advanced by various analysts over one hundred-thirty years (see table below).

King, Williams, and Davis included the categories of measurement advanced by early researchers (along with many others), but their standard for identifying the threshold of pelvic contraction—the point where

Table 8.1
Threshold Standard of the Normal Pelvis

Physician	Date	Conjugata	Diagonalis*
Jean-Louis Baudeloque	1781	4"	10 cm
Carl Litzmann	1851	4"	10 cm
Hugh Hodge	1866	3"	8 cm
King, Williams, Davis	1905	5"	13 cm
Joseph DeLee	1913	5"	12.5 cm

*An internal measure, defined in 1905 as "between the middle of the sacral promontory and the point in the upper border of the symphysis pubis crossed by the lines terminalis."

SOURCES: Jean-Louis Baudeloque, *L'Art des Accouchements* (Paris: Mequignon, 1781); Carl Litzmann, Die Formen das Beckens, insbesondere des engen weiblichen Beckens, nach eigenen Beobactungen und Untersuchungen,hebst einem Anhange über die Osteomalacie (Berlin: Georg Reimer, 1861), translated by the late Douglas Woken; Hugh Hodge, *The Principles and Practice of Obstetrics* (Philadelphia: Henry . Lea, 1866); A.F.A. King, Edward Davis and J. Whitridge Williams "Report of the Committee Appointed at the Previous Meeting to Consider 'Uniformity in Pelvic and Cranial Measurements,'" *Transactions of the American Gynecological Society* 30 (1905) 80–82; Joseph B. DeLee, *The Principles and Practice of Obstetrics* (Philadelphia: W.B. Saunders Company, 1913).

danger in birth theoretically began—was markedly wider than their predecessors, an inch (three centimeters) at least in the internal measure. External measures such as the "interspinous diameter" reflected a similar expansion. In other words, the committee in 1905 chose numbers making contracted pelvis—and the attendant need for obstetrical intervention—far more typical. It is very difficult to believe the determination was entirely the product of dispassionate scientific evaluation. Like so much else in this era of medical "revolution," the aura of science obscured some very dubious fact-finding. A genuine effort to ascertain the threshold defining contracted pelvis should have considered the growing body of reports indicating that many women diagnosed with the condition in fact gave birth without problem. A truly scientific investigation would have sought more data, encouraged further studies to determine the pelvic diameters of women who did experience difficulty. The committee reporting to the American Gynecological Society advocated none of this. Instead, the three physicians did no more than consult recent obstetrical texts, arrive at what looked to be reasonable figures. No bibliography was attached to the report; there is no way of knowing the texts reviewed. No statistical evidence was presented. Inexplicably, the conjugata diagonalis threshold identifying a woman in danger of obstructed delivery had increased by an inch, 25 percent or more over nineteenth-century estimates. A very convenient result, if the goal is to justify increased surgical intervention in childbirth. The report looked like science; that was enough. The larger specification was readily accepted; Joseph B. DeLee adopted essentially the same conclusions in a massive text published in 1913. Summarizing the various estimates of the frequency of contracted pelves advanced by various researchers in Europe and America, DeLee could only sigh: "These figures carry the stamp of unreliability on their faces."[61]

* * *

How much of the research and study of the contracted pelvis was based on verifiable pathology? How common was rickets among the general population? Did the disease predominate to such a degree as to support the rising practice of Caesarean section? Answers to these questions are not absolute and often lead to other questions. Evidence indicates that the condition was real, that complicated births happened. Evidence also shows that cultural, political, economic and social factors were part of the history of childbirth at the turn of the century and the decades following. In the vast majority of cases, the event of a birth was not medical; birth did not often involve sickness.[62] Childbirth was a rite of passage, imbued with meaning as much spiritually emotional as physical. The environment of birth and the culture of those giving birth influenced the outcome at least as much as physiology and anatomy.[63]

Obstetricians came to birth from an entirely biological point of view. Though the profession saw itself as value-neutral and objective, research rested on a history of racial and sexual discriminations shaping physiological interpretation. The occasional encounter with pelvic distortion opened a door: if women were endangered in childbirth, the duty of science was to save them. Whatever the cause, contracted pelvis was a pathology to be treated, even if the condition most often resulted in birth without complication. Obstetricians developed a surgical response, a burgeoning practice of Caesarean section, an increased use of anesthetic. Diagnosis of contracted pelvis inflated notably as the interpretation of measurement altered, despite considerable evidence to the contrary. Operative midwifery became the culture of birth in the western world, a culture built solely on anatomy and physiology, on medical science alone. Birth was reduced to a cold, clinical experience.

Writers of the early twentieth century—medical, anthropological, and various male pundits particularly—reduced the image of society to a discourse comparing the savage to the civilized (white, English-speaking, upper and middle class). Holdovers from the race science of the nineteenth century continued to inform medicine. Childbirth reflected this discourse in a complicated way, presumptively endowing the savage—the "Other"—with the primitive strength to achieve easy birth, while the weaker and less able yet privileged white woman required relief. Accepting this privilege, the so-called civilized white middle class and wealthier women began to expect freedom from pain. Operative midwifery was seen as a benefit of civilization. The relationship of doctor to patient came to involve more than the use of surgical procedures and instruments, the efforts to establish a new normative standard of childbirth. The delivery of a child was well on the way to becoming a completely mechanical process, as envisioned by Hugh Hodge a half century before. Issues of race and sexuality, as well as gender and class, shaped this history.[64]

* * *

Common ground existed among white obstetricians. The prejudices were all too evident at an invitational presentation delivered at the annual meeting of the American Gynecological Society in 1911. J.M. Munro Kerr, Chair of Obstetrics and Gynaecology at Glasgow Anderson College, Scotland, came to America to lecture on Caesarean Section and contracted pelves. Kerr's obstetrical text, published in 1908, had won international acclaim; Glasgow was viewed as the hub of medical research and treatment of rachitic pelves in the British Isles and throughout the western world.[65]

Eight. Intervention in Childbirth 143

Kerr's presentation offered no surprises. Subsequent discussion touched on issues rarely discussed at the meetings. J. Whitridge Williams boasted of bettering Kerr's rate of spontaneous delivery in cases of contracted pelves, for the moment taking the position that spontaneous delivery was the preferable outcome. A Doctor Gordon questioned Williams on the side issue of how women's muscles affect labor. Williams answered that the second stage of labor depended on the mother's muscles, that Black women were more muscularly capable of giving birth. Gordon expressed doubt. Another doctor argued that "American" women were 75 percent more nervous and thus exerted pressure to speed up labor. Doctor R. Norris noted that more and more deliveries involving a pelvic conjugate diameter of 8 centimeters or less were done by Caesarean section, and that Caesarean section was becoming an elective surgery. A Doctor Frye of Washington, D.C., offered that the majority of his Black patients exhibited minor contracted pelves, though not generally contracted or rachitic.[66]

Then the group began to relax. Edward P. Davis suggested that muscles came to play in the expulsion of the placenta. He broke into levity: "I do not know what happens to the negro when he comes North, but his head swells in many ways, and we see in Philadelphia a considerable number of negro infants whose crania are not small; they are not as small as they ought to be. (laughter) They have intrauterine rickets and political megalocephalus and the results are disastrous."[67] In such a context, who among these obstetricians and gynecologists could imagine women using muscles to give birth, never mind brains? Obviously neither African Americans nor women were present, unless the transcriber of the discussion was a woman. The discussion turned to white women, or well-to-do women. Having won the support of his audience, Davis charged the elite women with heavy over-eating during pregnancy and lamented the inability of the physician to limit their diets, consciously or unconsciously echoing the observations offered by Doctor Effa Davis six years before.

And so it went. Sensing the advent of their own power, America's medical midwives were finding an atmosphere conducive to a denigrating portrayal of the patients they saw as passive and dependent subjects. Intervention was plainly a necessity.[68]

* * *

Surgical intervention was a double-edged blade. Advocated by the obstetrical profession as a means to save lives, the procedures were themselves dangerous, promoting infection, the risk of hemorrhage, or other life-threatening repercussions. Surgeries were still largely experimental; inexperienced practitioners were not immune to tragic mistakes. Campaigns promoting middle class birth, the protection of infant and maternal life, actually created risk. Using informed mathematical approximation, Judith Walzer Leavitt posits that in the early twentieth century "one in every thirty women" faced possible death in childbirth over the course of their childbearing years.[69]

Enlarging on this grim evaluation, medical historian Irving Loudon compiled maternal mortality rates for the United States from 1915 to 1953. Dividing his statistics into white and nonwhite categories, Loudon calculated a rate of 60.1 deaths per ten thousand white births in 1915, compared to 105.6 among non-whites. Over the next fifteen years the numbers grew considerably. The overall rate in 1920 was 68.9; nearly triple the rate of European countries such as Denmark, the Netherlands, and Sweden. England's rate was 43.3. While obstetricians refined and increased their operative interventions, intent on saving lives and consolidating medical control, the rate of maternal survival in America was actually sinking.[70]

The issue became increasingly controversial during and after World War I. In a study released in 1921, Robert Morse Woodbury (1889–1970), Director of Statistical Research for the Children's Bureau, presented tables claiming that "the mortality from puerperal septicemia actually decreased throughout the period from 1900 to 1920." Loudon's exhaustive research clearly demonstrates otherwise. Though mortality dropped somewhat after 1920, the rates remained well above sixty per ten thousand into the 1930s.[71]

An analysis of childbirth in New York City published in 1933 clearly demonstrated the culpability of obstetricians and hospital settings as the origins of the greater part of maternal mortality, particularly from puerperal infection. Directed by Doctor Ransom S. Hooker (1873–1957), the study examined 2,041 maternal deaths; determining sixty-one percent were the responsibility of physicians, 36.7 percent the fault of the patient, just 2.2 percent resulting from traditional midwifery. Almost two-thirds of the deaths were preventable. Of the deaths in operative delivery, more than two-thirds were considered avoidable; the operating surgeon was responsible 86.6 percent of the time. The report expressed concern over the "surprisingly high degree of technical incompetence." New York's hospitals were widely regarded as among leaders in the advance of surgical technique. Responding obstetricians largely condemned the Hooker report as scandalous, in essence dismissing the findings out of hand.[72] By then, roughly a quarter of all American infants were delivered in hospitals; more than seventy percent in urban settings. Operative midwifery had come to define childbirth.[73]

Associated with eight different hospitals in Chicago, Joseph B. DeLee focused concern on the practice of housing maternity wards in general hospitals, noting that the standards of antisepsis in the delivery room were too often far more careless than other areas. Speaking out in a series of papers published 1926 and 1927, he condemned hospital practice, finding that "the peril lies in the infective influences which emanate from the wards devoted to medicine, surgery, gynecology, pediatrics, the laboratories, and the autopsy room." The consequence was the deaths of thousands of women from infection and puerperal disease each year. DeLee's concern drove him to advocate extreme isolation of maternity patients in separate hospitals designed specifically for the purpose. As might be expected, his efforts met a "stormy" response; repeated denials of the maternal mortality rates, coupled to disquiet over the expense. "All those who took part emphasized the financial aspect of the situation—segregation was too costly, in money." Returning to the subject in 1933, DeLee invited Doctor Heinz Siedendorf of the University of Liepzig to address the issue of maternal mortality in hospitals; the findings more than sustained DeLee's position. As to the issue of expense, DeLee observed "I will say only this: Nothing compares in value with human life."[74]

J. Whitridge Williams unsurprisingly argued against the plan for separate hospitals, observing that the isolation ward housing infectious patients at Johns Hopkins Hospital had been in the same building as the maternity wards before a new building, the Woman's Clinic, opened in 1924. Williams's experiences in the old building led him to dismiss DeLee's proposal out of hand. "It is a matter of indifference what types of patients occupy the floors above or below the maternity." Williams died in 1931. Studying the Johns Hopkins Hospital reports, DeLee discovered "one of the highest morbidity rates in the United States." DeLee claimed Williams once informed him of an outbreak of puerperal disease among his patients—sixty-two sick women.[75]

Home birth was giving way to a hospital experience. Innovations in antisepsis and anesthesia provided the justification; the hospital supposedly offered a safer, healthier, more convenient environment. At best, the claims of medical science remained dubious; maternal death remained a profound concern. There were no guarantees.

NINE

Pediatricians' Progress

By the early twentieth century, rickets had become a commonplace ailment in the minds of American physicians, most of whom were general practitioners. Many continued to believe race an essential factor in the origin and incidence of the disease. This belated recognition of rickets in many ways coincided with the growth of pediatrics, a concentration practiced by relatively few. The field—"the dependent dwarf of ordinary medical practice"—grew into a medical specialty by separating itself from obstetrics, which was emerging still more slowly. If the locus of growth in obstetrics lay in Baltimore inceptive developments in pediatrics were centered largely in New York City.[1]

Critical in the history of pediatrics was the need to rally society behind the saving of infant lives. An important voice was Doctor Abraham Jacobi (1830–1919), an immigrant from Germany well trained in the developing medical sciences. Jacobi was in many ways the father of a separate professional pediatric emphasis in the United States. Settling in New York City in 1853, Jacobi established a practice specializing in the medical treatment of children, taking on a number of positions before his appointment as Clinical Professor of Diseases of Children at the College of Physicians and Surgeons in 1870.[2]

The emergence of a pediatric specialty involved convincing medical practitioners that children needed a specific care based on physiology. Jacobi wrote forcibly about the need to address infant mortality, trying to rally social forces to address what he saw as wasteful, even uneconomic, loss of life.[3] In a time when so many babies died, he had to convince his audience of the value of a newborn infant. A contemporary of Rudolf Virchow, Jacobi shared Virchow's idea that medical care should be made available to all children. The newfound obstetrical determination to protect the infant's life as well as the mother's in childbirth helped to make Jacobi's campaign viable.[4]

Among Jacobi's many professional positions was chief of staff at New York City Nursery and Child's Hospital, where staff member Mary A.

DuBois felt called upon to defend the institution's ability to further the welfare of its residents. Jacobi traveled abroad to study comparatively the effectiveness of various children's institutions. He returned to the United States damning the current institutional facilities for children as death traps. "I want to draw but one conclusion," he noted "that the attempt to raise babies in great institutions even with large means to aid you cannot be justified. These institutions must be given up and reserved for other purposes."[5] Jacobi was expelled from the staff after refusing to resign.[6]

In his capacity as leader in the growing field of pediatrics, Jacobi was eventually associated in one role or another with every hospital in New York. He initially believed the care of infants had to begin with finding an alternative to institutionalizing foundlings. His hope was to place children individually in what amounted to foster or adoptive homes. The work went hand-in-hand with the efforts of child savers of the period. Along with many others, Jacobi believed that young children needed a mother or surrogate who could nurture them into good health and prosperity. His influence grew; in 1880, he was instrumental in the creation of the American Medical Association's Pediatric Section. Eight years later, he was elected first president of the newly formed American Pediatrics Association. Strongly influenced by German medical science and clinical practice, pediatrics had become a recognized specialty in American practice. (Although Jacobi contributed chapters to several medical works, he never wrote a book devoted to pediatrics.)[7]

Jacobi's very long career featured the innovative treatment of several childhood diseases, including diphtheria, croup, gastrointestinal afflictions, and dental disease, turning to their study as they appeared in his environment. Rickets was one such disease, drawing his attention early. Recognizing the prevalence of rachitic disease in European populations, noting arguments that rickets was reported more frequently in American children, Jacobi considered the condition a critical element in the development of pediatric medicine. He was one of the first American physicians to investigate craniotabes—the unusual softness found in the closing cranial sutures of some newborns, initially described by Edward Jenner. Jacobi interpreted these as a symptom of a specific kind of rickets, rickets of the cranium. Well aware of the ongoing debates regarding both the etiology of rachitic disease and the range of possible treatments, Jacobi recommended the use of cod liver oil and milk diets to combat the condition. Jacobi made the not uncommon mistake of associating the condition known as Laryngismus stridulus—spasmic crowing inhalation—with rickets. This was eventually identified as tetany, an entirely separate disorder.[8]

Later in his career, as Jacobi accepted the benefits of infant and children's hospitals, he argued that rickets had become one of the most common children's diseases, necessitating the establishment of separate facilities. Giving the first presidential address to the American Pediatrics Society in 1888, he argued, "ninety-nine cases out of every hundred of rachitis need not exist." Pediatric engagement in education and public health could help prevent the disease. Physicians pointed to the growing presence of rickets in children as part of the context to advocate increasing pediatric institutions and care.[9]

* * *

The visibility and presence of pediatrics as a separate study in medical schools came about slowly. Improvement in children's health depended upon separate institutionalization of child care. Students were required to gain experience in pediatric hospital settings to obtain the specialization, but facilities were less than ideal. Throughout much of the nineteenth century, few medical establishments pursued in-house medical care for infants and young children suffering from communicable illness. Lacking the knowledge or means to halt the spread of disease, contagion persisted as a problem for institutionalized children; often a sickly child was turned away.[10] Jacobi relented in his criticisms of hospitals late in the 1880s, lending support to new and more specialized institutions emphasizing treatment intended specifically for infants and children. The rise of children's hospitals and the medicalization of orphanages helped to further pediatric research, including the study of rickets.[11]

Children's hospitals and dispensaries gave doctors a place to acquaint themselves with child and infant sicknesses, providing an opportunity to learn treatment. Dispensaries were particularly important because they offered medical care to the poor and presented a wide range of diseases to the fledgling physician. Pediatric science developed in this context but also became business-like. Some pediatricians sought to make the dispensary method of health care provision economically sustainable, but issues of efficiency came foremost, mirroring the thrust of industrialization. Published studies make it clear that once children became patients in dispensaries or hospitals, they often became experimental subjects as pediatricians tried various chemical therapies, testing patients' blood and sometimes urine in the investigation of disease.[12]

Such hospitals gained ground in the United States more slowly than in Europe. Echoing Jacobi's early stance, many Americans saw children's hospitals as life-threatening institutions, especially for children under two. The advent of germ theory and antisepsis made children's hospitals more acceptable, aiding the rise of pediatric practice. Part of the trend led by Jacobi, medical culture began promoting the institutionalization of sick infants and children, as long as the hospitals were not too large and embraced a research approach.[13] Even as the numbers of children's hospitals increased and artificial infant nutrition improved, widespread campaigns continued to flare in opposition to orphanages and homes for foundlings. Hospitals specifically serving children remained fairly uncommon. So many children died.[14]

Allusions to rickets became an assumed background for proponents of specialized children's medical care and institutions. As Doctor John Holt, a medical student at Johns Hopkins in the 1920s, remarked, "It is hard for us to realize how important a problem rickets was in those days."[15] Rickets was significant both because of the rising incidence in children and the reputed effect on development of the female pelvis. Jacobi argued that the emergence of rickets established the need for separate children's hospitals.[16]

Emerging leaders in the new pediatrics tended to turn away from race as a significant determinant in rickets. Clinical and laboratory studies led to new horizons, more rigorous than late nineteenth century theorizing attached to domesticity, world geography, and sunlight. Efforts to discover the origin of rickets took root in biochemical research conducted at pediatric institutions. Eventual discoveries became part of the discipline's maturation as a medical specialization. As medicine became more authoritative, mothers and children gradually assumed new cultural and social roles, shaped by pediatric expectation. The lives of women and children grew distinct in new ways.[17]

* * *

In 1887, The Babies Hospital became the first institution in New York City founded for the exclusive treatment of infants and children. Established in a brownstone building at the corner of Manhattan's Lexington Avenue and 55th Street, the hospital was originally staffed solely by women physicians. The majority of the early cases were found to be rooted in malnutrition. Doctor L. Emmett Holt was appointed Director in 1889, ushering in an era of scientific medical exploration.[18]

Originally from Webster, New York, Luther Emmett Holt (1855–1924) obtained his medical degree at Columbia University in 1880, opening a general practice in Manhattan. Choosing to concentrate in pediatrics, he gained experience at New York City's Foundling Hospital while serving as consultant to the New York Infant Asylum in Mount Vernon. Devoting himself to the discipline, he assisted in establishment of the first journal devoted to the field, the *Archives of Pediatrics*, in 1884. Traveling to Europe, Holt enhanced his specialization in discussions with pediatricians from eleven different countries. Recognized by Jacobi and others as an assiduous young man showing enormous promise, Holt became one of the forty-three charter members of the American Pediatric Society in 1887. He began teaching pediatrics at the New York Polyclinic and Medical School in 1891. Under Holt's direction, Babies Hospital became a model institution devoted to research. Holt's star rose accordingly.[19]

Poorly funded initially, the hospital could not maintain adequate nursing staff. To supply the lack, Holt took on student nurses, offering "A Catechism for the Use of Mothers and Children's Nurses"—originally a booklet comprising twenty-three questions and answers covering all aspects of child care. Lengthened to sixty-six pages, *The Care and Feeding of Children*, first published in 1894, became a widely read guide to parenting, making Holt a powerful figure in the medical world. Holt was a no-nonsense disciple of disciplined motherhood; the guide insisted on regular meals, a daily schedule of activities, and no playtime for children under six months—he believed play made the little ones cranky. The guide engaged mothers in the science of pediatrics, though frustrating some with its inflexibility.[20] Holt's pediatrics text, appearing three years later and periodically revised, became the standard for the three decades following. Holt was elected president of the American Pediatric Society in 1897, began teaching at Columbia in 1901.[21]

A close association with oil magnate John D. Rockefeller (1839–1937) and his family did not hurt his opportunities. Holt and the Rockefellers attended the same Baptist Church on Fifth Avenue, became closely acquainted. In 1900, Rockefeller funding provided a new ten-story building to house the Babies Hospital, a complex featuring the very latest in child care facilities. The year following, discussions for the nation's first biomedical research organization came to fruition at a dinner party hosted by L. Emmett Holt. The Rockefeller Institute for Medical Research began with a two hundred thousand dollar check written to Holt, signed by John D. Rockefeller, Jr. (1874–1960). Simon Flexner (1863–1946), brother of Abraham, became the first director of laboratories.[22]

* * *

The rise of pediatrics faced a grim truth. Children's institutions were often harbingers of early death. Doctor Philip Van Ingen (1875–1953) in 1915 analyzed the rate of infant mortality in New York State, breaking down the numbers of deaths among children under two years of age. Estimating the state's total number of children under two, Van Ingen found from 1909 to 1912, 87.5 per one thousand children died. Hospitalization was a desperate choice. From 1909 through 1913, the eleven large institutions for child care in the state treated 28,210 children under two years of age. 11,918 died. In two of those institutions more than 50 percent of the children under two perished. The younger the child, the greater the threat of death. The largest percentage of infant mortality came from the lower and most vulnerable strata of society.[23] More sobering still was the fact that child mortality rates in the early twentieth century had actually *improved* over earlier decades. Response to a diphtheria epidemic in late nineteenth-century New York demonstrated the considerable influence of social status on the actions of public health authorities.[24]

To varying degrees, medical scientists were inured to infant death, expecting the worst, viewing the occurrence as commonplace. In a lengthy treatise published in 1898, Holt wrote of the difficulty working in a children's hospital, where death was so pervasive and inevitable. Especially troubling were the problems the facilities themselves seemed unable to avoid—the starvation and death of young patients, so often social outcasts—orphaned, abandoned, or committed by local government. Very few had contact with their mothers. Holt's solution was to limit the number of children admitted, create more room between patients to encourage better circulation, and focus on issues of nutrition. Citing the high rate of infant mortality that accompanied admission to hospital, he was especially concerned with helping infants who lost weight after admittance. Rickets was often part of their vulnerability. He took pride in the falling infant mortality rate at the Babies Hospital.[25]

The first and foremost challenge for children's hospitals was the effort to keep infants alive. Nutrition offered a new avenue of exploration. Specialists grasped the necessity of fully understanding the unique physiology of pre- and peri-natal fetuses and infants, the development of children from babies to adulthood. As so many of these infants had no contact with their mothers, doctors were first concerned to find a way to help them survive in lieu of breast milk. Attention centered on alternative or artificial infant feeding, along with a shift to medical control. Suspecting proper ingestion of calcium could be a factor in rickets, nutrition in pediatric hospitals specifically addressed the persistence of the disease among infants and children under two.[26]

* * *

Nutrition was not medicine's long suit. Until the late nineteenth century there had been little viable alternative to breast milk. Not understood completely in its biochemistry, breastfeeding was a contentious issue, made worse by research into infant feeding. Upper- and middle-class babies were often nursed by working-class women, deemed susceptible to disease and instability in their lives. Beginning in the late nineteenth century and persisting through the 1920s, medical scientists strove to manage wet-nursing, seeking the best alternatives to a mother breastfeeding her own child. Hospitals for children occasionally hired live-in wetnurses, guaranteeing the lactating woman's health. In the meantime, in a contradictory direction, pediatricians began to give mothers choices in infant nutrition—infant formulas. The alternatives involved complicated recipes for ratios of ingredients; doctors urged mothers to seek medical supervision in their use. Though the components varied from formula to formula, one ingredient was a constant: cow's milk.[27]

L. Emmett Holt was much concerned with the quality of milk in New York. Obtaining a grant from the newly established Rockefeller Institute, he undertook a study of the city's tenement districts, disclosing a connection between infant mortality and high bacterial accounts in the milk available. Citing the data, Holt pushed for higher standards of cleanliness in production, transportation, and delivery of the product, leading to the establishment of "certified milk." Milk commissions and advisory boards at the New York City Health Department eventually came to oversee the quality of what had become an essential in the modern home. The pediatric emphasis on artificial feeding formulas and the sanitization of cow's milk gradually led to a shift away from breastfeeding as the be all and end all of infant care.[28]

* * *

Holt maintained strong ties with Johns Hopkins University. He had studied pathology under William Welch, now the head of pathology at Hopkins, responsible for the emergence of the medical school as the nation's premier laboratory for bacteriological study.[29] As laboratory work became established at the heart of medicine, projects in various locations reached out to similar activities in other places, fostering a kind of community. Rickets persisted as a universal concern. A rhythm of competition and cooperation among institutions sustained scientific research aimed at discovery of proper treatment or tests of immunity. That spirit intensified with the opening of the Harriet Lane Home for Invalid Children at Johns Hopkins University in 1912. Once established, the institution was to set a new standard for pediatrics.[30]

The Harriet Lane Home brought laboratory analysis and clinical study—the direct observation of sick children—together under one roof. The patients were largely from East Baltimore—many African American, poor and in need of medical care for diverse maladies. The institution followed the trajectory already established by the first pediatricians, looking at contagious disease and nutrition as key areas of research and practice. Many articles, including several on rickets, emanated from research undertaken during the first decade at the Home.[31]

Harriet Lane (1830–1903) was the niece of bachelor President James Buchanan, serving as first lady throughout his term. In 1866, she married

Henry Elliott Johnston, a well-to-do Baltimore banking tycoon with lucrative interests in the railroad industry. Dying in 1883, Johnson's will stipulated funding for a memorial institution dedicated to his wife, to be established upon her death in memory of their two sons, who died young of rheumatic fever. Harriet Lane died in 1903; legal complications delayed the bequest. The funding amounted to four hundred thousand dollars, an amount too small to do much of anything meaningful. Negotiations ensued. Johns Hopkins was the obvious choice, a nationally recognized institution which had somehow neglected pediatrics in development of the medical school. The sticking point was a stipulation in Johnston's will requiring "a permanent residence for crippled and chronically ill children."[32] His trustees agreed to interpret the term very loosely; "invalid" morphed into "sick." A charter was signed incorporating the Harriet Lane Home as part of Johns Hopkins Hospital in 1906. A secondary purpose, outlined in Harriet Lane Johnston's will, was to establish "a training school for nurses."[33] The children were to be white only, and of all nationalities. Gaining authoritative control, the medical school soon overrode the racial requirement, offering care to children of other races. The Harriet Lane Home emerged from the charter a children's hospital, housing pathology, biology and laboratory chemical research.[34]

The medical faculty began a world-wide search in 1908 for an outstanding physician to become the first "Head of Pediatrics and Physician to the Harriet Lane Home." Several of the medical faculty at Johns Hopkins had trained in Germany; German medical expertise was held in the highest respect. Doctor Clemens von Pirquet of Vienna, the premier pediatrician in Europe, became the initial choice.[35] Search committee members had heard the doctor speak at an international congress on tuberculosis and hoped to import someone like the Austrian to Baltimore.[36] Negotiations proved difficult. Von Pirquet accepted the position and spent a year in Baltimore, but chose ultimately to return to Europe.[37]

Even as he withdrew from the appointment, von Pirquet influenced the children's hospital intensely, submitting architectural plans that guided construction of the Harriet Lane Home building. The original bequest proved too small to meet the ever-expanding dreams of the medical school; there was not even enough in the budget to finance an adequate structure. Administrators turned to the Rockefeller Institute and other philanthropic sources to cover construction and related costs. Constructed on University grounds south of the main hospital, the Harriet Lane Home emerged as a five-story building, divided into four isolated pavilions in the hope of containing outbreak of epidemic disease. The wings were small. Medical personnel had to walk outdoors to get from one pavilion to another, sterilizing their clothing before entering a separate department. The floor nearest the roof was intended for tuberculosis patients, but was initially unused.[38]

Money continued to be a problem; the hospital could offer just twenty-four beds to patients at the opening. The institution was segregated, with separate wards for African Americans and whites.[39] A student of the early years remarked on the stern and hierarchical structure of the lecture amphitheater. Students were not allowed to sit. The floor was hard concrete, the lighting poor, heating non-existent. Steel rails stood at the front of each row; students could lean if necessary. This punishing expression of medical hierarchy, the lowly status of students, stayed in place until after the Second World War.[40]

The search for a director reopened. Despite the renewed hope of finding a regarded German practitioner, the eventual choice was an American, Doctor John Howland (1873–1926), a native of New York City. Graduated from the College of Physicians and Surgeons at Columbia University in 1901, Howland served internships under Simon Flexner at the Rockefeller Institute and L. Emmet Holt at the Babies Hospital. He had left New York in 1910 to become Professor of Pediatrics at Washington University in St. Louis. Unhappy with the position, Howland resigned after just six months to accept the opportunity of a lifetime at the Johns Hopkins Medical School.[41]

Before moving to Baltimore, Howland traveled to Europe for a year, preparing for the position through a course of study under Doctor Adalbert Czerny (1863–1941), reputedly the most distinguished children's practitioner in the world. Czerny's specialization was pediatric nutritional disorder, including research on infantile diarrhea and rickets. His approach emphasized chemical analysis; Howland gained considerable practical experience serving in the German doctor's clinic.[42] He came to Baltimore prepared to focus his own research on infant feeding and diarrhea, as well as the study of rickets. Fully cognizant of the importance of laboratory research, he made chemistry an essential component of the medical curriculum, insisting students undertake their own chemical analyses. He gathered around himself a group of talented physicians and scientists who made great strides for the medical school and the professionalization of pediatrics, very quickly spreading the influence of the Harriet Lane Home across the United States.[43]

The official dedication of the Harriet Lane Home took place on November 21, 1912, though the facility had begun operations in late September. A dispensary was advertised in Baltimore newspapers early in October; the first patients were admitted to the wards in mid-November. An address by Abraham Jacobi (then age eighty-two) began the celebration appropriately.[44] L. Emmett Holt followed, offering a series of sober statistics to demonstrate the value and importance of such a promising new facility. In 1892, 41 percent of all deaths in New York City were children under five years old. Twenty years later, that same age group still accounted for a third of the city's deaths. Turning to the Baltimore environment, Holt pointed to a mortality rate the seventh highest among cities in the United States. The Harriet Lane Hospital was essential, a "modern" hospital, a site of specialized care for children, training for students and doctors, research laboratories for the furtherance of medical knowledge.[45]

Holt then turned to the issue of mortality itself, asserting that the public and all concerned with the institution must expect a high rate of death. Very sick infants were most likely going to die. Rather than protect the infant mortality rate by refusing such desperate cases, society benefited from the hospital taking in such infants. "Nearly one-fifth of the deaths in the Babies' Hospital, in New York, are in patients who live less than twenty-four hours after admission. But if such children were not received, in many instances, they would have died in the mother's arms while walking the street."[46] Vivid in its impact, at an obvious level the image re-enforced society's obligation to care for the poor and homeless. More deeply, the trope characterized the hospital's function as a center established to analyze mortally-ill infants while treating their afflictions. The work of the new hospital would improve the health of middle and upper class families while protecting them from exposure to disease and death on the public streets.

Emphasizing the benefits the new hospital offered to the general public (those outside the medical world), Holt stressed the need for parents and relatives to surrender their dead child's body to the hospital for autopsy.[47] Science needed the ability, the right to examine the child postmortem. Medical practice occupied a space separating the public from the great unknown, the final phenomenon of death. Just as childbirth moved towards birth in the hospital, removed from the home and common participation, pediatricians began to urge parents to bring sick children to the hospital to die. Medicine was to be the arbiter of life and death.[48]

* * *

Brought to operation, the success of the Harriet Lane Home rested on John Howland's ability to identify and recruit researchers possessing the wanted scientific methodological skills and the ability to work in teams. Sounding a too-familiar theme, Howland had little use for women doctors, and had difficulties even with nurses and the secretarial staff. Doctor Kenneth Blackfan (1883–1941), clinician and first resident, specialized in pathology and bacteriology. W. McKim Marriot (1885–1936) and Benjamin Kramer, two gifted chemical researchers, contributed heavily to several path-breaking studies in pediatric chemical research. Brought to Johns Hopkins one by one, Howland supervised and assisted the efforts of this entirely male staff of assistants, establishing a well-defined routine.[49]

In 1912, Howland recruited another Emmett Holt protégé, Edwards A. Park (1878–1969), a native of Gloversville, New York, educated at Columbia University. Park specialized in the microscopic study of bone growth; the study of rickets, scurvy, nutritional diseases in general, and lead poisoning were of particular interest. His work in bone histology complimented Howland's emphasis in the emerging field of biological chemistry. At this juncture, Park's service was brief—volunteering for the Red Cross with the outbreak of World War I, he was sent to France, where he directed an orphanage for Belgian children. Returning in 1919, Park remained only a short time before moving on to Yale.[50]

Like Holt and several other practitioners of the new pediatrics, John Howland and Edwards Park were much concerned with the problem of infant feeding. Howland developed his own formula, rich in protein, prepared each day by student nurses working in two basement rooms at the Harriet Lane Home. The research necessary to compound such a formula proved to be a kind of prelude to a determined investigation into nutrition in the search for the source of rickets.[51] Doctor Tom Rivers, who studied medicine at Hopkins under Howland and Park in the 1910s, recalled the involvement in infant nutrition:

> Feeding and infections were two of the major problems we faced.... I remember that in those days there were intricate formulas for diluting milk. Dr. Howland didn't follow the straightforward rule used in most places, and Ned Park frequently fought with Howland on the subject of dilution. Park always thought that a child could take whole cow's milk, as well as whole human milk, without any untoward effect, and when Park was in charge of the wards in the summer he would feed a child whole cow's milk instead of diluting it. That battle continued for a long time among pediatricians.[52]

Rivers eventually became Director of the Rockefeller Institute, specializing in virology. Looking back to the beginning of his career, he found the medical practitioners' absorption with the chemistry of infant feeding distant, almost unfathomable.[53]

The Harriet Lane Home was shaped from the beginning to become a thoroughly modern research hospital, a far cry from the home for invalid children originally envisioned. As a thoroughly integral part of the Johns Hopkins Medical School, the primary purpose of the Home was to pursue teaching and research, impervious to public scrutiny. Municipal hospitals for children enjoyed no such immunity. Something of a martinet, Howland drew strict lines, rigidly separating the laboratory and its staff from the hospital wards and the dispensary.[54] Medical students, residents, interns and physicians would be assigned one realm, have nothing to do with the other. Blackfan supervised the clinical side of the unit, working closely with patients; laboratory researchers were not to involve themselves with the children directly. Blackfan worked with physicians and scientists in the wards, while Marriot and Kramer overlooked the laboratory analyses.[55] Howland was remembered as "a one man's department," both supervising the care of the children on the hospital wards and pursuing biochemical research. Such organization isolated the laboratory work and analysis from the process of drawing blood, sampling tissues, taking the needed cultures from children. Though the operations were intimately interdependent, subsequent research publication furthered the dissociation of the laboratory from the hospital. The inflexible separation objectified the patients.[56]

Laboratory research resulted in several discoveries pivotal to the development of pediatric care. Confronted with several cases, rachitic disease quickly became an important focus of study. Working with Marriott, Howland first took on the grave problem of diarrhea in children, an extension of his work in Germany. A prevalent and often fatal condition, infant diarrhea is to this day the greatest killer of infants around the world. Their research, published in 1916, demonstrated the significance of acidosis in the digestive intoxication associated with diarrhea.[57]

The pair then moved on to biochemical investigation of tetany and rickets, two diseases long conflated. In an important laboratory breakthrough published in 1918, the two physicians identified a distinction between the diseases in the low phosphate and high calcium serum levels found in tetany afflictions. The discovery enabled them to identify eighteen cases of tetany (ten were identified as "coloured") and twenty-one children (thirteen African American) manifesting symptoms of rickets ranging in degree from "very severe" to "mild." Rickets patients often exhibited normal levels of calcium in the blood, while tetany sufferers' calcium levels were consistently low. Both groups benefited from treatment with calcium chloride. Definitively separating the two maladies while establishing a clinical therapy for tetany was a step forward; one disease was indisputably identified; the etiology of rickets grew clearer.[58]

The research continued. Howland joined forces with Benjamin Kramer on what came to be regarded as the most significant breakthrough for the department. Recognizing that the essential symptom in rickets was the lack of calcium salts in the bones, Kramer and Howland examined the ratio of calcium to phosphorus in the blood. Their study, published in 1921, found the "concentration of the inorganic phosphorus of the serum to be low in rickets. The amount was definitely increased following the administration of cod liver oil." At long last, they had identified a measurable symptom of the disease. The discovery was critical, first of all providing a possible test for rickets through analysis of the blood serum, eliminating the confusion of symptoms cited up to this time. Confirmation of the efficacy of cod liver oil was equally important, though the authors could offer no chemical explanation for the therapeutic value of the stuff. Working with the laboratory staff, Kramer by this time had devised a technique analyzing the significant ions in blood serum, enhancing the ability to undertake minute analyses.[59]

* * *

In 1911, the sixth edition of Holt's much respected text, *The Diseases of Infancy and Childhood*, appeared, for the first time bearing the name of an additional author on the title page. John Howland was recognized with the words "assisted by." The acknowledgment was a sign of a growing import among Howland's peers in the pediatrics profession. The seventh edition, issued in 1916, listed Howland as co-author. The text included a long discussion of rickets, examining the etiology, distribution, pathology, symptoms, prognosis, and treatment of the disease. Holt and Howland defined rickets as "a disorder of nutrition, the result of some disturbance of metabolism in which calcium plays a very important role."[60] Noting that the widespread frequency of rachitic disease had become apparent very recently, the authors firmly stated that rickets was present in all the world's populated regions, in all the races of humanity. Children of "southern races" (African Americans and Italians) apparently suffered in temperate climes, and in cities especially. Seasonality played a role; children born between January and June were twice as susceptible. Holt and Howland were willing to entertain the possibility the disease was hereditary, though the suspicion had proven immune to absolute proof. Environment perhaps played a role: "poor ventilation, filth and lack of sunlight have been regarded as potent factors in producing the disease. Their exact influence is difficult to determine."[61] The eighth edition, published in 1922, stated more emphatically that the role of sunlight was not proved.[62] What did seem to be absolutely essential was the role of nutrition:

> Three theories have been advanced in explanation of the deficiency of calcium in the bones, which is the most striking characteristic of the disease. The first one, that rickets is due to a lack of calcium in the food, is not supported either by clinical or experimental evidence. The second theory is that the disease is due to an increased excretion of calcium as a result of disturbances of digestion. It is very likely that the increased excretion of calcium occurs only in rachitic children. Diet alone or disturbed chemical processes are not sufficient to account for it. The third theory advanced is that although sufficient calcium is furnished in the food, it is excreted in excess because the bones are incapable

of absorbing it. This is the theory that has the most clinical and experimental evidence in its favor, though what produces the incapacity of the bone to retain calcium is quite unknown.[63]

Despite the determined efforts of both authors to develop an artificial infant formula based on cow's milk, the chapter granted that the comparative lack of rickets in the countryside could be due to the fact that mothers away from the cities were more likely to nurse their babies.[64]

In sum, the text issued by Holt and Howland offered a review of all that was known, suspected, or theorized regarding rickets as matters stood two decades into the twentieth century. Their own perspective was plain: despite the vast amount of ink spilled on the possible role of sunlight, urban environments, race, heredity, and the like, what mattered was what could be measured precisely, scientifically, experimentally. Something to do with calcium, how the body absorbed the element into the bones. The eighth edition of *The Diseases of Infancy and Childhood*, published in 1922, reproduced the discussion from the previous work almost verbatim. One significant paragraph was added, outlining the laboratory discovery determined at the Harriet Lane Home the previous year. Phosphorus levels in the blood serum measured very low among rickets patients. Administration of cod liver oil brought significant improvement. "When the phosphorus becomes normal, evidences can be recognized in the radiogram. This offers an explanation for the failure of calcium deposition in the bones during active rickets."[65] Much was suggested in that one simple paragraph. Cod liver oil needed further investigation. Radiograms—x-rays—were becoming an important (if unfortunately much abused) tool in the evaluation of rachitic cases. A solution to the riddle of rickets was perhaps close at hand.

* * *

Beginning with Abraham Jacobi, continued by the work of L. Emmett Holt, John Howland, and the researchers they encouraged and supported, the growth of pediatric science created conditions conducive to a more exacting understanding of rickets. More apparent than ever, the ultimate answer seemed to lay in the chemistry of the human body. Establishment of specialized, well-equipped children's hospitals provided the human children necessary to carry out the test analyses critical to the understanding of biochemistry. The laudable goal was the eradication of childhood disease, be it diphtheria or tuberculosis or scarlet fever. Or rickets. The reality of the moment, more often than not overlooked by the analysts, was the fact that helpless patients—malnourished, sickly, most often orphaned—became test subjects, the fodder for medical experimentation. Science demanded rigor and accumulated increasing power, while orphaned infants and children, better seen but not heard, were unable to articulate their needs or their experiences of pain and suffering. Even as scientific knowledge of disease increased, actual medical treatment remained limited. The paradox stands out in relief, that in an era newly devoted to pediatric care, orphans and children of the poor remained unprotected in the advanced medical setting, subjects of science, voices unheard in the march of pioneer discovery.

Ten

Case Records at the OOS

Under the supervision of J. Whitridge Williams, the importance of contracted pelves became a guiding principle at the Outdoor Obstetrical Service. Case records surviving from the early years indicate that the process of identifying the condition was much more easily prescribed than effected. Doctors, medical students, and staff looked carefully for indications of rickets and contracted pelves, anticipating their significance as a cause of obstetrical problems. With the passage of time, the records reflect changes in medical perception, the categorization of the bony pelvis in relation to birth. Williams kept his own separate records, the grist for statistical analyses presented in several different studies. The original OOS records suggest the science was far less exact than the published essays intimated.[1]

The Outdoor Obstetrical Service at Johns Hopkins helped to set historical precedent by establishing a prenatal routine for patients. Largely anonymous staff, perhaps nurses in many cases, filled out forms for each patient visit to the Dispensary, ideally recording results of a prenatal consultation, followed by the actual birth. Typed sheets delineated the required information and included space for diagnosis and comments. (This standard patient form derived from the work of French medical clinician Pierre Charles Alexander Louis [1787–1872], developed between 1823 and 1854.)[2] Preliminary questions began with the woman's name, address, race, age, number of children, marital status, miscarriages, history of pregnancies and labors. Previous attendance by doctors or midwives, complications of labor and birth (with outcome), pelvic shape, six pelvic measurements, history of any disease, and previous recourse to the Obstetric Service all found a place. Patient perspective appears on the record in their responses to questions from the form, such as, "when did you first walk as a child?" (Walking late—the time was not specified—was a symptom of rickets.) In the early records, patients very occasionally provided information for self-diagnosed small or contracted pelves.

The examiner wanted truthful histories as a foundation in anticipation of the coming labor. Responses helped to shape the attending physician's own expectations, the subsequent examination, and the resulting diagnosis.[3] Individual records reveal the texture of the experience, the relationship between caregivers and patients. Each case brought its own unique situation. Language barriers and religious differences were common; at times communication was difficult. Some patients were noted as Hebrew; Doctor Goldborough interpreted their Yiddish. A Polish immigrant woman spoke no English; it was "difficult to get accurate history through interpreter." Quite often, the examiner tended to doubt the patient—words could be filtered through a lens of disbelief. For instance, the patient "denied lues," (syphilis), or a patient with a small conjugata diagonalis might fail to recall previous trouble giving birth. Occasionally, disparaging remarks appeared: "seems especially unobservant, even for a negro." "Doesn't seem to be strong mentally." "The hygiene conditions were extremely poor." (In each of these instances, the patient was African American.) Records of the Outdoor Obstetric Service hold rare glimmerings of family and kin, involving a few mothers of the birthing woman, very rarely and only obliquely partners or husbands. The OOS served people who could not afford health care, shifting and broadening definitions of the "worthy poor," yet brought to bear alienation and constructions of "other" in the physician's views of his patients.

The latter half of the form recorded the actual birth of the child. The typewritten page provided space intended to note various aspects of the delivery, including the presentation, the duration of labor, the fetal size, any complications or signs of infection, surgical intervention, drugs employed, subsequent hospitalization, and most importantly, the outcome—hopefully both mother and child alive and healthy. Again, the information collected was a combination of measured precision and haphazard observation. The duration of labor might be exact to the minute, the child described as "small and rather puny," the outcome "very good." Birth was a very complicated event, difficult to encompass in pre-determined categories. Personal observations crept in: "Mother was very obstreperous." "Non-compliance" was noted, a medical term indicating refusal to follow the physician's orders. Medical students sometimes signed in as the attending physician during labor, indicating they had met a requirement for the medical degree. A student doctor's notes might describe a specific operative intervention, approved by the superior attending doctor with a signature—those who worked directly under Williams were always men.

The form included a space for five different measurements of the newborn's head. These numbers were part of an effort to determine the degree of cephalo-pelvic disproportion. Williams and others tied the disproportion closely to contracted pelves, making them one and the same. Before birth no one could ascertain the precise size of the fetal head. In a complicated case, physicians sometimes intervened during labor, trying to discover manually how the infant head fit in the pelvis as the birth progressed. Measurement of a woman's pelvis challenged the inexperienced practitioner when a patient called the OOS for the first time, already well into labor. "Called" is used in the records but these patients had no telephone technology. Rather, a friend or relative walked to the dispensary to get dispensary staff to come to the dwelling place. Most often in such cases, medical staff took measurements after the birth, intended to extend obstetrical knowledge through statistical analysis.

Control of the patients and the consistency of the records by staff increased over time. Fairly often in the 1890s and early 1900s, patients neglected the preliminary examination, showing up on the records only after giving birth. The OOS eventually disallowed service to patients who refused the preliminary. Regulations also tightened control of patient contact with midwives. In the notes and archives from the first decades, the laboring women themselves appear only formally, part of the statistical count or patients observed by others in case records. African American women particularly lacked voice. Williams mentioned women giving birth at the OOS essentially as subjects in his medical research, not as full human beings.

Multitudinous historical aspects of gender—roles and status of women, the relations between men and women, and the relations among races—are critical to the history of childbirth, the OOS, and The Johns Hopkins Medical School. The patients of course were women—both an expression of the biological nature of reproduction and a reflection of social and cultural values. Ethnic diversity was prominent; J. Whitridge Williams reported and repeatedly emphasized that nearly fifty percent of his patients were African American. Medical students, some of whom were women and none of whom were African American, had to spend a term visiting the Dispensary and supervising at least two births. Only white women were nursing students. Assisting physicians were exclusively male.[4]

* * *

Williams brought his belief in pelvimetry as a key to obstetrics to bear from the beginning, making pelvic measurement mandatory for each patient during the prenatal visit. The standard form asked for six different measurements of the mother's pelvis, external and internal, including Baudeloque's Diameter for the former, the conjugata vera and the conjugata diagonalis for the latter. The categories reflected the model established by Michaëlis and Litzmann. Pelvimetric data became the foundation for continued discussion regarding the definition of contracted pelvis. Data collection was good but not entirely consistent, especially in the early years. Occasionally a number would be omitted. Women refusing the preliminary examination could not be measured. A major obstacle to pelvimetry proved to be the discomfort engendered by the process of measurement.[5]

To determine the conjugata vera (the "true conjugate"—the diameter of the pelvis), the physician required the patient to lie on her back with her hips on a pillow. With forearm pressing on the bed, he slipped middle and index fingers into the vagina; the other fingers folded against the palm and pressed against the perineum. Pushing down, the examiner made every effort to reach deep inside to the sacral promontory. Pressing the nail side of the fingers against the sacrum, the distance between the thumb and the fingers pushed against the pubic symphysis, at the very front of the woman's sexual organs, defined the length. After the hand was removed from the vagina, the left index finger rested at the symphysis to ascertain the length of the conjugata diagonalis.[6] Williams remarked, "This method ... is usually more or less painful."[7]

Universal measurement intruded upon sexual privacy—especially during late pregnancy or labor—in an era still holding to vestiges of Victorian expectations of privacy. Some patients refused measurement. As time went on, dispensary staff warned these women there would be no help with their births if they did not submit to examination, and recorded the refusal on the standard form.

Enforcing examination and measurement illustrated medical dominance and assertion of power over patients. Undoubtedly rumors of examination spread among patients and prepared them to resist. As pelvic measurement appeared increasingly in obstetrical discourse, reflecting a medical determination to proceed, physicians alluded to measurement under anesthetic. This was part of an increasingly routinized use of anesthetic, most commonly chloroform.[8]

After a few years in the OOS, Williams discontinued reliance on the conjugata vera, substituting a method he found easier to obtain and more accurate: a measurement of the conjugata diagonalis (the distance from the promontory of the sacrum to the lower portion of the symphysis pubis). A less intrusive yet still invasive technique. Williams argued that physicians should measure the internal diagonal and subtract 1.5 centimeters from the result to estimate the conjugata vera. Howard Kelly, head of Gynecology, supported the preference for use of the more easily effected measure. Despite the modification of Carl Litzmann's original approach, the OOS universally-mandated internal measurement continued to overrule patient comfort—especially for the typically working class or impoverished dispensary patient.[9]

Williams's method became a model for obstetric practice generally, and the standard at the OOS. He strongly criticized physicians at other institutions who embraced the framework of contracted pelves but failed medical science by not collecting patient data to substantiate incidence of the condition. According to Williams, some might have said, "What is the use?," to which he answered, "these numbers will simply represent scientific data to prove contracted pelves cause complications of labor." Williams insisted on pelvic measurement's importance for the forthcoming birth, but also for science—to show that Michaëlis and Litzmann's insights and methods suited American medicine. He drew heavily from the history of medicine, recognizing the strengths and weaknesses of the past and his predecessors, but relied most upon what was at hand to establish obstetrical knowledge, or truth, derived from patient measurements and counting case records. His dictum for students was plain: know the measurements and be prepared for their impact on the birth.[10]

* * *

By the close of the nineteenth century, textbooks and articles generally assumed that contracted pelves were at the root of myriad complications in childbirth. Following Litzmann, obstetricians agreed that dystocia,[11] malpresentation of the fetus, *placenta abruptio* (premature separation of the placenta from the uterine wall) and other difficulties stemmed from a contracted pelvis. Litzmann had identified the "simple flat rachitic" pelvis as the standard template for the effect of rickets. Williams believed that "anyone, who will regularly pursue [the use of pelvimetry], will be amazed to find how many moderately contracted pelves do exist, and will then be able to explain, in a rational way, many difficult cases." A pelvis found to be contracted presented "a rational and sufficient cause" for medical intervention. A diagnosis of contracted pelvis meant there was a physiological block to the birth that only a doctor could handle.[12]

An analysis of the process of collection and the nature of the records of the Outdoor Obstetric Service at the Johns Hopkins Dispensary offers a panorama of evidence about medicine and the format of patient/practitioner relationship. Narrowing the focus to the contracted pelvis and comparing the very first years of OOS records with 1904 discloses the ambiguities of obstetrical categories used to diagnose patients. The OOS staff's accounting of individual pregnancy and birth underscores the perceived connections of race, rickets, and birth.

J. Whitridge Williams began instruction in pelvimetry by educating students and medical staff in the various shapes of bony pelves, working with cadavers. Next came the training necessary to properly measure the pelves of living patients and categorize them in diagnosis. Central to this process was an emphasis on recognizing the effects of rickets. In his *Obstetrics*, and likely in classroom lectures, Williams taught students to approach childbirth according to the patient's pelvic category, emphasizing above all the degree of contraction. The OOS patient records reveal a tentative quality in the actual assignment of pelvic category, and the challenge attendants and examiners faced fitting the condition of individual patients to the highly regarded framework advanced by Carl Litzmann.[13]

Muddying the waters of the diagnostic process was the fact that doctors, not only within the institution, but across the country, diagnosed or measured differently. Over time, patients experiencing multiple births at the Dispensary sometimes exhibited marked change in pelvic diameter. A pelvis considered normal at the first birth could be seen as contracted at the next, leaving unanswered questions. How flexible was the pelvis during birth? Did the rachitic contracted pelvis have a different flexibility from other types of pelves? Did the adult pelvis change in dimension as life wore on?[14]

The records collected at the OOS between 1895 and 1898 include thirty-six cases noting pelvic abnormality, most often some form of contracted pelvis. Summarized in Table 10.1, these cases encompass a variety of imprecise pelvic classifications, indicating a degree of disorder without committing to specific diagnosis. Means of identification varied; designations were vague (see table right).

From the beginning, the OOS staff recorded cases of contracted pelves, diagnosed rickets, and assigned abnormality in the pelvis—hopefully before, sometimes during, or occasionally after the birth. The spectrum of cases catalogued almost every conceivable type. In addition to the rachitic and contracted, pelvic shapes included what Williams designated "irregular forms"—a case of spondylolisthesis, along with an instance of coxalgic hip [pain in the hip joint], and a single instance of Justo Major [giant pelvis].

Judging from the dispensary case records, the influence of rickets took many forms. Medical scientists could not fully account for the variety of effects; the uncertainty persists to this day.[15] In the cases charted in Table 10.1, notations of so-called deformed pelves apparently included seventeen designated as rachitic, four declared generally contracted, and three simply contracted (likely including some pelves shaped by rickets). The "flat rachitic pelvis," Litzmann's largest category of pelves narrowed by childhood rickets,[16] appeared in just three cases in the eyes of the Dispensary staff. Employing contracted pelvis as a general designation, the obstetrical service dodged the question of rickets as causation. Investigation of the disease was left to other specialties.

Table 10.1
Pelvic Abnormalities at the OOS
Case Records from the Johns Hopkins
Outdoor Obstetrics Service, 1895–1898

Table 10.1a: All Pelvic Abnormalities Identified

	Patients		
	White	*Black*	*Total*
Cases Diagnosed by Pelvimetric Measurement	9	22	31
Cases Diagnosed by Description Only	3	2	5
Total Cases with Description	9	19	28
Total Cases of Identified Abnormality	12	24	36

Table 10.1b: Categories of Pelvic Abnormality

Abnormality	*White*	*Black*	*Total*
defined solely by measure	3	6	9
contracted rachitic[1]	3	1	4
flat rachitic[2]	1	2	3
signs of rickets[3]	1	9	10
contracted[4]	2	1	3
generally contracted	1	3	4
irregular forms[5]	1	2	3
Total Cases	12	24	36

1. Recorded descriptions include "contracted, rachitic, rachitic abnormal, rachitic first degree."
2. "flat rachitic, typical flat rachitic"
3. "rachitic taint by measure, looks rachitic, old symptoms of rickets, decided signs of rickets, suggests rickets, osteomalacic"
4. "contracted, no rickets"
5. "coxalgic hip, spondylolisthesis, justo major"
Total Births, OOS, 1895–98: 322
Percentage exhibiting contracted pelves: 10.25%

SOURCE: Medical Records Division, The Alan Mason Chesney Medical Archives, The Johns Hopkins Medical Institutions, Baltimore, Maryland. Survey of microfilm records undertaken by Deborah Kuhn McGregor, 2005.

Probably the word most appropriate to describe the records maintained in the early years would be ambiguous. By design, the case forms reflected a desire for scientific precision; execution fell remarkably short. Williams and his assistants readily accepted the causal link between rickets and contracted pelvis, but diagnosis of the disease remained an uncertain proposition. The verbs and adjectives employed reflected equivocation: women perhaps recalled having the disease as a child, walked several years late, or spoke of "narrow hips." Physical examination led staff to nebulous conclusions; phrases such as "taint of rickets," "suggests rickets," "signs of rickets," or "symptoms of rickets" imply hesitancy. In most cases, the patient was unable to help, lacking sufficient memory of early childhood. Other variables affected the accuracy of the records. Some patients arrived already in labor, with no previous examination at all. In other cases, a physician was called to the home of a registered patient, the labor well advanced.[17]

Of the thirty-three cases of pelvic contraction interpreted as troubling, every last one of the conditions may very possibly have originated in rickets. Essentially half looked more or less rachitic. Four were defined as "generally contracted"—presumably the condition Williams believed to derive from congenital inheritance. The remainder were identified solely on the basis of pelvimetric measurement, with no attempt to explain the resultingly ominous figures. The threshold points in those figures were themselves arbitrary. At best, the categories of pelvic abnormality were extraordinarily fluid. Scientific certainty was elusive.

Of the 322 total cases recorded between 1895 and 1898, roughly one patient in nine exhibited a pelvis deemed problematic enough to impede birth. Of the thirty-six women, twenty-three (twenty-one Black, two white) proceeded to normal, spontaneous delivery. No intervention necessary during labor. Six women were delivered with instrumental assistance (five cases mentioned forceps specifically). Just seven labors necessitated more serious measures: three craniotomies, two symphysiotomies, and one resource to traction. There were no Caesarean sections. (Nothing was recorded of the one birth remaining; hopefully the delivery was uneventful.) Numerous births occurred without medical assistance, almost entirely among Blacks, before or immediately upon arrival of dispensary staff. This phenomenon, frustrating and limiting for medical personnel, persisted into the early twentieth century. Nearly two-thirds of the cases defined as problematic (65.7 percent) in fact posed no problem in delivery at all.

How to interpret such a result? Discretionary precaution might be one explanation. A desire to inflate the numbers might be another.

J. Whitridge Williams regarded these early OOS cases as a proving ground, editing the composite records at an unknown time for statistical evaluation in future publications. In doing so, he eliminated the evident ambiguity of classification in the records. Categories became specific and exact. The process of keeping records altered with time. Uncertainty diminished as staff became more adept and, more importantly, definitions shifted to fit a more fully established perception of the contracted pelvis. Procedures for identifying the condition grew more consistent. Where in the 1890s pelvic morphology descriptors proliferated, by 1904 the designations were reduced to six—three being variations of the generally contracted. Published articles nonetheless employed the early data, adjusted to agree with the definitions established by the twentieth century.[18]

Table 10.2
Pelvic Abnormalities Identified
Case Records from the Johns Hopkins
Outdoor Obstetrics Service, 1904
(All cases underwent pelvimetric measurement)

Abnormality	White Patients	Black Patients	Total
contracted rachitic	0	2	2
flat rachitic[1]	2	2	4
borderline[2]	2	5	7
generally contracted	1	11	12
generally contracted rachitic	0	2	2
generally contracted borderline	0	1	1
irregular forms[3]	3	1	4
Total Cases	8	24	32

1. "flat, simple flat, simple flat normal"
2. "borderline normal, borderline"
3. "justo major" [giant pelvis]
Total Births at the OOS, 1904: 243
Percentage Exhibiting Contracted Pelves: 11.5%

SOURCE: Medical Records Division, The Alan Mason Chesney Medical Archives, The Johns Hopkins Medical Institutions, Baltimore, Maryland. Survey of microfilm records undertaken by Deborah Kuhn McGregor, 2005.

Table 10.2 reflects a changing distinction in diagnosis by race at the OOS, superseding the focus on rickets. Between 1895 and 1898, staff tentatively identified seventeen of thirty-six patients as rachitic. Five were white, twelve Black. Half the Black patients exhibiting abnormal pelves were deemed victims of rickets. In 1904, of thirty-two total cases, just eight were declared rachitic. Six were Black women. Two of these were diagnosed as "generally contracted rachitic"—women who had endured rickets in addition to a pelvis generally contracted. The category of "generally contracted pelvis" had assumed fundamental importance.

In the earlier cases (Table 10.1), just four pelves were considered "generally contracted," three Black, one white. Cases of generally contracted pelves among Black women grew to fourteen of twenty-four by 1904, identified in three separate categories: generally contracted, generally contracted borderline, and generally contracted rachitic. By this reckoning, generally contracted pelves accounted for more than half of all pelvic abnormalities among Blacks. Just one white woman was diagnosed as generally contracted; she was a Jewish immigrant. Generally contracted pelvis—the condition Williams believed to be congenital—had become the predominant diagnosis for African American women at Johns Hopkins.

Observations of flat pelvis, identified in various terms on the record, foreshadowed an eventual obstetrical standard identifying white women as the most frequent exemplars. Cases encountered at the OOS offered few clues; in the early years (Table 10.1), examiners firmly identified just three cases. Two were Black women. Just four such patients appeared in 1904; two Black, two white.

In the earlier records, "borderline" was not a designation. As the name implies, a borderline case identified a pelvis measured to be within the parameters of pelvic contraction, but on the edge of normal, or lying between two categories. (This was perhaps a subtle acknowledgment of the ambiguity inherent in pelvimetric measurement.) Litzmann had emphasized that borderline cases were the most important for attending physicians to assess and observe, the most liable to cause unexpected problems. Following the footsteps of his German predecessor, by 1903 Williams recognized the borderline contracted pelvis to be the most difficult to evaluate, requiring careful medical consideration as to the best way to proceed. Moderately contracted pelves, he maintained, had the potential to cause complicated births, though often they resulted in what medicine considered spontaneous deliveries.[19]

Two hundred forty-three women sought assistance in birth at the OOS in 1904. Roughly one in eight was judged to exhibit pelvic abnormality, a small but definite rise from the earlier years. Yet, the number of medical interventions actually diminished. Of the eight white women, one was delivered by forceps, one assisted with podalic version. The remaining six were normal births. Among the Black women, twenty-three delivered spontaneously; version aided the twenty-fourth. No symphysiotomies, no craniotomies, no Caesarean sections in any of the thirty-two cases. The rigors of thorough pelvimetric measurement may have resulted in more explicitly defined categories, an enhanced theoretical understanding of pelvic contraction, but the measures had not flagged a single truly problematic case.

What does seem to have changed with time is the use of drugs in delivery. Between 1895 and 1898, mention of drugs appears in just seven of the birth records—whether this was due to purposeful restraint or neglectful record-keeping is impossible to say. Ergot—employed to induce and speed labor—was mentioned twice. The two patients subjected to symphysiotomy were chloroformed, as were two of the women experiencing forceps delivery, along with the one case of traction. In 1904, ergot was administered in twenty-nine of thirty-two cases; anesthesia (generally chloroform) was employed in twenty-two deliveries. Morphine was used once, codeine twice. The greater reliance on medication seems evident—speed the delivery, reduce patient pain, eliminate patient interference. Whether women requested anesthesia was not recorded.

As birth moved toward a hospital setting, increasing medical supervision came to insist on the prone position for the laboring woman, the emblematic physical statement of an assumed and much desired passivity in birth. Physicians routinely forced women into prone positions, taking control of the woman's reproductive and sexual area, prohibiting any other positions or movement a laboring woman might seek. Women delivering at home with midwives and relatives in assistance walked around and squatted as part of their labor. In such births, the mother-to-be noted that the pains diminished as she got on her hands and knees. Williams and his colleagues occasionally played with the idea that squatting or repositioning a woman diagnosed with contracted pelvis might facilitate an easier delivery, but Williams could not bring himself to take the alternative seriously. Doctors and medicals students in the dispensary much preferred to put the laboring woman to bed and work with them as they lay flat on their backs. Sometimes they moved the patient to the extreme lithotomy position at edge of the bed, legs bent and feet against the buttocks, facilitating the use of forceps or other forms of intervention. Gynecological stirrups were another option. Often the attendants anesthetized the patient and carried her to the operating table. The drugs, the enforced passivity, the obstetrical interventions all contributed to playing a deity in the delivery room.[20]

* * *

Medicine offered assistance in birth, but at the same time accelerated the use of frightening forms of intervention. The OOS records show a different side to the changes taking place. Case histories and birth narratives charted experiences of pain by the length of labor, the nature of labor, and the medical response (or lack of response) to the laboring woman's situation—the language of male-dominated obstetrics. Several episodes revealed tensions over medical intervention. Occasionally the records note what was regarded as inappropriate patient behavior: hysteria—an outburst of uncontrolled, sometimes wild emotional anxiety. Hysterical women could be masculine in their aggression, at times uttering obscenities and using vile language, dismissing their newborn infants, refusing to play the part of mother. Hysteria represented a kind of resistance, at times an outright refusal to cooperate with gendered expectation.[21] Childbearing was supposed to be a mechanical, "natural" process. Psychological, emotional, or sexual components were unwelcome. Hysteria in birth, though unpleasant and disquieting, expressed the feelings of laboring women who apparently refused to accept a medical regimen predicated on obstetrical intervention.[22]

A diagnosis of hysteria expressed the physician's point of view. Judging a woman hysterical, rather than considering her behavior a natural reaction to an unpleasant experience, placed blame for any difficulty upon the laboring woman. Hysteria became a rationale for using anesthesia in larger doses and relying more fully upon operative techniques, a way to silence the patient. At some point the concept of hysteria in birth disappeared, smoothly replaced by the application of quieting, numbing drugs. Women's cries during labor were hushed.[23]

OOS case records describe and designate hysteria not as a specific diagnosis, but as an associated behavior, a regrettable adjunct to the process of birth. Fear undoubtedly dominated many OOS labors. Women, experiencing difficult labor, well aware of the possible instrumental and surgical interventions, could not envision a positive outcome and on occasion became hysterical, out of control.[24] The interpretation seems credible, given that at least one woman, described in the early OOS case records, became hysterical during an *external* measurement of her pelvis during a preliminary examination. Once labor began, the patient had little control over what happened should complications emerge. Expected to remain passive, she might easily lose emotional control. Becoming hysterical, she in turn put the responsibility for the birth's outcome squarely on the shoulders of the attending physician. She surrendered her own power in birth.

An OOS case from 1900 illustrates hysteria in delivery. The laboring woman was the married and white mother of three children born without complication. Her fourth labor simply stopped after the second stage began, at which point she became hysterical—delirious and exhibiting paralysis, resulting in halted contractions. From the birth notes, the hysterical symptoms suggest the woman may have been trying to push the baby out; changing her position might have brought about birth. Nothing of the kind was attempted; the notes simply indicate the contractions stopped completely while the woman manifested contortions and paralysis, complaining of pain in her back. The recording attendant entered the word hysteria on the form. Consistent with the accepted definition of the condition, the symptoms included "awful grimacing."

Having gone on for several hours, the labor seemed obstructed. The attending medical student called in a staff physician, who introduced small doses of chloroform. The second stage returned, to last a long time, thirteen hours in all. Though there was no explicit indication of pelvic contraction, the physician reported that the fetal head became stuck below "the spines" of the pelvis. The baby had come partially through the cervix, only to meet obstruction in the birth canal. The infant's head, the doctor observed, was simply too large to get through. After bringing the woman to the side of the bed on her back, in the lithotomy position—her legs wide apart and restrained from movement—the doctor resorted to a strong dose of chloroform and ergot to encourage birth. Subsequent use of forceps and version brought eventual success. The placenta took more than six hours to deliver; in all the labor lasted twenty-three hours.

The physician's narrative attached to the case record powerfully detailed his strategy. The anesthesia took away the woman's active participation in the labor, while the ergot brought an unrelenting rough beat of contractions, meaning the doctor had to manage the birth largely on his own. He tried various maneuvers with the forceps, only to have them fail. As an obstetrician, he drew on past education and experience, alternating between hand manipulation of the fetus and further experimentation with the forceps, seeking a way to get the baby born. Small wonder he crowed that after all his efforts, mother and child were fine. In the case record, the mother got no credit for her part in giving birth to a healthy child.

Many factors were at work in this hysterical birth. Complete frustration and impatience with labor on the part of the patient; a doctor's preemptive and, from his perspective *only* solution: operative intervention. In his notes, the physician did not explore the causes of the complication. Some form of contraction must have been at work, but the diagnostic warning signs so firmly posited by J. Whitridge Williams were not in evidence. The pelvic measurement recorded a conjugata diagonalis of 12.5 centimeters, well within the range considered normal. The attending doctor did his best to describe the obstruction, explaining that the pubic symphysis seemed to block the rotation of the fetal head, which did not quite reach the outlet. Faced with a hysterical patient, a protracted labor, and the inexplicable obstruction, the doctor felt he had no choice but to experiment. His choice was to anesthetize the mother, eliminate her participation, and proceed with instruments. Science supplanted the mother's ability to decide how the birth should proceed.

* * *

A decade later, J. Whitridge Williams would have diagnosed the hysterical woman's physical obstruction as funnel pelvis. Physicians in the early twentieth century credited Williams with discovery of a pelvic contraction Litzmann and his followers had missed. Since the 1860s, studies had focused primarily on the pelvic inlet, or superior strait. Williams identified a contraction of the pelvic outlet, a narrowing of the pelvic opening that could cause an infant's head to become stuck at the vulva, almost but not quite born. The angle of the sacrum, accompanied by constriction of the pubic arch, blocked delivery. In a pelvis seemingly normal, such a last minute obstacle proved a crisis indeed. Attempting to deliver the child with low forceps, the physician often fractured the skull. The forceps could slip terribly; birthing women suffered numerous lacerations, especially of the perineum. Such births struck Williams as unexpected and much more difficult than they appeared. Believing this to occur most often in white women, he developed his ideas in a series of three articles written between 1909 and 1911, examining the records of twelve hundred patients to determine the origin and frequency of the condition.[25]

Researching his subject, he found precedent in the works of Madame Boursier du Coudray and Baudeloque. He also declared that van Deventer's book, *The New Light for Obstetricians and Midwives*, had a copper etching on the cover showing funnel pelvis.[26] Thomas Addis Emmet in 1868 noted many such births among his vesico-vaginal fistula patients, but offered little comment.[27] William Turner's work on the structure and shape of the pelvis, published in 1886, proved especially instructive. Turner developed a sacral index, multiplying the breadth of the sacrum (the triangular bone joining the hipbones at the base of the spinal column) by one hundred and dividing the result by the bone's length to classify the pelvis. In the doliochohieric pelvis, the length exceeded the breadth, and in the platypellic, the breadth exceeded the length. The measure provided a basis for defining the funnel pelvis.[28]

Familiarity with rickets and maternity led Williams deeper into the development and growth of the pelvis in childhood. He turned his attention to specific pelvic bones—especially the pubis, the ilium and the sacrum—parts of the three bones transformed into the innominate bone at puberty. Indications of the "assimilation pelvis," verified by Austrian researchers Carl Breus and Alexander Kolisko, provided Williams a framework.[29] Williams credited German physician Michaela Klien with establishing a protocol in 1896 to measure for funnel pelvis.[30]

Williams focused on the fusion of the five vertebrae that formed the sacrum as a woman matured to adulthood, a process known to anatomists as assimilation. In a case of funnel pelvis, a sixth vertebra was assimilated at one of two places. Fusion at the sacro-lumbar joint affected pelvic shape in the formation of the sacro-iliac joint, a "higher" assimilation. Williams considered this "a fetal type," a childlike pelvic form.[31] Fusion at the coccygeal joint resulted in a "lower" assimilation at the end of the sacral formation. Not surprisingly, judging by its name, the higher assimilation was to Williams the more significant occurrence, as the condition purportedly could interfere with births among whites.[32]

Williams explored funnel pelves mostly as a way to address the problems of white women in childbirth. Unable to obtain cadaveric specimens of funnel pelves from whites, Williams resorted to estimation, concluding the condition must be quite common.[33] To verify the presence among patients at Johns Hopkins, he added a calculation of the width of the pubic arch and a measure of the inferior strait of the true pelvis to the list of standard measurements on the case form. Williams required the figures only when the preliminary examination indicated a probable funnel pelvis; the additions were still more challenging than previous intrusions. The physician either had to put his whole hand in the *anesthetized* woman's vagina or press deeply in the rectum. A measure of the transverse or antero-posterior diameter of the pelvic outlet between nine and eight centimeters or less indicated a funnel pelvis.[34] In such cases, the ischial tuberosities (an unusual elevation of the lower section of the hipbones) stood too close together, blocking the passage of the fetus.[35] Williams found that the relationship between the narrowing of the ischial tuberosities or the pubic arch and the posterior sagittal diameter (how much room there was behind these bones in the outlet) together predicted the likelihood of difficult labor.[36] Analyzing his twelve hundred cases, Williams identified this new contraction in a relatively high seven percent of white women, sustaining his argument for the significance of the condition.[37]

The difficulty with funnel pelvis lay in the fact that women diagnosed with the condition often delivered naturally. Williams suggested attendants allow the second stage of labor to proceed. Caesarean section was no longer an alternative if the fetal head met obstruction only upon reaching the vulva; the prescribed operative intervention in such cases was serious indeed: pubiotomy. The surgeon sawed through the mother's pubic bone to open the pelvic outlet, a procedure similar to symphysiotomy but perhaps slightly more favorable in outcome. Pubiotomy did not necessarily render a woman sterile, but did result in the likelihood of stillbirths, subsequent Caesareans, and chronic difficulties—vaginal tears and difficulty walking, among others. Williams began to rely on pubiotomy in 1906, before grasping the importance of the funnel pelvis.[38] The surgery became his preferred choice.[39]

Williams sought to develop a science of obstetrics and parturition, but his work—as a close examination of the original cases records shows—

repeatedly became an obsessive effort to reconfirm evidence of racial difference and evolution. He elaborated at great length upon the funnel pelvis in terms of racial comparison, seeking an explanation for the condition while assuming the answer was grounded in racial characteristics. Easing his dependence on clear race distinction and the perceived unique biological weakness of African American women, he identified one type of funnel pelvis more common among Blacks—the generally contracted funnel pelvis, possibly rachitic. His explanation for cases of lower pelvic assimilation among Black women fell in familiar territory. Mature women exhibiting the condition had inherited the characteristics of their species, never reaching a higher evolutionary stage of development. In Williams's perspective, whatever happened to the victims of lower assimilation was due simply to their rank in the order of evolution. Race trumped all other factors.[40]

Far more ominous to J. Whitridge Williams's way of thinking was the inescapable fact that pelvimetric numbers indicated funnel deformity occurred almost equally in white and Black women. While Williams was excited to discover and typify a new kind of pelvic distress, he struggled with the challenge to his assumptions of distinct racial pelves, clearly disquieted by the implications. Based on his own intellectual understanding of race and evolution, he was eventually forced to conclude that some white women suffered a form of degeneracy. They had funnel pelves. A sobering realization.[41]

The logic of the conclusion left him with the obligation to alter the situation as best he might, more than anything by limiting the reproduction of defective models. This was a line of thinking shared by many in the Progressive Era; the eugenics movement was aiming to purify the race. Williams's understanding of the funnel pelvis and most contracted pelves signified the possibility such abnormalities were passed on from generation to generation, though he could not be sure. Weighing his self-appointed responsibilities, J. Whitridge Williams took on the task of blocking the reproduction of defective, degenerative physiologies as best he could.[42]

* * *

The ongoing march of medical intervention, the more frequent resort to drugs, raised important questions. What was the impact of science on infant and maternal mortality? The hope of course, the justification, was to save lives. Developing his obstetrical regime, Williams felt his institution fared as well as any in keeping mothers and babies alive during and after birth, and better than most. For the record, he qualified mortality numbers, discounting those deaths involving infection or illness, as he did not feel either he or his colleagues culpable for them. Doctor Goldsborough, OOS physician and instructor, published an article on maternal mortality at Johns Hopkins in 1908, finding forty-one deaths in five thousand cases—roughly 0.8 percent. Women, for the most part, seemed to survive childbirth in the OOS. Williams's first concern was the survival of the mother.[43]

Attendants at the OOS generally recorded the condition of the child at birth and sometimes ranked the degree of asphyxiation apparent. Case records noted stillbirths, referred to as macerated births, the craniotomies, and the deaths of infants following birth. In an article analyzing the first one thousand maternity cases under his supervision at Hopkins, Williams reported 82.44 percent of the children were born alive, an infant mortality rate better than the United States as a whole. By the standards of the time, the mortality rates at Johns Hopkins were not a concern.[44]

Focused primarily on the pathology of birth, Williams for the most part did not concern himself with mortality issues. In 1901, he published an essay urging obstetricians to embrace Caesarean section as the most viable approach to obstructed birth, relying on a specific range of conjugata vera as the determinant. Caesarean section should replace what he saw as needlessly more dangerous uses of high forceps, version, induction, and symphysiotomies, especially for contracted pelves. Except in cases involving infection, Caesarean had a better mortality and morbidity record (Williams placed the mortality rate at 3 to 4 percent), with ever better outcomes than the other choices—or so he maintained. Accompanying tables provided the basic framework for his argument. Race figured heavily; his figures indicated that "the variety of the deformity varies markedly in the two races." Among white women, more than half fell into his categories designated as "simple flat" or "rachitic," while two thirds of Black women exhibited the "generally contracted" pelvis.[45]

* * *

The original case records make it clear that the diagnoses of patients examined at the OOS deviated substantially from the theoretical model Williams imposed on the data. If he did measure every patient, his students failed to apply a consistent diagnosis, or one relevant to the pelvimetry so fundamental to his system. More to the point, the vast majority of the cases in some way designated abnormal were not problematic at all, nor did the cases break down by race in the manners anticipated.

Eleven

An Obstetrical Definition of Race

J.T. was a young woman, twenty-two years old, in the ninth month of pregnancy, seeking assistance in the Dispensary at Johns Hopkins Hospital. She was African American; her appearance suggested a deformed pelvis. J. Whitridge Williams found her physical presence remarkable. He had a side view of her naked body drawn, showing the extent of the spinal curvature in her lower back, the pendulous pregnant belly and a protuberance at the base of her spine, plus the generous curve of her hips. Hers was a very rare case of spondylolisthesis, the forward displacement of the fifth lumbar vertebra, resulting in curvature of the pelvis. On top of this, the patient disclosed a fall that hurt her hip, eventually causing a limp. She denied a previous pregnancy. Concerned about the extent of pelvic obstruction, Williams, in consultation with another physician, planned a Caesarean section. Apparently, J.T. belonged to a group of people who looked out for each other; supported by friends, she flat out refused the surgery. J.T. understood that her health and prognosis for childbirth was not good; she felt a need to seek medical help. Yet, the Black fear of white doctors, so common at the time, proved evident. When she entered labor, the attending physicians elected to perform a symphysiotomy—the pulling apart of the bones comprising the pubic joint. Williams did not record whether the staff honestly informed her of the nature of the surgery, or offered a choice. For her part, J.T. refused to be honest with Williams about her past experiences in childbirth.[1]

Her pregnancy came due while Williams was on vacation; the case fell to the hands of an assistant, Doctor George Dobbin. J.T. "confessed" to Dobbin that she had had a previous birth without operative interference. The child had lived. Dobbin's intervention was successful; the child "was born asphyxiated, but was soon resuscitated."[2] The patient went into shock following the surgery, but recovered quickly. Then, seven days later, quite suddenly, the surgical wounds became greatly infected. J.T. died. An autopsy revealed the stitches applied to mend the symphysiotomy incisions had torn away.

The case became one more study, grist for the mill of obstetrical articles emanating from the Outdoor Obstetrical Service. Williams published the highly unusual case of spondylolisthesis in 1899. The tone of the article suggests his enthusiasm rested more with acquisition of the woman's pelvis than concern over her death. J.T. either lived without family in a Baltimore neighborhood or had traveled a long way for help in her birth. Williams had little interest or patience with the presence or lack of cultural response to her death. He lamented that her relatives lived at a remote location on Maryland's Eastern Shore, out of immediate contact. The autopsy had to wait four days, by which time much had decomposed.[3]

Williams's prize was her skeleton; he carefully preserved the pelvis and the attached spinal column. Over several pages, he recorded the measurements acquired from the bony pelvis, typified the pelvis in its particular qualities. Most significant appeared to be the point where the spinal column met the pelvis, the spondylolisthesis causing the sacrum to curve under, a downward and forward displacement of the lower lumbar vertebrae into the pelvis. Williams thoroughly reviewed the history of such cases and the possible explanations of the origin. Some thought the condition congenital; others ascribed it to pressure on the back from hard activity.[4]

Williams compared his subject to the Hottentot Venus. The ordered drawing of J.T. from the side closely resembles various nineteenth-century artistic renderings of that legendary exhibition.[5] The skeleton of Saartjie Bartman, preserved by George Cuvier in 1815, remained on display at the French Museum of Natural History nearly a century later, a horrid example of race science at work. J.T.'s subjective status paralleled that of Bartman. In life, both were treated as creatures with little to no mental ability.

The preservation of their remains epitomized the fascination with the greatly sexualized traits attributed to women of African descent. The quality of life for both was of no matter to the scientists examining those remains.[6]

Like Saartjie Bartman, J.T. too became an exhibit of sorts, her pelvis carefully preserved with the lower vertebrae intact, quite possibly displayed somewhere in the obstetrics lab. The black and white ink drawing of her exposed body was published professionally at least twice, emphasizing a tail. Williams valued her bones, representative of a rare but telling example of pelvic distortion, proof of a connecting link to the "lower races," a scientific legitimation of his assumption of racial hierarchy, white over Black.[7]

The case of spondylolisthesis was rare, an extreme example of pelvic disproportion, yet emblematic of the underlying assumptions guiding operations at the Outdoor Obstetrical Service. The patients were poor, as many as half the women African American. Much the same conditions prevailed at J. Marion Sims's hospital in Montgomery, Alabama, in the early 1850s, at the Woman's Hospital in New York City decades later. Those institutions provided real medical assistance to needful clients, but in the eyes of the practitioners, the women were not simply patients lacking wherewithal. They were experimental subjects, human bodies come available for exploratory research. In each case, the story was the same; the indigent and defenseless, representative of the lower classes of society, bore the brunt of medical exploration intended to assist their social betters. Williams was strongly aware of the difficulties Black women suffered in childbirth, including high maternal and fetal mortality rates. He knew these women often experienced rickets. His adherence to race distinctions diminished his concern for their suffering. He saw them as patients but primarily as subjects for research whose observed experiences provided advances in obstetrics—a way to bring American medicine to the level of European practice.[8]

* * *

Johns Hopkins Hospital was extraordinary in offering care for what we know today as outpatients, or ambulatory patients.[9] Baltimore's booming population, the neighborhood setting, and the new medical school helped to shape the Dispensary and in turn the OOS.

In his first publication based on records of the OOS, published in 1899, J. Whitridge Williams reviewed the examination reports and measurements made by his assistant George W. Dobbin and argued, " in almost every case mentioned in this article the examination was also controlled by me, so that there is no reason to attribute any of the cases to faulty pelvimetry."[10] Several factors in the context of obstetrics at the Dispensary compromised the perfection numbers might have granted to the pelvic types. Yet Williams remained confident of the accuracy and validity of his presuppositions and went further, boasting of his control of all the records, the infallibility of his measurements. Williams found one hundred thirty-one of his first one thousand patients (650 OOS patients plus 350 at Johns Hopkins Hospital) to exhibit contracted pelves, a figure he included in his subsequently published obstetrics text. Condensing the cases to four categories of contraction, he proceeded to demonstrate that "generally contracted pelves" were far more prevalent among Black patients, whereas white women more often exhibited "simple flat pelves," sustaining his racial interpretation of the condition. Williams used statistics to buoy his argument, showcasing models of the contracted pelvis and detailing the actual experiences in the OOS as evidence. Of the total, he categorized seventy-nine as generally contracted; sixty-five of these patients were Black. All very precise, very neat, very scientific.[11]

Williams thought Baltimore's large African American population made the city unique. This, he argued, accounted for the results of a study published in 1901, disclosing a frequency of 12.1 percent contracted pelves at the Johns Hopkins Dispensary. "Contracted pelves were observed 2.6 times more frequently in colored than in white women; .... every fourteenth white and every sixth colored woman in Baltimore has a contracted pelvis."[12] "The race of the patient is not only of importance in determining the absolute frequency of contracted pelves," Williams declared, "but our observations have shown that the variety of the deformity varies markedly in the two races."[13] By way of explanation, he continued

> Anyone who is acquainted with the colored people in the large cities of the South cannot fail to be impressed with the marked prevalence of rhachitis among them, and at first thought would suppose that the rhachitic pelvis would be the variety most frequently observed.[14]

Williams underscored the common perception that rickets ran rampant among Southern and urban blacks. The prevalence of rickets among Southern African Americans in the post-Civil War years was accepted as common knowledge, needing no further elaboration. Physicians frequently referred to the notion, offering little or no medical evidence. Historian Edward H. Beardsley wrote that one could commonly see the effects of the disease in Black bodies; rickets among these people was normal, visible in their gait and posture until the condition remitted.[15]

Despite the acknowledgment of rickets as a factor in the incidence of contracted pelves among Black women in Baltimore, Williams was more than certain additional factors were at work. In his early publications, he established a grouping of four kinds of contracted pelves: the flat pelvis, the rachitic pelvis, the generally contracted pelvis and the asymmetrical pelvis. Morphology helped to define the categories, calling for precise attention to measurements while allowing for inclusion of diverse types of deformity in certain cases. The rachitic pelvis, for instance, was heart-shaped, but was not the only contracted pelvis that might originate with rickets. The categories resembled those established by Carl Litzmann in their emphasis on shape rather than etiology. For obstetrical practice, the question of etiology, specifically the impact of rickets, no longer mattered. To Williams, the disease was an essentially irrelevant descriptor of origin, becoming the somewhat ambiguous "rachitic" in his pelvic categories.[16]

Early cases at the Dispensary no doubt confirmed his belief that contracted pelves were critically important signifiers of difficult birth. In the hand-written copy of his first edition of *Obstetrics,* Williams observed that the obstetrician would find "the greater the contraction the greater the difficulty of the birth of the child.... In women with rachitic pelves I generally notice that severity of the labor pains is greater than is normal, as uterine muscles are less developed as is also the pelvis." The statement simply and clearly summarized the bottom line of his medical science. Contracted rachitic pelves caused difficult births. His words effectively separate "women" from their labors and the "severity of labor pains"—that mechanistic comprehension of labor.

The obstetrical system established and recorded at the Johns Hopkins Outdoor Obstetrical Service under Williams's supervision lay at the very heart of his investigations. He moved quickly to application of numerical methods; the gathering of statistics provided a framework with which to develop and assess operative technique. Pelvic measurements defined a statistical determination of the normal pelvis, the abnormal pelvis and the incidence of the various deformities.[17]

In a hand-written version of *Obstetrics*, Williams discussed the incidence of contracted pelves, entering the subject of race into the equation:

> On analyzing our cases ... the generally contracted pelvis occurs three times more frequently than the rhachitic [sic]. The explanation for this is to be found in the fact that the colored people in the large cities are in great part physical degenerates, as is shown by their generally faulty development and the readiness with which they succumb to various diseases.[18]

In the published edition of the text, Williams insisted that the high incidence of generally contracted pelves among black women "is undoubtedly a sign of degeneration, and is a manifestation of the imperfect development which characterizes Negroes living in large cities."[19] Williams and other obstetrical writers from Hopkins often referred to generally contracted pelves as undeveloped or "retarded development." J. Whitridge Williams believed that African Americans carried a constitutional affinity, a degeneracy making them susceptible to disease of all kinds. To his way of thinking, "generally contracted" pelves—a category not ruling out the influence of rickets, but different from the classic rachitic pelvis, derived from a different origin. Race, not rickets, was the causative factor.[20]

Conflating nature and nurture, Williams drew from an evolutionary concept that among the lower races the afflicted woman's body never grew out of childhood in the process of maturation. Here again was the notion that Blacks stood low on the evolutionary scale, a proposition supposedly demonstrated by the morphology and physiology of the skeleton. As Williams wrote, the eugenics movement was gathering strength, recapitulating the argument that the "lower races" were degenerating, verging on extinction.[21]

Williams was doing his best to explain the indisputable fact that despite the presence of a contracted pelvis (as defined by mathematical measure), Black women exhibiting the condition generally gave birth without difficulty. In the article published in 1901, he elaborated: "It is generally considered that the comparatively easy labors of the colored women are due to the fact that they approach more nearly a primitive and normal physical condition, as they have not been long subjected to the deteriorating influences of civilization."[22] Williams linked Black women's purported ease of birth not to lack of exposure to civilization, but to a more profound and biological factor—their own physical wants as African Americans. Their bodies were smaller, as were the heads of their babies, hence lacking in a scale determined by "survival of the fittest." Because of its subjective nature and cultural bias, race obfuscated the obstetrical approach to childbirth.[23]

Internal measurements for the African American women giving birth at Johns Hopkins proved surprisingly abnormal. Black women were different in their measurements, but the upshot often was that they were able to give birth without operative interference. Implicit in the interpretation is the underlying fact that the standards of pelvimetry defined the white race as normal, the Black as abnormal. (Williams was not the first to make this supposition; German research had set the standard.) Discussing the process of measuring pelves at considerable length, he noted,

> Had I employed external pelvimetry alone I should have concluded that at least one-half of my colored patients possessed contracted pelves, as it is a matter of experience that one rarely sees colored women whose external pelvis measurements are normal.[24]

* * *

In 1904, Theodore F. Riggs (1874–1962), an intern serving at the Outdoor Obstetrical Service at Johns Hopkins University, published an article contrasting the pelves "of white and negro women." Riggs was well qualified for the assignment. A student of the anthropological literature biologically differentiating the races, he listed five authors who contended aboriginal women experienced "easy labors," and another eight maintaining that "the pelvis of the less civilized races is narrow and deep as compared with the low and broad pelvis of the European."[25] Among his sources were Samuel Gache and George Engermann. This collection of material became the foundation for a comparative analysis of the disparities in Black and white birth at Johns Hopkins. Riggs's study sought to establish a definition of race based on the incidence of contracted pelves—an effort

J. Whitridge Williams subsequently cited as pivotal in numerous publications. Of the numerous articles produced under his guidance, Williams extolled this effort in particular.[26]

At Williams's behest, Riggs embarked upon a statistical analysis of the relationship of the fetal head to the maternal pelvis, seeking to uncover indications of racial difference in the Johns Hopkins obstetric cases. His experiences growing up in the Dakota territory with Native Americans nearby may have assisted him in the task—exposure to interracial contact perhaps prepared him to consider a connection between birth as racial experience and the concept of cephalopelvic disproportion. Generating ten tables of comparative statistics covering fourteen pages, his measurement of fetal heads became a means to demonstrate the significance of race in birth.[27]

In part, the project came about in response to an article published in London by physician Clayton Arbuthnot Lane (1868–1949) in 1903, comparing the childbirth experiences of Bengali, European, and Eurasian women in Calcutta, India. Lane had derived a law asserting that within each race, the fetus *in utero* naturally grew in proportion to the dimensions of the maternal pelvis, facilitating a trouble-free vaginal birth. Though Lane offered no citations, his theory essentially mirrored conclusions offered by anatomists Gerardus Vrolik and Moritz Weber in the early years of the nineteenth century.[28]

Lane believed his law an example of natural selection at work, a hereditary mechanism promoting survival of the fittest. As such, the law operated successfully only within the confines of each race—a mixing of races resulted in a mismatch of the mother's pelvis and the fetal skull, fostering often mortal difficulties. A series of tables demonstrated the close relationship between the size of the woman's pelvis and the size of the child within each of the three races under examination.[29]

Lane's study motivated Williams, and in turn Riggs, to analyze birth patterns at Johns Hopkins. Familiar with pelvimetric anthropology, Riggs undertook a statistical survey of deliveries at the institution, focused on the differing experiences of Black and white women. Patterned after Lane, the research addressed conditions rising from the relation of the calculated size of the female pelvis to the size and shape of the fetal head.

The first task was to define race. Riggs was entirely open in his perspective, explicitly detailing the assumptions shaping his analysis. The small numbers of mixed-race mulattos and quadroons would be treated as Black. There would be no attempt to identify whites by nationality, as the majority were born in America. His analysis would comprise just two categories: white and Negro.[30]

Riggs identified 1500 births suitable for study, "779 white and 721 negro." Employing the categories established for the OOS by J. Whitridge Williams, Riggs sorted the cases in each group into categories of normal and abnormal pelvis. So tightly defined were the classifications they became tautological: race seemed to define the pelvis and the pelvis race. Much depended on the definition of "normal." Established statistically, the term described "all pelves having normal external measurements and a diagonal conjugate of 11.5 cm. or over."[31] The latter was internally measured, following standard practice at Johns Hopkins. Riggs reduced the multitudinous descriptions of pelves not meeting this standard to three basic categories. The definitions were fluid—Williams firmly believed rickets was a heritable disorder in the Black race; encountering deformed pelves in whites, he tended to ascribe the condition to some other cause.[32]

Reflecting conclusions Williams had previously ascertained, Riggs found that more than one-third (34.82 percent) of Black women manifested pelvic measures deemed abnormal. Nearly one-fourth were "generally contracted," a category especially significant to Riggs, who declared "it is well-known that this variety of pelvis is a sign of degeneracy and is associated with poor development of the rest of the body."[33] Painting his figures as statistically accurate determinations, he concluded African American women patients suffered nearly four times as many contracted pelves as whites.[34] His definitions of pelvic abnormality categorized a great many Black women as different, inferior, partially deformed. They stood in sharp contrast to the more than ninety percent of white women exhibiting "normal" pelvic proportions. Riggs concluded that overall, "the pelves in women of the lower races are narrower but relatively deeper than in white women."[35] While there were obvious differences among the many women classified as Black patients, one pelvic characterization served to describe them all. Riggs devised such a definition to support and rationalize perceived differences in the races. Declaring the typical white women's pelvic measurement the standard of normalcy was nothing more than an *a priori* assumption, an unquestioned bias distorting all subsequent analysis.[36]

There was much to explain away. If the Black pelvis was in some way deficient, why did white women suffer more and need more help in childbirth? Riggs found "a higher percentage of spontaneous labors among the negroes than among the whites." (The difference was not great; 80.23 percent of whites delivered spontaneously, 84.46 percent of African Americans.)[37] The problem was to explain why so many African American women gave birth easily despite the high percentage of contracted pelves. Riggs answered that Black babies were a "lower grade," smaller and less developed, more often female.

Unsurprisingly, Riggs determined that contracted pelves were a significant obstruction in childbirth. Fully committed to the tenets of racial hierarchy so prevalent in the anthropological science he studied, Riggs shaped statistical findings to fit theories of racial adaptation. Recorded measurements indicated there was less difference in the skulls of Black babies than in the size of their mothers' pelves, leading to the conclusion that "the negro child is materially smaller than the white."[38] The infant heads were smaller and more malleable.[39] What seemed a weakness was really a gift: "The small size of the child is a conservative provision of nature; for were its size to approach that usual in the white race serious dystocia would be almost a daily experience."[40]

The revelation seemed to explain the seemingly easier spontaneous birth among Black women, conveniently overlooking the fact that their maternal mortality and morbidity rates were at least twice as high as whites. Masked as statistical science, Riggs advanced an unsupported pathology delineating supposedly inherited phenotypical traits. The Black women he encountered became a single anthropological type, representative of "the lower races."

Sticking to his declared focus, Riggs argued that the relationship of the fetal head to the maternal pelvis during birth depended upon a number of complex variables, and could not be assigned to any single factor. Therefore, he could not support Clayton Arbuthnot Lane's contention that within each race, a rule of nature promoted harmonious proportion between the fetal head and the maternal pelvis. "We fear that such a hope cannot be fulfilled."[41] But Riggs did feel he could discern a reason explaining why Black women had larger numbers of deformed pelves, yet fewer operative interventions in childbirth. The answer was simple: white women gave birth to bigger, healthier babies with larger skulls, more often male. "The higher the grade of the race the greater is the proportion of males to female children."[42] One more well-known assumption entered the analysis: the greater the size, the greater the intelligence. Committed to an interpretive tradition reaching back to Paul Broca and Samuel George Morton, Riggs considered head size undeniable evidence of racial superiority. White women produced more male babies; male babies had the larger, more intelligent heads.

Riggs believed the proof to be in the hospital records; white women at Johns Hopkins birthed more male babies than Black women, thereby empowering the Anglo-Saxon race. Mothers were the vessel for the generation of civilization; white women suffered greater cephalopelvic disproportion because evolution made them the vehicle to reproduce a superior race. (Even as Riggs offered this assessment, biometrician Karl Pearson was casting doubt on the relation of head size to intelligence, pronouncing the idea false and unscientific. Anthropologist Franz Boas would demolish the claim in 1911.[43])

Eleven. An Obstetrical Definition of Race

"A Comparative Study of White and Negro Pelves" pleased J. Whitridge Williams immensely, furthering his own work on the female pelvis. As Riggs's introduction notes, there had been little research comparing the pelves of whites and Blacks, little work on measurements of the fetal heads of each race. The sheer bulk of his statistical analysis buttressed a racial framework conditioning Williams's approach to the science of childbirth. Seeking to avoid long discussions of racial difference in his own essays, Williams cited the paper frequently, referring to Riggs for clarification of contrasting biological traits. Though Riggs returned to the West after completing medical education, his study of white and Black pelves continued to influence obstetrical research throughout the profession for years to come.[44]

Twelve

The Learning Curve of Alfred F. Hess

With the increasingly disparate developments in the obstetrical and pediatric sciences, publicly conscious medical practitioners found themselves in a binary world, pitting the environment against the biological. Pediatricians most often tended to weigh the influence of environmental factors in the framework of their investigations, while obstetricians such as J. Whitridge Williams and his many of assistants believed biological inheritance grounded in race a critical consideration. Contrasting perceptions impacted the disciplinary approach to issues ranging from personal hygiene and proper nutrition to the reform of public health policy. What the specialties shared was an unbounded faith in their ability to shape the future, to resolve the challenges facing their spheres of medical practice. Childbirth was controllable, the insalubrious practices of the past swept away in the development of rigorous scientific procedure. The children brought forth would no longer be haunted by the specter of infant death, the scourge of rickets. The practice of obstetrics was steadily gaining ground. Pediatricians had much to figure out.

* * *

The influence of Luther Emmett Holt extended well beyond his own research, his efforts to promote public health, his connections to John Howland and the Harriet Lane Home. The myriad problems beckoning pediatric investigation created an atmosphere conducive to cooperative study in the City of New York. In addition to the work of Holt and Howland, studies undertaken by Doctor Alfred F. Hess (1875–1933) did much to shape the understanding of nutritional disease in children.

Alfred Fabian Hess was an independent New York City physician with strong German ties; his parents were wealthy German immigrants. Achieving his medical degree at the College of Physicians and Surgeons at Columbia University in 1901, Hess served an internship at Mount Sinai

Hospital before traveling abroad for further study. Two years of clinical training in Prague, Vienna, and Berlin made him familiar with scurvy and rickets, as well as other childhood diseases. Returning to the United States in 1905, he undertook further internships under Simon Flexner at the Rockefeller Institute and Emmet Holt at the Babies Hospital before entering private practice. His practice was very small; unlike most pediatricians of his time, Hess did not need to rely on the income. Family wealth enabled him to pursue medicine without an all-consuming commitment to any given institution. Relatively free of financial concerns, Hess threw himself into scientific research. Among other opportunities, he became Director of Pediatrics at the Beth Israel Children's Hospital, originally established as a dispensary by Abraham Jacobi in 1891. (Though the two were friends, Hess never cited Jacobi in his extensive writings.)[1]

The association with L. Emmett Holt was strong. Hess had studied under him at Columbia, served at the Babies Hospital, worked alongside at the Rockefeller Institute, at various children's medical centers around town. Holt was everywhere. His essential role in the development of public health policy provided Hess the opportunity to assist Doctor William H. Park at the New York City Bureau of Laboratories, where he learned from a master the practical benefits of public health treatment and bacteriology.[2] Hess eagerly entered into research on childhood infectious and chronic diseases, including infant diarrhea, childhood tuberculosis, mumps and a long list of further conditions. Always aware of his surroundings, Hess came to see his work at various institutions as an opportunity to benefit from consistent and controlled environments for patients, providing a basis for scientific studies of childhood disease. Unusual for such a remembered and productive figure in the early twentieth century, Hess never held a faculty appointment at a major teaching institution. With a growing reputation for careful and exacting research, his relative independence helped to create a model for the aspiring medical scientist.[3]

Professional peers came to regard Alfred Hess as a premier practitioner of children's medicine, on a par with L. Emmett Holt. Hess practiced independently of major medical institutions, but strove to attain a new and deeper insight, sometimes putting that desire before the health and well-being of the infants and young children in his charge. Though involved with several different medical institutions, Alfred Hess's experimental research was initially confined largely to patients at Beth Israel Children's Hospital. A new opportunity developed in 1911, when the Hebrew Infant Asylum appointed Hess to their governing board as medical director and attending physician. Described by Abraham Flexner as "a well-meaning but old-fashioned institution," the asylum originated in 1860 as a home for Jewish "children under five years, made orphans by the death of one or both parents; children left without proper guardianship; and children whose parents are too destitute to care for them properly."[4]

The medicalization of the Infant Asylum rode the line of public trust. Like the Harriet Lane Home, Hess's work rested on palatable justifications. First, that medical science benefited children's health: a closed setting such as an orphanage facilitated laboratory-based studies that tracked the progression of symptoms of disease as they appeared. Second, that medical science needed human bodies to determine a more precise diagnosis of seemingly related diseases, as well as to determine the viability of various inoculations, injections, and tests of immunity.[5] Alfred Hess oversaw a carefully crafted regimen designed to make efficient use of his experimental subjects. The system was much the opposite of the Harriet Lane Home, where John Howland maintained a rigorous division separating laboratory research from clinical practice—laboratory specialists never entered the wards. At the Hebrew Infant Asylum, researchers moved freely between the floors and the laboratory, interacting with patients in the light of biochemical results. The practice promoted a fuller comprehension of the pathological aspects exhibited with treatment.[6]

Hess realized that a separate group of patients not receiving the treatments intended to ameliorate suffering was central to any study of disease treatment. Facing a puzzling outbreak of scurvy at the Asylum in 1911, Hess set about testing the virtues of pasteurized milk and orange juice, providing a daily allowance to a specified group of children, leaving a second group untreated. Tracking the course of the disease in each group demonstrated the relative efficacy of the therapy under study. The study was a stark illustration of experimental science as practiced on infant children devoid of protection.[7]

Affecting bones and teeth, scurvy was long thought to be a variation of rickets. Sir Thomas Barlow established the difference between the two conditions in 1883, identifying scurvy as a hemorrhagic disease afflicting the sufferer in various forms—bleeding under the skin, from mucous membranes. The disease was long known, most infamous for the staggering mortality among sailors on long exploratory voyages. The benefits of citrus fruit were recognized as early as the sixteenth century, though no one could explain the underlying biochemical reason. Fresh milk seemed another preventative.[8]

Removal of orange juice from the children's diet at the Hebrew Infant Asylum had resulted in the scurvy outbreak; pasteurized milk proved insufficient to eliminate the disease.[9] Determined to trace the cause, Hess enlisted the help of staff Doctor Mildred Fish to analyze the chemistry of blood drawn from the afflicted children. Was it a quality in the blood that caused the bleeding, or something else? The careful hygiene and precision of nutritional preparation at the orphanage provided ideal conditions for a study. The sizable number of patients provided a control group, essential for the validation of subsequent results.[10]

Hess and Fish tested a new method of pasteurizing milk, purportedly preserving anti-scorbutic properties. The product was given to some infants while withholding orange juice. A series of blood tests followed—drawn from the jugular vein (a prick of the finger was insufficient), measured to determine coagulability, platelet levels, leukocytes, erythrocytes, hemoglobin. Analysis demonstrated departures from normal blood chemistry, sometimes suggesting anemia, but not nearly enough "to account for the hemorrhages associated with the disease."[11] Healthy patients in the control group actually contracted scurvy while consuming the formula. Only the substitution of raw, untreated milk reduced the symptoms, often to the vanishing point within two weeks. Servings of orange juice, or even squeezings from the rind, restored children to health. Recovery was rapid and conclusive. Though the defining symptoms of scurvy included subcutaneous bleeding, spongy gums, and anemia—all signs of internal hemorrhage—the condition seemed in some inexplicable fashion a disease of nutrition.[12]

Pasteurization effected the chemical composition of milk; some essential component was boiled away. Recognition that absence of a nutritional substance brought the onset of scurvy posed larger implications, strengthening the hand of those who argued rickets, a disease exhibiting similar symptoms, also derived from a dietary deficiency rather than environmental conditions.[13]

As Hess worked with Fish to prepare an article on the scurvy research for publication in 1914, his attention was drawn to the work of Casimer Funk (1884–1967), a Polish scientist in London researching nutritional deficiency illnesses such as beriberi, a weakening disease endemic to Asia. (Funk's work built on long years of research conducted by Dutch physician Christiaan Eijkmann [1858–1930] in Indonesia.) Recognizing that substances providing protection from various diseases must exist in natural foods, Funk isolated such an anti-beriberi quality in rice in 1912. The year following, he coined the word "vitamine" (vital amine) to specify the substance. The label was a misnomer; Funk mistakenly believed he had found an amine (an organic compound containing nitrogen). Eventually realizing his error, Funk explained that he had employed the phrase as a catchword denoting a group of chemical compounds providing resistance to nutritional diseases such as beriberi, pellagra, scurvy, and rickets. Although nitrogen did not actually figure in any of these substances, the name was attractive. Shortened to "vitamin," the name stuck. Composition of the various vitamins proved elusive; identification continued well into the 1920s. Research continues to this day.[14]

The discovery came to the attention of Hess far too late to have much bearing on his study of infantile scurvy. Summarizing Funk's research in a paragraph added to a 1914 article, Hess described vitamins as "substances which are essential to the health and life of the body, the lack of which produces a group of diseases which he has termed the 'avitaminosen." Absorbing Funk's descriptions, Hess initially envisioned vitamins as "crystallized nitrogen containing bodies of very complicated structure which are chemically defined, but concerning the exact structure of which we as yet know little. They are essential to life, although present in very small amounts."[15] The explication captured the mysterious quality this vitamin factor suggested. Hess referred to the "marvelous" orange which in so many forms, even heated, had stopped scurvy. Apparently, a vitamin was at work.[16]

In the six years to follow, Hess published forty-two articles in various medical journals, ranging in subject matter from tuberculosis, rubella, mumps, scurvy and rickets to "Institutions as Foster Mothers for Infants." Fifteen examined aspects of scurvy, including several devoted to dietary experiments on guinea pigs. The work culminated with the doctor's first monograph, on scurvy, published in 1920.[17] He wrote little on the subject thereafter. His attention turned to rickets.

* * *

Cod liver oil had fallen out of fashion, neglected as a successful treatment for rickets by much of the medical world. Doctors generally believed the fatty oil to be a waste of money, that the better plan was to provide milk to children. Drawing on medical literature extending back to the eighteenth century, Alfred Hess considered the potential curative worthy of exploration. In 1915, he and co-practitioner Lester J. Unger (1888–1974), physician at New York City Bureau of Laboratories and an assistant at the Infant Asylum, began a study to determine the effectiveness of cod liver oil in preventing rickets.[18] They would dispense prophylactic therapy in an African American community in New York called Columbus Hill, a "black spot" suffering the highest mortality rate in the City. Also known as "San Juan," the district stood low on the social and economic scale—"high rents and low wages" ruled the day. The largely African American population numbered nine thousand people, mostly immigrants from St. Kitts, the Barbados, and St. Croix in the West Indies.[19]

Two Progressive reform groups, the Henry Street Settlement House operated by Lillian Wald (1867–1940), and an organization known as The National League for the Study of the Urban Conditions of the Negro, had investigated the area just previously, identifying an especially high rate of mortality among infants. Three hundred fourteen per one thousand infants died in 1915. (White infants in the city died at less than half that rate.) Hess and Unger noted that these infants often died of respiratory failure, pneumonia, pulmonary tuberculosis and whooping cough. Weakening muscles, rachitic disease predisposed infants to such conditions, often leading to death. Interest in saving lives and bettering health conditions combined with opportunity to employ scientific methodology to address the underlying cause of the child mortality at Columbus Hill.[20]

The doctors hoped to explore several variables hypothesized as leading to rickets, concentrating on habits of nurture and lifestyle that might contribute to the disease. There was also the matter of race. Hess and Unger plainly stated, "Our main reason was the fact, agreed to by all, that of all races the negro is most subject to rickets. This tendency is so marked that it may be safely stated that over 90 percent of the colored babies have rickets, and that even a majority of those that are breast fed show signs of this disorder."[21] The study would consider the role of race as a cause of rickets while determining whether cod liver oil could prevent or cure most cases of the disease. The scientists selected "about fifty babies" to receive varying doses of the treatment, all between four months and one year old, to the extent possible living in homes where other children already suffered from rickets. The hope was to catch infants vulnerable to rachitic disease, providing a test of the preventive qualities of the oil. (The study consistently supplied a Norwegian variety.) No other treatment was offered; the dosage varied with each infant. Hess and Unger weighed the effects on infant digestive process and the prevention of rickets. More than a few mothers could not or would not cooperate; a number of these were counted as control cases not receiving treatment.[22]

The study involved close work taking staff into the homes of participants. The physicians noted that "we were fortunate in having the services of a nurse who had worked in this district for many years, and who was able to facilitate our access to the homes of these people."[23] The acknowledgment understated the depth of this (unidentified) woman's contribution. Accompanied by Hess or Unger, preliminary visits required a physical examination, a case history of the infant and mother, an examination of diet, "the economic condition of the family, the length of time they had lived in the North, and many other data."[24] Subsequent duties included oversight of breast feeding, examination of the infant for craniotabes, beading of the ribs, and swelling of the epiphyses—the telling symptoms of rickets. The nurse's social skills and familiarity with the people in the neighborhood won Hess and Unger the confidence and trust of the mothers who were the linchpins of the study.[25]

The results were conclusive for the value of cod liver oil. As expected, Hess and Unger found a high presence of rickets in the Columbus Hill population, determining that "all most all the colored babies developed rickets even though they nursed."²⁶ Presenting six richly-detailed tables of data presenting results derived from forty-nine cases, the scientists were able to graphically demonstrate the prophylactic effects of the oil. Among the thirty-four breastfed infants, twenty-nine did not develop rickets; of the five who did, four had received a minimal dose. Twelve of fourteen artificially fed babies exhibited no signs of the disease. The control group, those not given oil, numbered sixteen cases; all but one developed rickets. (There was no public outcry regarding the existence of a control group.) Further examination broke down the results according to the variation in symptoms and the amounts of oil administered. The conclusion was plain: cod liver oil was effective, the more the better. In "four fifths of the infants who received the oil for six months, and in more than one half of those who were given it for four months," rickets did not appear.²⁷

Word of the symptoms of rickets and the efficacy of cod liver oil for both treatment and prevention spread among neighboring mothers. Initially, the oil was dispensed to individuals in the home; staff ultimately moved provision to a central location at the neighborhood's settlement house. Requests for the oil grew; in time a neighborhood rickets clinic took shape. One question regarding cod liver oil was answered absolutely: supposed difficulties in administration were imaginary. The study went on for several years, resulting in an article reporting findings published in 1917, with a second article examining diet in the study households appearing a year later.²⁸

Armed with knowledge of the treatment's success and the accompanying interest spreading so rapidly throughout the community, the authors advocated rickets dispensaries "be provided in large cities in the negro and the Italian districts, for rickets is almost as prevalent among the Italians as among the colored people."²⁹ The expense would not amount to much; cod liver oil could be distributed at existing milk stations or health centers. Doctors objected. When Hess offered an oral presentation of the research at a meeting of the American Medical Association in 1917, one physician argued that ethnic food habits caused the disease. Another insisted that milk would better serve poor neighborhoods. A government-funded study successfully treating rickets in a poverty-ridden population, employing cod liver oil?³⁰

The study at Columbus Hill did nothing to dispel the perception that race was somehow involved in the etiology of the disease. In the eyes of Hess and Unger, the factor was not some quality of biological inheritance, but perhaps a trait to be found in cultural behavior. Continuing the study of cod liver oil, the scientists turned their attention to this question, enlarging the research to examine patterns of diet. Gathering further data regarding dietary habits of seventy-five Columbus Hill families, they sought exacting detail—types of food, protein, carbohydrate, and fat content, quantities of meat and vegetables. Weekly analyses included the food for every member of the household, examined in terms of the number and age of those eating. Not surprisingly, the physicians discovered inadequacy in the diet when compared to a standard defined as normal. Not only was there less provision than needed, but the food was not well-prepared, considered by the authors to have been boiled too long.[31]

Hess and Unger demonstrated a respect for the people they studied, an unwillingness to label the diet insufficient due to any stereotyped "ignorance" such as that advanced by audience members at the American Medical Association presentation in 1917. Hess may well have identified food ways as cultural expressions of race.[32] Curious about the environment, life style and food culture in these seventy-five mothers' places of origin—most were from the West Indies, a few from the American South— the researchers interviewed the women regarding foodways in their native lands. The contrast was telling. In their former homes, fresh fruit and vegetables abounded, often eaten uncooked, providing a much higher nutritional value than the limited produce available in New York City markets. Life on Columbus Hill paled by comparison. Meat became the essential ingredient at meals, very possibly affecting the metabolism of mother and child.[33]

The findings added yet another dimension to the unsolved etiology of rickets. Writing to various physicians in the Caribbean, Hess and Unger sought to determine the incidence of rachitic disease. There was essentially none. While acknowledging the possible influence of climate and the alteration of lifestyle, the physicians argued that the nutritional value of the food available contributed to the great numbers of Black immigrant children contracting rickets in New York. The two recognized that "the nature of rickets and the cause of this racial susceptibility remain illusive and unsolved problems. It is known, however, that the negro in the tropics does not suffer from rickets." Most pediatricians were more than prepared to accept the idea of racial susceptibility; the virtual non-existence of rickets among the Black populations of the Caribbean was a fact difficult to comprehend. The implications seemed obvious to Alfred Hess. Racial hereditary was not a factor in the disease.[34]

* * *

Alfred Hess never entered directly into any anthropological discussion on the meaning of race. Despite the conclusions drawn at Columbus Hill, ambiguity remained. Discussing the Caribbean backgrounds of the district's families, Hess showed an inclination to do his own field work, shying away from flatfooted statements regarding the influence of race in the etiology of rickets. Never pausing to qualify definitions of Black versus white, he failed to acknowledge the categories of race themselves were wanting. Designation of the majority of Columbus Hill residents as a specific ethnic group with a discrete migration history distinguished them from other African Americans, yet Hess lumped the entire Black population under the term "negro" in his summaries. He persisted in the practice despite long association with Franz Boas (1858–1942), renowned pioneer in the study of physical and cultural anthropology.

Boas, a German immigrant resident in America since 1887, pursued a wide variety of cultural studies before embracing an academic career. Appointed Full Professor of Anthropology at Columbia University in 1899, he spent more than forty years researching and reshaping the concept of race. Employing the anthropometric methods championed by Paul Broca and too many others, Boas examined growth patterns of immigrant children for the Federal Immigration Service in 1911, demonstrating that head size and shape among various nationalities altered with the change in environmental location.[35] There was no skull shape endemic to any group; racial classifications based on such assumptions were demonstrably untrue. A vigorous opponent of the scientific racism embraced by J. Whitridge Williams and countless others, Boas challenged the concept of racial inferiority, arguing there was not the slightest proof of any pattern of progress toward "higher forms," within species or among species. Human nature was culturally relative, behavior shaped by social tradition in response to environmental conditions.[36]

Among his many interests, Boas researched Hebrew children extensively. Corresponding with Alfred Hess, he arranged to expand his studies to include orphan children at the Hebrew Infant Home (the name had changed; the considerable numbers of children had not).[37] Boas wanted to use records of these infants to compare their growth with other Hebrew infants growing up in homes rather than an institution. An exchange of letters lasting several years ensued. Hess once wrote to Boas requesting information regarding the growth patterns of African American children. Boas cautioned him, stating, "Of course, it must be understood that figures for Negroes always include a great many mulattos and quadroons."[38] From an early point in his career, Boas had paid special attention to the taboo topic of racial mixture, recognizing the widespread blending of people of varying color throughout human history. As a category of human classification, race had no real meaning. Racial purity was a myth, as was the contention that mixing of the races led to degenerative offspring.[39] Referring to a much-cited study by Robert Woodbury charting growth patterns in urban children, Boas noted the simplistic categories of Negro and white the author employed.[40] Every child not seen as purely white was considered

Black. In reality, there was almost endless variation. The report was meaningless. The anthropologist's own research showed that the living environment—conditions of the home, the degree of poverty—impacted body size and shape a great deal more than any supposed influence of race.[41]

Boas maintained a long exchange with Hess, suggesting a kind of common ground between them. Yet Hess continued to tread the same worn path, adhering to the racial classifications so fundamental to American culture—the metalanguage of race. Though fully recognizing the cultural differences among the various families living on Columbus Hill, he regarded all simply as Black—the report on the cod liver oil study was in part titled "Therapy in a *Negro* Community." In his book on rickets, published twelve years later, nothing had really changed: "the negro may possess an inherent racial tendency to rickets—a tendency shared perhaps by other races."[42]

Exploring the subject further, Hess wrote, "My personal opinion ... is that the negro, as well as some other southern races, evince a racial susceptibility to rickets when they migrate and live in a northern climate."[43] He perceived the epidemiology of rickets in terms of racial groups—the Italians, Greeks, and African Americans. In a footnote entered later in his text, Hess observed "The signs of rickets in the negro are so exaggerated that, from a clinical standpoint, it is virtually a distinct type of disorder."[44]

Yet he eschewed the idea of rickets as a hereditary affliction. Studies of diet convinced him beyond doubt that the disease came from migration and an extreme change of lifestyle.[45]

In the seventh edition of The *Diseases of Infancy and Childhood*, Luther Holt and John Howland again emphasized the susceptibility to rickets among Blacks and Italians, observing "it is exceptional to see in a dispensary or hospital a child of either of these races who does not show, to a greater or less degree, the signs of rickets."[46] The disease was universal. Along with many others, the writers concluded that the only explanation was "a race peculiarity."[47] Hess recognized the ubiquity of the disease among Blacks and Italians, but detached himself from identification of race as a critical factor, continually minimizing the possibility.

* * *

America's entry into the Great War did much to drive home the fact that rickets was a widespread and ruinous disease. Instituting a military draft in June of 1917, the health of young men between the age of eighteen and thirty became a burning issue. David Paul von Hansemann's essay "On Rickets as a Folk Disease," published in 1906, had anticipated the problem, rightly predicting rickets would leave a considerable percentage of German youth unfit for the military. The same would prove true for the

United States. Of the first one million men examined for service in 1917, over 290,000 were rejected. Of those, more than one in five suffered poor physical health. Afflictions ranged from poor teeth and spinal curvature to flat feet. Doctors evaluating inductees attributed all three debilitating conditions to rickets.[48]

The physical classifications—labeled "the mechanical"—were "far and away the most common defects found in the examination for military service, constituting the most important group from the military point of view." Assessments after the War found that "numerically the most important item in this group and indeed in the whole list of defects found in young men, is that of weak feet."[49] Doctors most often identified bow legs and knock knees as specifically rachitic, but generally included flat feet in the same category. Although those identified were not necessarily rejected by the draft, they were often classified as eligible for noncombatant positions only. The primary requirement for fighting men was the ability to walk.[50]

Because so many men were found physically and mentally limited in their draft exams, a great deal of analysis after the war highlighted the "defects found in drafted men." The post–War report, authored by the infamous eugenicist Charles. B. Davenport (1866–1944) and Lieutenant Colonel Albert Love, described the problem sketchily: "the feet are badly adjusted to the demands made upon them in modern civilized life."[51] In their estimation, war was an essential aspect of modern civilization; these men fell short of their obligation to fight. Surprisingly, the authors found that most of the flat-footed draftees were white, coming from the urban industrial Northeast—thought to be the victims of long hours spent standing in poorly made shoes. Draftees from the Pacific Northwest were also numerous. There were few flat-footed cases in the South, a finding unanticipated. Davenport and Love concluded this was "due to the comparative absence of shoes in the rural population," especially among African Americans. A further possibility was the "anatomical and physiological peculiarities" thought prevalent in the Black population. (The irony in that statement surpasses belief.) Race was an ever handy explanation in early twentieth-century America.[52]

Alfred Hess noted the conflicted opinions on the etiology of flat feet. In the volume on rickets published in 1929, Hess held rickets to be a probable cause, stemming from muscular weakness, a rachitic symptom identified by Francis Glisson three centuries before. A wave of flat feet among young men in Germany and Austria following the world war provided the perfect example. Famine swept through the vanquished countries, resulting in an epidemic of rickets among young adults. "Weak musculature and lax ligaments" developed accordingly. Such weakness led "to the development of the various curvatures of the spine, to knock-knee, flat foot and other deformities." Studies conducted in the immediate postwar period were useful to researchers such as Hess, confirming long-established hypotheses regarding the disease, though contributing little to understanding of the bone disorders increasingly viewed as central to the etiology of rickets.[53]

* * *

The studies conducted by Alfred Hess and others, combined with the indicative discovery of vitamins, offered new direction to the investigation of rickets. The Great War added impetus to their work. If anything could add fuel to the already burning concerns of race suicide, the fact that 6 percent of America's young men—almost all of them white—were weakened by rachitic disease would certainly serve. The nation was thoroughly modern, increasingly urban. Industrialized. Civilized. Tame. Diseased.

Measures were necessary.

THIRTEEN

Control of American Birth

On September 25, 1916, Julia C. Lathrop, Director of the Children's Bureau, submitted to the U.S. Secretary of Labor a report researched and written by Doctor Grace Meigs, director of the Bureau's Division of Hygiene. A long-winded title encapsulated the content: "Maternal Mortality from all Conditions Connected with Child Birth, in the United States and Certain Other Countries." A two-page summary informed the Secretary that "in 1913, in this country at least 15,000 women, it is estimated, died from conditions caused by childbirth; about 7,000 of these died from childbed fever, a disease proved to be almost entirely preventable, and the remaining 8,000 from diseases known to be to a great extent preventable or curable." Despite the advances in germ theory and sanitation, death rates in childbirth had not fallen appreciably over the previous thirteen years. Only tuberculosis brought more death to women of childbearing age.[1]

The first decades of the twentieth century witnessed a proliferation of statistical record keeping; public attention turned to statistics of maternal and infant mortality as registration spread across the United States. The Children's Bureau was instrumental in the development, lobbying the Government to establish a National Birth Registry, a measure adopted in 1915. Registration enabled Bureau educators to track births and provide educational assistance to new mothers, as well as keeping tabs on birth rates. Death records improved as well. Bureau statistician Robert Morse Woodbury noted that in 1900 "the death-registration area included 40.5 percent of the population of the United States; in 1920 it included more than twice as large a proportion, 82.2 percent."[2] The numbers were seriously flawed by inconsistent documentation; states varied considerably in methods of categorization and the collection of data.[3] Sometimes doctors' reports of deaths listed a cause of death as tuberculosis when the woman died in childbirth. Or, a poor child born of immigrants may have died with no record kept at all. Despite the issues, an overall trend became alarmingly clear. During and after World War I, the rate of American maternal mortality grew demonstrably greater than that of several European countries. The increasing numbers most probably resulted from puerperal fever, tied to the growing practice of Caesarean sections, still very risky in the hands of the inexperienced. Questions pertaining to various aspects of reproduction—abortion, women's health, women working and the status of the child—all turned to statistics for answers. Doctors created and often manipulated statistics in order to defend their reputations.[4]

Shielding their own lack of knowledge and experience, doctors blamed midwives for the mortality, portraying them as unschooled, ignorant, "un-American" and by inference uncivilized, lashing out at them for the loss of women's lives, though the great majority were not their fault. Professionals damned traditional midwifery for flawed and unhygienic practice. Joseph B. DeLee vehemently attacked midwifery, maintaining "the midwife is a relic of barbarism."[5] J. Whitridge Williams found midwives beneath contempt. State legislatures, state regulatory commissions listened. Medical professionals and social reformers turned public attention to births supervised by midwives. Studies of midwifery popped up all over the country, focusing largely though not entirely on urban areas. State laws targeted midwives throughout the 1910s and 1920s; practice diminished radically. Hospital birth, supervised by an obstetrician, almost certainly male, was well on the way to becoming the norm. Midwives became criminals.[6]

* * *

Any definition of midwifery must include an understanding of the social, economic and even political environment of historical practice. Childbirth in the early twentieth century was most often at home; the care of a midwife common.[7] Problems were few; a physician could be brought in should difficulties appear. The relationship was often uneasy. Knowing medical practitioners disapproved of their efforts, many midwives remained hidden from view, disappearing before the doctor arrived. By the turn of the century, physicians never failed to deprecate the midwives.[8]

While scholars can only estimate numbers of midwives and births among African Americans in the post–Civil War era, evidence mounts that African American midwives garnered power in the South after the collapse of slavery. Black women developed a strong tradition, taking control of their own reproduction in surprising and unrecognized ways. Use of the cotton plant as an abortifacient and tool of birth control exemplifies an often-unrecognized aspect of self-protective invention that outsiders saw as folk medicine and superstition. Black midwifery escalated in importance as poverty grew amidst social, political, legal and economic changes wrought by white supremacy. By the early twentieth century, granny midwives (as Black midwives were called) played a singularly central part in childbirth of the rural South.[9]

The campaign against Black and immigrant midwives serves as a painful reminder of the serious growth of color lines during the Age of Reform. Some reformers did point out that midwives were often the only available care for pregnant and laboring women. The African American midwife often represented the sole recourse in rural areas, as well as overcrowded urban areas ridden with poverty. Reform efforts grounded in white middle class values at times brought hardship to those most in need of assistance. Though midwives of all races were in practice, including many immigrants, medical practitioners aimed in particular at African American women bearing the double stigma of race and midwifery, stinging them with "a language of shame, stigma and pollution tied to racial difference."[10]

Historian Valerie Lee uncovered statistical evidence from the turn of the century through the 1920s showing that the number of African American granny midwives grew significantly. Many practiced in rural Southern areas. A Federal public health survey in 1925 found 43,627, practicing midwives (not medically trained); most were Black.[11] Black midwives served Black and white women alike. With increasing governmental and medical regulations and extensive suppression, these midwives suffered the greatest loss of practice and identity. In Lee's analysis, the forces let loose on African American midwives targeted both their practice and their race. Medical and governmental excoriation of Black midwives resulted in the obliteration of their memory in the minds of African Americans, so forceful and hateful was the campaign.[12]

* * *

In 1914, J. Whitridge Williams was elected president of the American Association for the Study and Prevention of Infant Mortality (AASPIM). The national headquarters of the new group was centered in the Medical and Chirurgical Faculty Building at Johns Hopkins University. Founded in 1909, the organization grew out of discussions regarding maternal mortality occurring at a meeting of the American Medical Association. AASPIM would be controlled exclusively by male physicians; the University hosted the first national meeting in November of 1910. Among the participants were William Welch, Dean of the Medical School, Abraham Jacobi, the nation's most revered pediatrician, and Williams. Doctor J.H. Mason Knox, instructor in pediatrics at Johns Hopkins and director of a sanitarium for infants, became the Association's first president.[13]

In his presidential address, Knox articulated the focus of the organization and emphasized education as the core.[14] "The pivotal point is the mother," he insisted.

Thirteen. Control of American Birth

She is the natural caretaker of her baby. She must be instructed in the absolute necessity of providing her baby during its dependent and helpless state with such food and surroundings as are compatible with health and life, and we who know and have must see to it that we share with her our knowledge and means until her baby as well as ours really enters into the possession of its birthright, namely, the right to live, now so often denied it.[15]

Knox could not have articulated a clearer image of the elitist assumptions defining the organization. Certainly an expression of Progressive Era sentiment, the speech underlined the desire to supervise, to regulate, to make the necessary decisions on behalf of the nation's mothers. AASPIM was an association framed by physicians, sensing the advent of their own power, desiring more. No one could deny the benefits of promoting proper hygiene, urging a better diet. The underlying presumptions were much darker.

Contemporaneous with the campaign to reduce infant mortality was a drive to not merely prevent race suicide, but to improve the white race through elimination of the "unfit"—those deemed biologically ill-equipped to forward racial survival and improvement. Eugenics, the concept adduced by Francis Galton in 1883, had attracted a large and powerful body of support, both in Britain and the United States. In essence, eugenicists maintained that race was a definable and heritable trait, that races could be ranked in definable terms of superiority, that a mixing of races brought inferior children into the world, that a regulated supervision of reproduction would bring about racial "progress." (Recall, this was a "Progressive" era.) Human beings could accelerate the process of Darwinian natural selection through selective breeding. The first step was to identify the estimated ten percent of the American population deemed undesirable, mentally and physically. Prevent their reproduction. Pass laws eliminating miscegenation. Eventually, the superior race would achieve purity. Already strongly established in race systems around the country, race prejudices slipped easily into the eugenic frame of the fit and the unfit—the need to purify the race and strengthen whites.[16]

In 1904 Charles Davenport, director of a biological laboratory on Long Island, obtained a grant from the newly formed Carnegie Institution to open and direct a research laboratory for the study of evolution at Cold Spring Harbor, Long Island. Fascinated by the work of Francis Galton, Davenport would pursue eugenics in an American context, focused heavily on race characteristics—race in the old race science sense of polygeny. His influential book, *Heredity in Relation to Eugenics*, appeared in 1911.[17] Deeply involved in the study of family pedigrees, he linked eugenics to the study of heredity and the renewal of interest in Mendelian chromosomal genetics, tracing the fitness or unfitness of individuals and families through genealogies. Davenport was a founding member of AASPIM.[18]

Moderate followers of eugenic theory argued that in the face of "race suicide," education ought to teach the mothers of all infants how to care for their children. In the vernacular of public health and social reform, the word hygiene came to sport a double meaning—a science of sanitation coupled to survival of the fittest. While eugenics categorized humans as fit or unfit, emphasizing inheritance as almost exclusively the cause of any deformity, educating mothers in hygiene—especially the poor mothers—became the thrust of the reform effort. As historian Richard A. Meckel observed, AASPIM's members saw themselves "as involved in both a philanthropic effort to save infant lives and a scientific endeavor to advance human welfare by improving the mental and physical quality of humanity."[19]

The leaders of the Association, along with many in the membership, promoted the goals of the eugenics movement, holding to an ideology of social efficiency. The prevailing belief was that "racially unfit" infants, or offspring with hereditary disease, would die naturally. Not all infant mortality was unwanted. Abraham Jacobi promoted barring the unfit from marriage, and sterilization of the unfit. William Welch, charter member of the American Eugenics Association, gave a lecture at AASPIM's first meeting, delineating which childhood diseases should concern the members as part of the plan to strengthen the race.[20]

In 1911, the Association passed a resolution urging the states adopt legislation legalizing use of surgical procedures to prevent the begetting of unfit offspring. Speaking before the Association in 1913, Emmet Holt made the point plain. "We must eliminate the unfit by birth not by death. The race is to be most effectively improved by preventing marriage and reproduction by the unfit, among whom we would class the diseased, the degenerate, the defective, and the criminal." AASPIM would promote medical science to save the babies born; employ the same science to eliminate births among the unfit.[21]

AASPIM was a private organization organized by medical practitioners—obstetricians and pediatricians. Education was essential, but an education extending well beyond the lessons of sanitation and caring for baby. The proper approach to child care in the twentieth century would begin with birth: the modern woman would deliver under the care and instruction of a physician, preferably in a hospital. Midwifery was to be discouraged, outlawed if possible. Seizing control of birth, doctors could then proceed to the next essential step: deciding which people should be allowed to produce children at all. They would reform American society in a far more comprehensive fashion. They would save America from race suicide.[22]

Williams served as AASPIM's president from 1914 to 1916.[23] In the first volume of the organization's professional journal, published in 1910, Williams contributed an essay titled "What the Obstetrician Can Do to Prevent Infant Mortality,"[24] framing his ideals for the professionalization of obstetrics. Defining the steps in the process of supervising a proper obstetrical birth, Williams argued that educational reform was essential, both for the expectant mother and the doctor supervising the delivery. The call for prenatal care as a measure to prevent infant mortality was innovative and perspicacious.[25] His vision for the future held little for midwives:

> We hear a great deal of the necessity for improving the status and mode of education of the midwife; and while I am perfectly willing to admit of all her imperfections, I am, somewhat skeptical of the good which may be accomplished in this respect in this country. I am inclined to believe that in the larger cities her gradual annihilation should be our aim, although I am not so certain that it would be advisable in poor and sparsely settled country districts. On the other hand, judging by my own experience, I believe that the ordinary midwife does no more harm, if as much as the poorly trained doctor.[26]

Obstetrical reform rested at the heart of Williams' ambition for AASPIM. Asked to undertake a study of the "Midwife Problem" for the organization's 1911 meeting, Williams instead used the opportunity to examine the state of obstetrical education. Dismissing any hope of training midwives sufficiently, he prepared a survey sent out to medical schools across the nation, seeking information on current medical education programs. Forty-three responded. What emerged became a famous exposé; Williams declared "most of the ills of women ... are the result of bad obstetrics,"[27] damning the profession's poor embrace of modern medical science. His ideal obstetrician and teacher built a career based not in private practice, but clinical experience in a hospital setting, combined with laboratory research. Medical students needed practical exposure to birth in dispensary settings such as the Outdoor Obstetrical Service, where they could gain experiential skills in obstetrical operations ranging from forceps to Caesarean section. His schema subordinated the reduction of infant and maternal mortality rates to the reform of medical education, strengthening the specialization and authority given to obstetrical science. Loathing the appellation of obstetricians as man-midwives, he descried poor salaries for practitioners. There was no time nor possibility, he declared, to better the practice of midwifery. Best to let it go along until it died. Participation in AASPIM was one way to move in that direction.[28]

* * *

Maryland proved no exception to the established predominance of African American midwives in the South. Middle-class white reformers fussed over the state's midwife population. A study published in 1905 descried the failure to execute legal control over midwives. The author, Doctor Guy Steele of rural Maryland, saw the practice of African American midwives as criminal, yet essential to the rural areas. Like Williams and DeLee, Steele sought to establish legal control of midwives.[29] His survey concluded that African American women provided the only pool for midwives. Lack of education and age limited their abilities; not one in ten was under fifty years old. Some truth may be found in the older age of rural midwives; elderly Black women were often left behind by the migration of young Blacks to the cities. Still, the presumptive bias in Steele's analysis was plain: among Black midwives, age was representative of ignorance.[30]

In 1925, the Journal of the American Medical Association published a study of midwives in Baltimore, written by Doctor Mary Sherwood, chair of AASPIM's Obstetrical Section and the Midwifery Committee. Sherwood had traveled abroad to earn a medical degree at the University of Zurich, specializing in the new field of bacteriology. Returning to the United States, she was refused residency at the newly opened Johns Hopkins Hospital on the basis of sex. Lilian Welsh, Sherwood's lifelong companion, also a graduate of the medical school in Zurich, joined her in Baltimore. Appreciating the women's skills even as they refused to advance their careers, the medical faculty at Hopkins employed the women in the laboratory.[31]

Struggling to support themselves, Sherwood and Welsh eventually left the hospital to partner in private practice. Attracting few cases, they assumed control of the Evening Dispensary for Working Women and Girls of Baltimore, holding late hours to better serve the needs of their patients. Women doctors such as Sherwood and Welsh increasingly defined their careers through reform activities, educating the lay public. Their assessment of the lives of the poor and the working class followed a familiar pattern governed by standards grounded in social hierarchy.[32] Despite their own discriminatory treatment at Johns Hopkins, both women treasured their affiliations with the medical facility. Each joined AASPIM at the organization's inception. Sherwood and Welsh could not bear the thought of midwives practicing without medical education or license while female physicians experienced ongoing social and economic restraint in their careers. Of necessity, doctors would supplant midwives. Placed in a subsidiary position, Sherwood's task was to educate the public in the presumed benefits of the new obstetrics—medical science and governmental certification were to be the *sine qua non* of reformed childbirth.[33]

Sherwood's study mirrored a model developed by Elisabeth Crowell in New York. Crowell, a social worker and staff nurse at the Rockefeller Foundation, joined with the City's Association of Neighborhood Workers to undertake a survey of the "Midwives of New York," published in 1907. Crowell's study became a prototype for several subsequent studies of midwives. She sent investigators, sometimes sheriffs, into the neighborhoods to find midwives, interview them thoroughly, and subsequently shadow their practices with detectives. Just 10 percent were deemed qualified or reliable.[34] The predominant tone cast the midwife in the role of criminal. The study found the midwives' bags filthy. Opprobrium grew among white middle class reformers; many suspected midwives of performing abortions.[35]

In perspective and in tone, Sherwood's approach was similar to Crowell's. A committee of three female doctors, including Welsh, undertook the Baltimore study. They began with an examination of data collected from the Evening Dispensary for Working Women and Girls, supplemented by materials from the Mothers' Relief Society.[36] Employing a social worker to interview the one hundred-fifty midwives found in Baltimore, the study uncovered "intolerable" conditions while determining that midwives took responsibility for 40.7 percent of the city's births. Sherwood condemned the midwives' lack of training and their 24.7 percent illiteracy rate.[37]

Regulations taking effect in Maryland in 1910 required midwives to register. Those already in practice were not required to take an examination, but beginning midwives were to be examined by the State Board of Health. The ability to read and write was a necessity. The applicant had to earn a certificate from a maternity hospital or a qualified medical practitioner, confirming competence in attendance at five or more births. The regulations further stipulated that midwives could not conduct a vaginal examination or intervene mechanically or technologically in any way during a birth. If an unusual situation in labor arose, the midwife was to alert a physician. Sherwood's report lamented the deficiencies in registration, as well as the inadequacy of the qualifications for midwifery. A regulation considered especially important mandated midwives apply silver nitrate eye drops to all newborns to prevent the blindness possible from venereal disease. Sherwood found just three midwives observed the requirement.[38]

The published report featured two rich tables breaking down the data on the midwives interviewed. Length of practice, ethnic origin, and criminal behavior, along with standards of hygiene and antisepsis, were listed by ethnicity—15 total groups, including "American." Seventy midwives were immigrants, including twenty-seven Germans. Of forty-five Black midwives, twenty-six had practiced more than twenty years—a longer duration than any other ethnic group. Thirteen were between sixty and seventy years old, ten between seventy and seventy-nine. One was over eighty. Thirty of the forty-five could neither read nor write.[39] The report adjudged about twenty-four percent of Black midwives guilty of what was labeled criminal behavior, implying the practice of abortion. More likely, the criminality was the failure to use eye drops. None had earned a diploma; just one was registered with the health board. Yet, in an unusual but telling category, Sherwood admitted nearly all the midwives examined scored very well in caring for the mother.[40]

Sherwood graded most of the Black midwives' methods as "poor," exhibiting a lack of hygiene in the care of infant eyes and the umbilical cord. Just thirty-one percent employed antiseptics. Midwives' bags, which Sherwood judged to be dirty, contained the tools of birth, what midwives kept by their sides, carried from labor to labor. Sherwood and later reformers sought to educate midwives by demonstrating what should be in the bag and what should not, according to the regulations and medical standards.[41]

Sherwood's study confirmed that midwives practiced widely in Baltimore; many had practiced a long time. AASPIM regarded these midwives as professional and economic competition, yet the study left crucial essentials of their work unexamined. "The Midwives of Baltimore" was an exercise in judgment. Sherwood was at least more tolerant of the presence of midwifery than the physicians practicing at the Outdoor Obstetrical Service.[42]

A companion study conducted in Maryland's rural Anne Arundel County in 1912 found midwifery still more integral to the community, the lack of trained physicians making the practice a critical necessity. The population was far too small, too scattered to support more physicians to supersede the midwives. There could be but one solution: "Since the midwife seems to be a necessary evil in these southern districts the problem resolves itself into one of education."[43]

* * *

If residents of Maryland paused to ponder the issues of childbirth early in the twentieth century, they had good reason. Still another examination followed AASPIM's efforts in Baltimore and Anne Arundel County. The Children's Bureau conducted a field study of infant mortality in Baltimore in 1915, based on records of birth for that single year. Why Baltimore? The final report explained that "in its population, the variety of its industries, and the rate of infant mortality prevailing, Baltimore may be regarded as a typical city with a typical problem in relation to infant mortality." (The report did not mention the presence of the nation's most prestigious medical school.) Of the eight cities the Bureau surveyed beginning in 1912, Baltimore was the only one to include a large percentage of Blacks, a population ranking fourth in the United States in 1910.[44]

Published in 1923, the study featured numerous charts and lengthy analyses portraying a diverse city populated by immigrants of several nationalities, as well as Black and white native born. Dissecting the data, author Anna Rochester, child labor activist and reformer, time and again found the origins of infant mortality in disease and poverty, evidenced by income, residential location, employment of the mother, legitimacy of the infant, breastfeeding vs. artificial feeding, levels of hygiene. Statistics on attendance at birth were relegated to an appendix: the women agents found that physicians attended at 67.4 percent of the city's deliveries, midwives were present at 47.1 percent (a figure seven percent higher that Sherwood's determination). Four-fifths of all births occurred in the home.[45]

The highest rate of infant mortality was among the Polish, who suffered the loss of 163.2 infants for every 1000 births, followed by African Americans at 158.6. For native whites, the rate was 95.9.[46] Among the less fortunate, living conditions in Baltimore had not changed much in a quarter century. Rochester's study carefully delineated areas densely populated by one racial group or another. Blacks paid high rents for substandard facilities often lacking sewer connections, family toilets or bath tubs. Prescribed hygienic measures proved difficult to implement. Polish families had the lowest level of dwellings of all; twelve percent had no sanitation provision.[47] Foreign born immigrants suffered the highest number of deaths from tuberculosis[48]; Black infants experienced higher rates of infant mortality from infectious disease such as tuberculosis, syphilis, and whooping cough than any other population. These diseases often accompanied or proceeded from rickets. Much of the infant mortality occurred in the late winter and spring, similar (and perhaps related to) the seasonal pattern found in rachitic disease.[49]

The study showed poverty was "an important factor in infant mortality." Weighing the problems of the different populations, Rochester concluded the economic barriers facing African Americans seemed the greatest. Blacks were paid the lowest wages, kept in the least paying jobs, and forced to pay the highest rent. "The sheer absence of means with which to supply the necessities of wholesome living seemed to be itself a factor in mortality."[50] The death rate reflected "a real difference in conditions and care."[51] Rather than the ignorance often labeled a racial trait, the high morbidity and mortality of Black infants and their mothers came from factors related to poverty—race prejudice and exploitation.[52]

African American women experienced a tragic anomaly in the high rates of infant mortality they endured. Black mothers cared for their infants as well as circumstances would allow, but they were among the groups most often employed outside the home. Fathers earned little, or worse, nothing. Blacks were excluded from better paying jobs; women worked most commonly as chars—domestic servants or laundresses. Bureau agents found breastfeeding without artificial supplements was surprisingly common among these women. (Most physicians at this point maintained that such a regimen was best for the infant—often reiterated as a way to prevent rickets.) Lacking alternative means of feeding, infants left at home by a working mother too often failed to thrive in her absence. Rochester closed a discussion detailing the impact of mothers working with a cogent observation: "In general then, the baby whose mother works away from home during pregnancy or during the baby's first year pays dearly for the physical strain to the mother and for the lack of a mother's care."[53]

Rochester's study, having conclusively demonstrated that the roots of infant mortality lay in poverty, substandard living conditions and discrimination, nonetheless placed the onus on the mother to stay with the infant. The Children's Bureau could offer few answers to the problems facing Baltimore's poor families. The pamphlets, magazines and films intended to teach proper mothering were perhaps helpful, but could do nothing to alleviate the socioeconomic realities thwarting much of what the Bureau recommended. Domiciles without plumbing could not maintain the proper standards of hygiene; families with insufficient income could not afford for the mother to stay at home. The Bureau's response controverted those realities. Despite comprehension of the deep social roots at the heart of infant mortality, Rochester used the evidence she collected to promote a policy advocating mothers be at home. Working women were an aberration.[54]

Rochester's report mirrored the perspective of the Children's Bureau staff. Motherhood was to be privileged above all else; to the Bureau, a child's welfare depended on the traditional mother in the home. Creating and driving public policy, Bureau reformers used their positions to uphold a traditional social system giving little credence to women as workers. A widow with children should be given a pension rather than go out to work. The solution to infant mortality was mothers living domestic lives, cleaning house, bearing and raising children. Anna Rochester and Mary Sherwood failed to see the irony in the position they upheld.[55]

* * *

Rarely in American history have policy makers woven together issues of infant and children's well-being as one with maternal health care. The Great War and the accompanying burst of nationalism augured profound awareness of a future rooted in the survival and health of the next generation. That platform informed the efforts of the Children's Bureau through the 1920s. The perceived needs of the military assisted the Bureau in their efforts to press for new federal child welfare policies. In May and June of 1919, the Bureau sponsored a series of conferences to promote definition of the scientific approach to child care, culminating in a White House Conference on Standards of Child Welfare. Experts in the field gathered from across the United States, joined by several participants from Europe.[56]

The tumult attending the end of the Great War prevented the gathering of a single discussion forum, but the series of meetings did promote a productive exchange, resulting in a volume titled *Standards of Child Welfare*. The science of child care as understood by the Children's Bureau achieved definition.[57] The work delineated three areas of concern: the public protection of the health of mothers and children, the protection of children entering employment, and the needs of children requiring special care. Measures of expected physical growth were established; the norms of care described. For American families to meet the defined standards, fathers should receive an adequate wage; mothers could then remain at home. Though there was considerable talk of a scientific revolution in childcare, conference expectations painted a picture of a very traditional household.[58]

With one notable exception. The experience of childbirth:

> Maternity or prenatal centers sufficient to provide for all cases not receiving prenatal supervision from private physicians; the work of such centers to include adequate examination, instruction in the hygiene of maternity and infancy, adequate instruction and care in the home afforded by visiting public-health nurses and adequate medical and nursing care at confinement, whether in the home or in the hospital.[59]

Not a word about midwives. Motherhood was to remain entirely domestic; birth would be medicalized.

* * *

The Children's Bureau had always been careful to separate itself from medical practice, appointing social workers to administrative positions rather than physicians. Ongoing struggles with the medical profession characterized the Bureau's work in the 1920s. Attempting to provide women in rural areas access to proper health care, the Bureau in 1921 achieved passage of the Maternity and Infancy Protection Act (better known as the Sheppard-Towner Act), providing grants to states to establish maternity consultation centers, public health nursing programs, and childcare seminars.[60] Opposition from the United States Public Health Service influenced the shape of the legislation. The Service, responsible for federal research into disease and prevention, sanitation, sewage disposal and water supply, wanted control of Sheppard-Towner funds, arguing medical considerations should govern the intended programs. A compromise allowed medical authority to gain a foothold. Control of the budget remained the responsibility of the Children's Bureau, with the provision that the monies be dispersed for educational and preventative health programs only.[61]

The American Medical Association—an organization that did not admit women until 1915, formed a "women's auxiliary" in 1922—resisted passage of the act, maintaining the measure was an intrusion into medical practice. The stipulation that Sheppard-Towner funds not be dispersed for direct medical care brought grudging compromise.[62] Over the next eight years, some three thousand prenatal care centers opened across the nation, 180,000 infant care centers. Some states employed funds to train and license midwives. The efforts were remarkably successful, showing particular success in lowering infant mortality rates.[63] Yet AMA resistance gained steam, coupled to public protests resulting from fears of communism and feminism. The program came to a final end in 1929, just as the Great Depression struck. General practitioners and obstetricians eagerly converted several of the maternity and infant clinics to private practice.[64]

AMA lobbyists and conservative politicians sought to redefine and perhaps erase the entire Children's Bureau. Calling for a White House Conference on Child Protection and Health in 1930, President Herbert Hoover limited involvement in planning to physicians, shutting out participation from the Children's Bureau. Hoover conducted negotiations intended to turn the Bureau over to the Public Health Service, believing that medical professionals more properly should govern programs promoting child welfare. While a last minute campaign preserved the Bureau's future, the increasing power of privatized medicine became apparent.[65]

* * *

Unlike the Children's Bureau, AASPIM was a private organization, heavily influenced by the medical community. Though much of the association's work was educational, paralleling the efforts of the Bureau, emphasis varied. Elected president of AASPIM in 1914, Williams used the opportunity to present a paper further pursuing his particular brand of prenatal care. Drawing on the records of ten thousand births at Johns Hopkins Hospital, Williams charted 705 fetal deaths, finding syphilis the most prevalent, followed by "Unknown Causes." Dystocia—obstructed birth, most often caused by cephalopelvic disproportion—ranked third, resulting in 124 infant deaths—17.4 percent. Borrowing the language of eugenics, he later called these deaths "the unnecessary wastage of foetal life."[66]

Williams voiced surprise to discover that deaths attributed to "abnormal" pelves occurred more frequently among whites than Blacks, having long contended that deformed pelves occurred far more frequently in African American women. Unsurprisingly, his determined adherence to racial science provided an explanation. Recognizing African American women had more premature babies dying in the first week after birth, he attributed that statistic "to the lack of care and intelligence which so frequently characterizes that race."[67]

Having emphasized race as a significant factor in infant deaths resulting from dystocia, Williams lamented that prenatal care could have saved many lives. Such care was to his thinking entirely obstetrical, to be carried out within the confines of medical supervision. Recognition of dystocia was beyond the abilities of the most skillful nurse; expectant women should be educated to submit to an examination by a physician at least a month before delivery. If diagnosed with a deformed pelvis, "these women should not be delivered in their own homes by a doctor or a midwife," but only in a well-equipped surgical hospital.[68] Under Williams's tutelage, the AASPIM solution to every aspect of infant mortality was to be found in medical intervention.

AASPIM's stated purpose—the reduction of infant mortality—attracted multiple shades of participation. Reflecting Progressive Era reform, membership discussed and promoted programs ranging from health education to the suppression of midwifery, the necessity of operative obstetrics, the deadly pall of eugenics. The influence of hardline medical science emphasized by J. Whitridge Williams did not endure. Changing its name to the American Child Hygiene Association in 1918, the organization transferred headquarters from Baltimore to Washington D.C. four years later, determined to concentrate their efforts on raising public awareness of proper hygiene. Secretary of Commerce Herbert Hoover initiated consolidation with a similar group in 1923, establishing the American Child Health Organization in New York City.[69] Despite losing a pulpit for his views, Williams's career gathered strength at Johns Hopkins Hospital.

* * *

For years Williams had dreamed of a building housing more ideal facilities for the practice and teaching of obstetrics. The Women's Clinic—five stories high, offering sixty obstetrical beds, sixty-six gynecological beds in semi-private cubicles—opened in 1922. Williams became head of the newly established Obstetrics Department. Firmly entrenched in his own authority, he extended his reach, determined to bring every aspect of childbirth under obstetrical supervision.[70]

One such measure was birth control. Joined by Raymond Pearl

(1879–1940), director of biological research at Johns Hopkins, and Adolf Meyer (1866–1950), professor of psychiatry, Williams reached out to community reformers in Baltimore to establish the Bureau of Contraceptive Advice, opened in 1927. Unassociated with the University, the Bureau was headed by Doctor Bessie Moses (1893–1965), daughter of an influential local judge—one more underappreciated female graduate of the Hopkins Medical School, taking up a subsidiary position.[71]

Birth control offered an alternative approach to conditions Williams had isolated in obstetrical practice. Planned pregnancies presented the possibility of a more thorough monitoring by physicians, lessening the chance of an unfortunate outcome. Many reformers involved in the national campaign to better infant and maternal mortality rates participated in the growing birth control movement, headed by Margaret Sanger (1879–1966). Demands for access to birth control were an important component of the drive for women's rights, yet at the same time signified an expansion of medical authority over women's lives. Doctors would be in charge of the dissemination of contraception. Services at Baltimore's Bureau of Contraceptive Advice were strictly limited to married women.[72]

The "science" of eugenics permeated practice at the Bureau. Adolf Meyer, member of the supervisory board, was a formal associate of the American Eugenics Society; Raymond Pearl and J. Whitridge Williams were at the least fellow travelers.[73] Each tried to play down any affiliation, but eugenic tenets shaped their perspective.[74] Meyer helped to establish the concept of "mental hygiene," grafting eugenic notions onto psychiatric research. His essay, "The Right to Marry," laid out an approach to controlling reproduction by limiting marriage to those determined eugenically fit. Mirroring the oft-expressed Progressive contention that belief in individual rights was the product of an outmoded past, Meyer advocated a mediated involuntary limitation on reproduction. For Meyer and his associates, contraceptive planning was more than families deciding when to have children; the underlying purpose was to determine who should have little ones at all.[75]

Eugenics as a force in American politics and life reached an apex during the 1920s. The racial component was complicated. Many believed the Black race inferior; laws in thirty-eight states prohibited inter-racial marriage. Williams argued that miscegenation was in part responsible for the high overall maternal mortality of American women, writing in 1928 that "colored women may be constitutionally inferior to white women.... It has occurred to me that [the mortality rate] may be due to some constitutional inability to resist infection which has developed as a result of the admixture of races in this country."[76]

Others defined inferiority in terms of intelligence, maintaining the "feebleminded" had to be barred from reproduction, regardless of race, creed or color. Margaret Sanger and W.E.B. DuBois voiced eugenic theories; neither was racist. Several states outlawed marriage of those with physical or mental disabilities. Intelligence tests identified many defined as mentally unfit while becoming enormously popular as a tool for measuring child development.[77] Thirty-two states adopted legislation permitting sterilization for those deemed genetically degenerate, incompetent, or criminal. The United States Supreme Court upheld the constitutionality of such measures in 1927. Three years earlier, Congress had enacted laws essentially cutting off immigration of "inferior" peoples from southern and Eastern Europe. Eugenicists saw poverty and substandard hygienic conditions as products of genetic inferiority, an indication that Blacks and immigrants should be especially subject to control. Fearing race suicide, America was taking Galtonian pseudo-science to the illogical extreme.[78]

By 1928, Williams had become fully cognizant of his eugenic affinities, referring specifically in print to the concept for the first time. "I found I was brought into contact with many questions of eugenics which I could not face without sympathy, but whose practical implications I could not follow without doing violence to my inherited and acquired medical conscience."[79] The observation, offered at roughly the midway point of an article discussing "Indications for Therapeutic Sterilization in Obstetrics," prefaced discussion of fifteen sterilizations undertaken after psychiatric assessment. The diagnoses included dementia, epilepsy, psychosis, postencephalitic depression, and four cases of "pronounced feeblemindedness." Williams had performed a considerable number of sterilizations to protect the physical health of women, but these cases were different. The patients suffered with "maladjustments" and were "human misfits," "undesirable citizens."[80] Sterilization seemed to Williams the natural therapy. To his credit, he described thorough-going efforts to inform patients and gain permission to sterilize, emphasizing the need to contact a guardian in the case of a minor.[81] Yet his embrace of race explanation persisted. "The great majority of such cases have occurred in colored women, many of whom were of such rudimentary intelligence." Williams reserved the right to unilaterally sterilize a patient without her consent.[82]

He detailed a case exhibiting the qualities he considered sufficient to justify sterilization:

> A colored girl, aged 19, had a generally contracted rachitic pelvis of such degree as to afford absolute indication for cesarean section. She was referred to us with the statement that she had a mental age of 8 years and had several times been arrested for petty thievery ... we had abundant opportunity for observing her and the unanimous opinion was that she was the least intelligent

patient who had been in the service for years, and that it was improbable that she could care for her child.[83]

A case of rachitic contracted pelvis leading to a Caesarean section, followed by sterilization. Most obstetricians would have supported the Caesarean, a procedure that saved the life of both patient and child. The decision to proceed with sterilization, based on the woman's behavior and intelligence, was far more troubling. A second case involved "an imbecile white girl" brought to the attention of Johns Hopkins by the state's attorney. Her uterus was amputated.[84]

The article on "therapeutic sterilization" defended a practice long utilized. While Williams may not have made specific reference to eugenic considerations until 1928, sterilization was an aspect of his practice as early as 1910. In an article published in 1922, obstetrical associate John W. Harris analyzed the results of sixty-four Caesarean Sections performed at Johns Hopkins, concluding that "we have always taken the view that hopelessly deformed or mentally defective patients from the lower classes should be sterilized."[85]

The article revealed two important points. First, the position Williams put forth was an institutional, not an individual perspective. Sterilization of the "unfit" was the *practice* in the Hopkins Hospital and dispensary; the point of view cultivated among students and faculty. Secondly, by the early 1920s a defensiveness had surfaced, or at least an impulse to revisit and clarify a policy that had *always* been in place. There was no inclination to end the arbitrary sterilizations. Defense came through the mustering of statistics.[86]

Engaging criticism from a colleague in 1915, Williams stated that as a Southerner, "I do not have a Puritan conscience." He would continue his practice of arbitrary sterilization. Discussing the shift to tubal ligation in 1920, he superficially probed the ethics of the surgery. "In Baltimore we have the question of the ignorant colored woman, and whenever we got a colored woman who had had several illegitimate pregnancies required Caesarean section I took the uterus out for the good of the community."[87] A majority of his sterilization cases involved African American women with contracted pelves. J. Whitridge Williams was truly playing the deity, making women's reproductive decisions for them, bringing both medicine and eugenics to bear. Maryland was one of the few states to never pass a eugenic sterilization law.[88]

"Based on data derived from the ongoing record keeping at Johns Hopkins, Williams (working with Doctor Ko Chi Sun) believed incidence of rachitic pelves among Black women was increasing, stating in 1926 that seven African American women now presented rachitic pelves where four had previously."[89] Reminiscent of his address as president of AASPIM in 1914, Williams again interpreted the evidence for abnormal pelves through the persistent lens of race science, insisting the increase was a sign of degeneration. He did note that a greater percentage of white women also exhibited signs of rachitic pelvis, but maintained that few were extremely contracted. Analyzing conditions among whites, Williams determined that the most common form of contraction—the simple flat (non-rachitic) pelvis—carried probably the greatest implications for childbirth. Though the contraction was less severe, statistics showed that infant death occurred more frequently during or after the labor of white women with the condition.[90] His response was to further lower the standard diagonal measure defining contraction (established in 1905), from 13.0 centimeters down to 10.5 centimeters. More operative obstetrics for white women, more Caesarean sections. Among Blacks, the charts showed a greater number of spontaneous and healthy births, despite a greater degree of contraction. Williams explained the difference as a product of racial characteristics, reminiscent of the observations advanced in 1914:

> The generally contracted rachitic pelvis should be regarded as a manifestation of degeneration, and that the child takes part in the process, as manifested by its smaller size.... White women presenting flat pelves ... manifest no signs of physical degeneration, frequently exceed the average in height and weight, and have babies of more than average size.[91]

In Williams's view, white women could become victims of their own racial superiority. Destined to give birth to larger babies, larger skulls especially, a flat pelvis could pose serious problems. They needed greater supervision during birth.

The authors crowned their eugenic thesis by making one of the strongest and most expansive statements on the subject ever published:

> Small children are associated with all of the generally contracted types of abnormal pelvis, and relatively large ones with the simple flat and typical funnel varieties.... It would appear plausible to assume that the generally contracted types may be regarded as stigmata of degeneration, and that the imperfect development of the pelvis represents only one of the manifestations of the generally imperfect development.... The children would participate in the maternal characteristics and a certain plausibility is lent to this view by the fact that the smallest children in both races are associated with the generally contracted pelvis; and it would not require a great stretch of imagination to assume that that type of deformity may be regarded as a manifestation of extreme physical degeneration.[92]

The language of degeneration pervades the essay. Williams suspected that African Americans as a people were doomed, with or without prenatal care.⁹³ The editor of *The American Journal of Obstetrics and Gynecology* printed a disclaimer, accepting no responsibility for the views and statements contained in the study.⁹⁴

The inconsistencies in the article are striking. Determined to interpret contracted pelvis in labor through a racial lens, Williams and his co-author determined that Black women required more surgeries for birth and suffered a mortality rate two and a half times greater than whites, yet white women's cases cried for greater attention. Perceived racial distinctions proved so potent, the authors could not see the distortions read into their statistics. Beginning with an assumption of racial difference, the data took shape to the conclusions wanted. The sole piece of truly significant information was recognition that the impact of rickets was seen to increase in the 1920s.⁹⁵

Reflecting on his explorations of Caesarean section in 1921, Williams expressed measured optimism in a momentary consideration of the incidence of rickets. Underscoring the high presence of rachitic pelves among Black women, he suggested that "if the application of suitable dietetic and hygienic measures should eventually lead to the disappearance of rickets, Caesarean section would be very rarely indicated in the black race."⁹⁶

* * *

While J. Whitridge Williams responded to the growing frequency of contracted pelves by focusing on experimental development of Caesarean section, others looked to what was in many cases the root of the problem: the ever growing incidence of rickets. Pediatricians such as Alfred Hess and Edwards Park perceived a near universal incidence in some American populations. Doctor J.H. Mason Knox, inaugural president of the now defunct AASPIM, attended carefully to the subject. Writing as a faculty member at the Johns Hopkins School of Public Hygiene and Health and chief of the Bureau of Child Hygiene for the state of Maryland, his article published in 1924 demonstrated the dominant presence of rickets among rural children, Black and white. A study undertaken in the City of Baltimore released two years later found that 70 percent of Black children under age two suffered from rickets, and 30 percent of white children. Pelvic deformities were evident. Assumptions of degeneracy did not cloud the analysis; Knox explicitly denounced racial determinism in the health of Black children, emphatically stating, "there is no marked physical inferiority inherent in the negro race." He went on to argue that Blacks were reproducing at a healthy rate, that the "excessive morbidity and mortality rates among negro infants are due to conditions which are a menace to the whole population, white and black alike."⁹⁷ Knox devoted considerable time and effort improving the supply of safe milk to the poorer sections of Baltimore.⁹⁸

Working with the Pediatrics Department at Yale University, the Children's Bureau launched a study of rickets in New Haven, Connecticut, in 1923. Children's Bureau governance meant the demonstration would focus on the education of mothers. Emphasizing the idea that proper use of cod liver oil and sunlight could alleviate mild chronic rickets, The project's director, Martha May Eliot, labeled the project "the control of rickets."[99]

* * *

Control was a concept implicit in Progressive Reform. Actors in this history sought control of rickets, control of conception, control of midwives, control of hygiene, control of birth. At every turn, America was confronted by expert reformers, determined to reshape a nation's behavior in the name of science. The consequences reached into the most fundamental experiences in American life.

FOURTEEN

Solving the Riddle of Rickets

In Europe, physicians continued to follow the path established in the 1850s by Guztav Michaëlis and Carl Litzmann, exploring the physiology of rachitic disease. The work was imperative. A long line of analysts—Rudolf Virchow and August Hirsch in Germany, Armand Trousseau in France, Max Kassowitz in Austria, Leonard Findlay in Britain—repeatedly demonstrated the impact of rickets on European populations increasingly urban and industrial. In the early years of the twentieth century, studies employing new methodologies, built on preceding research, imparted a more exacting picture of the course and effects of the disease. Rarely alluding to race difference in the etiology of rickets, European research remained relatively unclouded by such constructions, while the vast number of cases provided the basis for numerous publications. Whatever doubts persisted regarding the connection between contracted pelvis and rachitic disease essentially evaporated.

The work of Austrian physicians Carl Breus and Alexander Kolisko expanded understanding of the symptomatology of rickets. After years of cadaveric research, the pathologists published a series of volumes in 1904, confirming perceptions of pelvic narrowing with the onset and progress of rickets. Few had examined the effects of the disease on infant pelves. Case studies numbering in the hundreds detailed the rachitic deformities found in the skeletal remains of babies, children, and adults—many twisted into contortions scarcely shadowing life.[1]

In 1909, Dresden pathologist Georg Schmorl (1861–1932) published data and analysis derived from the cadavers of 386 children aged from two months to four years, autopsied between 1901 and 1908.[2] The large number of subjects available reflected the high rate of infant death associated with rickets, 221 of the necropsies were of children under the age of eighteen months; death had been attributed to a variety of causes. Schmorl found an 89.4 percent incidence of rickets, with most dying before three months of age. The findings revealed the frequency of hidden rickets as well as different stages of the disease, some active, some inactive.[3]

Fourteen. Solving the Riddle of Rickets 221

Schmorl's study took medicine beyond the patient's skin, showing that skin color was not a defining factor. Histology—the minute study of the structure and composition of tissue and bone—provided the real evidence for presence of the disease. Exacting exploration of bone development and the process of healing contributed essentially to comprehension of the pathology. The work established anew that a high percentage of children, regardless of race, most presumably white, suffered from the disease, often without being diagnosed until after death. Rickets was an even more ominous presence in the general population than previously suspected. A landmark in rickets studies, Schmorl's study typified the strength of a German practice combining clinical and pathological methodology.[4]

Medical researchers throughout the Western world—pediatricians and obstetricians alike—cited the work of Schmorl, Breus and Kolisko for decades. The works became irreplaceable as the rate of infant death fell, the availability of children's bodies to autopsy lessened, and the Great War came, limiting European medical research of this nature. In Europe and America, physicians continued to regard the conclusions drawn from autopsy studies the most telling and reliable evidence for the etiology of rickets.

While physicians lauded the cadaveric studies of the early twentieth century, interest in the newly developed Roentgen ray attracted considerable attention. By the years of the Great War, physicians were using X-rays on living patients to diagnose rickets. German physicist Wilhelm Roentgen discovered the phenomenon during studies of the electromagnetic spectrum in 1895, describing the experience as "truly sensational."[5] An invisible ray allowing the viewer to peer through the skin at the shadows of bones seemed impossible: thus the X-ray—the incomprehensible. Initially, application was direct and basically without bounds; researchers maintained Roentgen rays were a form of natural light and hence harmless. Several years were needed to measure the strength of the rays and standardize their use, at least to a degree.[6] X-rays were a dangerous tool; the temptations fascinating. In the first decades of use, many doctors were unable to restrain themselves, producing untold harm. Some thought the ray's potential curative, though serious injuries quickly became obvious. Doctors eventually recognized the risk of sterilization. The study of rickets was an obvious application, offering the opportunity to diagnose and track the progress of the disease. Young children were radiographed far too often. Pregnant women too. In America, Yale University obstetrician Herbert Thoms developed X-ray methodology to measure prenatal pelves and identify contractions, a new and dangerous form of pelvimetry.[7]

* * *

The association between rachitic disease and contracted pelves was entirely clear to European eyes. In 1911, Doctor Amand Routh, gynecologist at two major London hospitals, reported on the results of a survey analyzing the growing incidence of Caesarean section throughout Britain. More than one hundred physicians responded, providing details of 1282 surgeries performed between 1890 and 1910. The widely-read study definitively linked the surgical practice to the presence of rickety contracted pelves. Of the twenty-eight Caesareans performed before 1891, all but two had resulted from contracted pelves; eight of the women died. Dividing cases over the next two decades into five year increments, Routh traced the considerable growth in use of the surgery. Eighty-three Caesareans were performed between 1891 and 1895 (sixty-two the result of contracted pelves); by the years 1906 to 1910, the total had grown to 711. Of the twentieth-century cases, 83.4 percent derived from contracted pelvis. Death rates dropped significantly as surgeons refined the practice, falling to 5.3 percent maternal death in the years 1906 to 1910.[8]

Undertaking a more detailed study of cases for the year 1904, Routh listed eighty-six Caesarean sections performed over the year. Descriptions of the condition dictating the surgery varied with the reporting physician, but the overall indication was clear. Forty cases reported a contracted pelvis, another twenty-five cataloged rachitic pelves, seven noted a "flat" pelvis. All told, 83.7 percent of Caesareans resulted from pelvic deformation. Unlike America, where mental gymnastics attributed varying degrees of contraction to racial characteristics, British physicians recognized that the vast majority of cases were the product of rickets. Of the eighty-six cases occurring in Britain in 1904, twenty-four developed in Glasgow, Scotland, the most industrially polluted city in the Kingdom.[9]

The British Medical Research Committee and Advisory Council, established by Parliament in 1913 to disperse funds allotted for research, granted support for a study of rickets in Glasgow. Conducted in 1917 by Miss Margaret Ferguson, who undertook house-to-house visits in "suitable districts," the study was directed by Leonard Findlay (and D. Noël Paton). In an introductory history of rickets accompanying the report, Findlay again propounded his theory of exercise and fresh air as the cure for rickets, initially advanced in 1908. Findlay drew heavily from Georg Schmorl's Dresden autopsy studies to define the physical characteristics of the disease.[10]

Ferguson's sociological framework substantiated Findlay's premises. Relying on a list of children identified by a Royal Hospital in Glasgow, Ferguson visited 450 families with a rachitic child, and 200 households free of rickets. Rickets was exceedingly common among children and pregnant women in Glasgow, as were contracted pelves. Findlay concluded rickets affected about fifty percent of "the general population" of children.[11] Surveys tracked the health of families and the household income, examining hygienic practice in a comparative model. Hygiene was flexibly defined, encompassing a family's blood inheritance, the design and cleanliness of the home, family income, health of mother, the individual child's health. Dietary considerations were limited to questions of the length of breastfeeding, artificial feeding, caloric intake, and fat consumption. There was no attempt to evaluate potential antirachitic factors in food. Ferguson found that "the actual conditions of the home" heavily influenced the development of rickets, that "the cleanliness of the house was distinctly better in the non-rachitic than in the rachitic family." Among the conclusions summarizing the findings of the study, Findlay reiterated his contention that "inadequate air and exercise seem to be potent factors in determining the onset of rickets."[12]

The report enlivened a growing debate among researchers seeking a solution to the problem of rickets. Many argued against the applicability of the survey, especially as contrasted with newly developed laboratory studies in nutrition and vitamins. If some nutritional lack was at the root of rachitic disease, the fresh air and exercise advocated by the Edinburgh School had to be a chimera.[13]

The long years of the First World War profoundly influenced the trajectory of research on the topic of rickets. In many ways, the war was fought over food supply. A global economy had made European nations increasingly dependent on foreign sources; cutting off an enemy's import of food and fertilizers became essential strategy. Neutral observers reported widespread war-oedema—swelled bellies, the result of malnourishment. The post-war era witnessed a catastrophic increase in rickets. War-time babies and young children in central Europe suffered especially, motivating a new scramble to uncover the origin of the disease. Late rickets appeared in great numbers among youth maturing on near starvation diets. Osteomalacia multiplied, many women endured bone weakening attributed to starvation. Researchers pursued the study of both diseases to better understand what they were, their relationship to one another and to malnutrition. In such a context, nutritional deficiency seemed an obvious answer.[14]

As early as 1901, English biochemist Frederick Gowland Hopkins had suspected that the recognized components of the human diet—the proteins, carbohydrates, the fats and so forth—inadequately explained the chemistry of nutrition. There had to be additional factors, minute substances critical to growth. Casimer Funk's 1912 discovery of what came to be known as Vitamin A proved an initial indication. Chair of Biochemistry at Cambridge University, Hopkins in 1912 published the results of a series of animal feeding experiments confirming "the importance of accessory factors in normal dietaries."[15] By 1920, Hopkins had demonstrated that heating and aeration could destroy Vitamin A, an essential step in the identification of further vitamins.[16] As an influential member of British Medical Research Committee, Hopkins played a significant role in Ferguson's Glasgow study, but his engaged and creative approach most importantly served his student, Edward Mellanby. In 1918, Mellanby was awarded a grant to conduct an investigation of rickets.[17]

Mellanby chose to experiment with dogs, feeding them exclusively on a diet of milk and oatmeal, seeking a nutritional factor. Keeping his subjects indoors, he inadvertently created conditions producing rickets, becoming the first to induce the disease in dogs.[18] The result unfortunately misled Mellanby to conclude cereal was a cause of rickets, prompting physicians to misinform patients and their families. Influenced by research from America, Mellanby continued his experiments through 1921, eventually concluding that a diet rich in animal fats such as butter, suet, and cod liver oil reduced or eliminated rachitic symptoms. Vitamin A—the fat-soluble vitamin—looked to be the cure. The Medical Research Committee credited him with having found what they called the "anti-rachitic factor," substantiating the contention that the dietary factor was the cause of rickets.[19]

While Mellanby studied dogs in England, Doctor Kurt Huldschinsky faced heart-rending conditions in Germany. Serving as a medic during the Great War, Huldschinsky, a pediatrician of Polish heritage, faced one of the many tragic conditions of the conflict's aftermath: as many as half of German children suffered from rickets. Aware of studies promoting the positive effects of sunlight, the doctor experimented with the various heliotherapies popular at the time, exploring different wave lengths, including X-rays. Trying newly marketed mercury-vapor lamps producing ultraviolet light in the winter of 1919, Huldschinsky found the lamps completely healed bone lesions from rickets within two months. His report could only add to the general consternation regarding the disease. How could a fat-soluble vitamin and an ultra-violet lamp both be cures?[20]

Britain's Medical Research Committee, in cooperation with London's Lister Institute for Preventative Medicine, determined to undertake a prolonged survey designed specifically to address the question. The study took place in Vienna, the once enviable urban center of the Austro-Hungarian Empire, hub of medical knowledge and innovation, now an occupied city. The epidemic of rickets among infants and children wrought by the war provided an opportunity to study the disease in the light of the newly published, critically important experimental research.[21]

Dame Harriet Chick, microbiologist and nutritionist at the Lister

Institute, headed the study, which treated as many as sixty children at a time at three different Vienna clinics. Despite the victory of the Allied Forces in the war, friendship, respect and deference persisted among the international team of doctors. German and Austrian influence remained strong in medicine and science. (Ironically, Clemens Von Pirquet, the star inaugural director of the Harriet Lane Home, headed one of the clinics in the study.) Dame Chick and her partners initiated competing therapies designed to test either the efficacy of cod liver or the effects of ultraviolet light. The studies, lasting from 1919 to 1922, involved intricate comparisons of light and diet, maintaining flexibility in treating the babies relative to their health. Based in part on the work of Hopkins and Mellanby, researchers assumed that a deficiency of fat was at work. Similar to other studies—those of Alfred Hess in particular—researchers varied the dosages of each to determine what amounts proved most effective. The greater success resulted from administration of cod liver oil, but exposure to ultraviolet radiation worked as well. Time series photographs of children progressing from sickness to health reflected the pleasure caregivers derived from the work. One byproduct of the study was visual demonstration of the falseness of the idea that race was a causative factor in rickets. These Austrian children were undeniably white.[22]

The Vienna study once more verified the presence of an anti-rachitic factor in cod liver oil. The work of Edward Mellanby, published while the study was ongoing, seemed to indicate that the accessory factor was Vitamin A, the fat-soluble vitamin. Moreover, there was the indisputable fact, conclusively demonstrated in Vienna, that ultraviolet light was an equally effective treatment for rickets. The mystery deepened with a report out of India.

Doctor H.S. Hutchinson, an English physician seasoned in the British colony, conducted a study in the Nasik portion of Bombay, modeled after the work of Margaret Ferguson in Glasgow. Assisted by an Indian researcher, Hutchinson strove to survey the presence of rickets objectively, focusing on social factors but adding groups to the analysis, controlling for the class and caste status so essential to Indian society.[23] His conclusion was startling: the chief victims of rickets were among the upper classes of strictly Purdah (face-covering) Hindu and "Mahomedan" (Islamic) people.[24] Examining hygienic practice and the impact of religious belief, Hutchinson found clear distinctions in daily habits. These people enjoyed a better diet by the standards of the time—meaning a diet of meat, fat, and milk—and far better hygiene than the poor. Obviously there was a sizably larger intake of the fat soluble vitamin, yet the onset of rachitic disease was far more common than among the poor. Exposed to famine, poor children were scorbutic but not rachitic. Interpreting his evidence,

Hutchinson argued that neither race nor diet caused the rickets, but rather the cultural practices among the upper classes that kept women and children indoors. Women in confinement following birth obeyed far greater restrictions of movement—with few degrees of difference among the religious cultures. Hindu women felt the greater restrictions, with strict confinement for months, the infant as well, and the enforced wearing of the purdah. Breastfeeding did not keep the infant from rickets. For well-to-do Hindu families, the incidence of rickets was 38.2 percent, while among the poor, 6.4 percent. For the Mahomedan families, where the cultural differences lessened, Hutchinson tallied 28.5 percent rickets among wealthier children, 24.6 percent in the poor. The result was clear—access to open air and exercise prevented rickets. The dark, smoky confines of the tightly constructed wealthy homes increased the vulnerability of infants to rickets.[25] Poorer women and children made do with a lesser diet, but enjoyed a far more active outdoor life. Hutchison concluded that "a deficiency of fat-soluble vitamin cannot be the principle cause of rickets," crediting the Glasgow School's identification of "fresh air, sunlight and exercise" as the correct theory to understand the disease.[26] His report was mostly neglected by medical researchers, his quiet insistence that race did not account for the origin of rickets ignored.

* * *

Interest in vitamins was by no means limited to European scientists. Not long after Casimer Funk isolated the "vitamine," Elmer McCullom, a biochemist at the University of Wisconsin, began a series of studies on cattle, experimenting with various grains to determine the optimal diet to encourage growth. The question of bone development led him to research the presence of vitamins. Beginning in 1912, McCullom and his team undertook a series of nutritional studies, employing a new experimental animal, the rat. Concentrating on food factors in butterfat, the team identified the characteristics of vitamin A, the fat-soluble vitamin. (This was the research drawing the attention of Edward Mellanby.) By 1915, McCullom had discovered what was initially deemed the water-soluble vitamin, later designated vitamin B, a factor found to promote growth.[27]

Johns Hopkins University took note. Obtaining a grant from the Rockefeller Foundation, the university opened a School of Hygiene and Public Health in 1916; William Welch successfully recruited Elmer McCullom to become Professor of Chemical Hygiene. Taking up the position in 1917, McCullom brought along several coworkers from Wisconsin. John Howland, Director of the Harriet Lane Home, pulled McCullom into rickets research, organizing a multi-faceted approach. Howland and his associates were constantly refining their research into bone metabolism and

Fourteen. Solving the Riddle of Rickets

the chemistry of the blood; McCullom provided a different dimension with his work on food factors. Working under Howland, Paul G. Shipley conducted pathological research; Benjamin Kramer remained the expert in micromethodology. Returning from France in 1919, Edwards A. Park renewed his position as a member of the research team. Nina Simmonds worked with McCullom in the Department of Chemical Hygiene.[28] The question to be addressed: did vitamin A treat rickets?

Alfred Hess did not think so. Following the Columbus Hill study of rickets, Hess had turned his attention once more to scurvy, further exploring the role of antiscorbutics. Studying the international medical literature very closely, he found what he read in 1919 profoundly disturbing. Frustrated with the recent research in nutritional deficiency, he observed "There is growing danger of attributing every explained growth impulse to the new, attractive but ill-defined vitamins."[29]

The source of his dismay was the British Medical Research Committee's pronouncement that the fat-soluble vitamin—vitamin A—was the long-sought anti-rachitic factor, as evidenced by the work of Edward Mellanby.[30] Renewing his interest in rickets, Hess began a series of experiments at the Hebrew Infant Home, designed to evaluate the efficacy of vitamin A.[31] The resulting essay, published in 1920, began with a discussion of his clinical experience with children exhibiting multiple symptoms suggesting scurvy, beriberi and/or rickets. Hess outlined the distinctions among the diseases, emphasizing the influence of climate, geography, and sunlight as unique to rickets. Ninety percent of the children at the Home showed some degree of the disease. Identifying one hundred infants, Hess dispensed orange juice to children with signs of scurvy, but did not give cod liver oil to infants developing rickets, providing instead a carefully balanced formula of milk and cottonseed oil. The substitution was intended to eliminate confusion over the nutritional factors involved; cottonseed oil was rich in the fat-soluble vitamin, but offered no known ameliorative for rickets. Despite a continued regimen of vitamin A, the rachitic children showed no improvement.[32]

Concluding the essay, Hess expressed his frustration with Edward Mellanby's research and the mistaken endorsement of the Medical Research Committee (MRC). The MRC had gone so far as to publish a list of foods thought to be anti-rachitic, foods that were nothing of the kind in Hess's estimation. "It is impossible to interpret the contrary conclusion which Mellanby came to, ... or to accept the term 'fat soluble vitamin' as synonymous with 'antirachitic factor,' as Hopkins and Chick would have us do."[33]

Fully committed to research on rickets by 1921, Hess reported experimentation on the subject in fourteen further essays over the next two years. The articles came monthly, from research at the Hebrew Infant Home or the College of Physicians and Surgeons, where Hess held a research appointment. Several considered the role of sunlight and ultraviolet radiation. Building on Huldschinsky's research, Hess experimented with carbon arc lights, which provided a stream of light more fully mimicking the sun's spectrum.[34] He found the curative power of the sun and the sources of artificial ultraviolet light "to be fundamentally the same."[35] This confirmation explained the long perceived seasonality of rickets; children born in winter were more prone to the disease due to lack of exposure to sufficient sunlight. Hess determined that the blood phosphate levels in infants rose with frequent exposure to the sun, a biochemical reaction attributed to ultraviolet radiation from the sun, rather than visible rays.[36]

Hess referred to work done by McCullom, Park and others, suggesting their conclusions were similar to his—"that light is able to exert a favorable influence on the experimental rickets of rats."[37] He had previously noted that research reported from Johns Hopkins supported his conclusion that the fat-soluble vitamin was not the anti-rachitic factor. Vitamin A could prevent beriberi; the substance had no effect on rickets. Cod liver oil had more than one accessory factor.[38]

A series of articles in *The Journal of Biological Chemistry* titled "Studies in Experimental Rickets" recorded the efforts of the Johns Hopkins group. Continued experimentation with rats was essential to the process. Guinea pigs had proven problematic in research on rickets because they did not show human-comparable symptoms. X-rays readily tracked the progress of rickets in rats; use of the animals added significantly to laboratory capabilities to investigate feed, nutritional chemistry and the pathology of the disease. The process was not without difficulties. Edwards Park wrote of the challenge of wild rats attacking the caged rats, and also the problem of the caged rats eating one another. The studies proceeded nonetheless.[39] Under Elmer McCullom's direction, dietary experiments with the rodents came to fruition in 1922.[40]

While McCullom and his associates proceeded with dietary studies, Grover Powers, Edwards Park, and Paul Shipley, with others, subjected rats to experiments based on ultraviolet light. Publishing their results in 1921, the team confirmed that the influence of radiation from a mercury-vapor quartz lamp (yet another form of heliotherapy) was nearly identical to that of cod liver oil. The interactive experiments among the large group of The Hopkins researchers, combined with the new understanding of the critical role of phosphorus and its ability to affect rickets, caused them to question "whether the antirachitic factor in cod-liver oil was identical with or distinct from Vitamin A."[41]

Edwards Park and Alfred Hess discussed the question at a meeting of

Fourteen. Solving the Riddle of Rickets

the American Pediatrics Society in 1921. Despite his profound skepticism and critical eye for the research of others, Hess's curiosity for the work of the Johns Hopkins lab team drove him to attend a paper on "The Function of the Organic Factor as Exemplified by Cod Liver Oil."[42] In the discussion after, Hess pressed Park to commit to distinguishing what they called the organic factor in cod liver oil from vitamin A. While Park agreed that it seemed possible that there was something different from the vitamin A, he remained cautious. "If two organic factors exist distinct from each other, we have not succeeded in finding them separate. When one is found, the other is present. Therefore, I am absolutely unwilling to commit myself to the view expressed by Dr. Hess."[43]

The studies by Frederick Gowland Hopkins demonstrating that heating and aeration destroyed vitamin A became an essential element in the Johns Hopkins research. Heating cod liver oil to near boiling point while bubbling air, McCullom and his co-workers removed all traces of the fat-soluble vitamin. The step was verified by the failure of the treated oil to cure xeropthalmia, a vitamin A deficiency disease causing abnormal dryness of the eye, prevalent during the Great War. Vitamin A removed, applications of the substance remaining nonetheless cured rickets in rats. A series of tests with further fatty substances yielded identical results. Researchers could now affirm there were in fact two fat soluble factors. Announced in Part XXI of the "Studies on Experimental Rickets," the Hopkins publication, submitted on June 20, 1922, concluded that the power of certain fats to initiate the healing of rickets depends on the presence in them of a substance which is distinct from fat-soluble A. These experiments clearly demonstrate the existence of a fourth vitamin whose specific property, as far as we can tell at present, is to regulate the metabolism of the bones.[44]

As the fourth vitamin to be identified, McCullom, following the pattern established, designated the discovery "vitamin D." In future publications, McCullom referred to the substance as the "organic factor." Edwards Park simply called the chemical property 'X,' reflecting the mysteries still surrounding its properties.

The discovery was front page news in *New York Times*.[45]

Prevention of rickets was at hand. Having conclusively demonstrated that prevention depended on consumption of vitamin D, McCullom and his associate, Nina Simmonds developed a popular guide to "the new science of nutrition." Published by the authors in 1925, the booklet began with an examination of the changes in American diet over the past sixty years. Foods were now commonly transported over long distances by railroad, refined to prolong shelf life. McCollum and Simmonds warned against the degermination of flour and rice, a process that removed essential vitamins.

Devoting chapters to each of the four vitamins discovered thus far, the authors began their discussion of D by noting that fifty to eighty percent of children suffered from rickets in some parts of the United States. As vitamin D was not abundant in most available foods, they urged regular doses of cod liver oil for all young children, and for pregnant and nursing mothers as well. Regular exposure to sunlight also helped. Cow's milk in any form would not prevent rickets. The chapter closed with a discussion of the purdah and the deleterious effects of shielding the body from the sun, acknowledging the research of H.S. Hutchinson in India.[46]

* * *

In 1918 Leonard Findlay had declared, "We have practically no real knowledge of the nature of causation of this widespread malady or of the factors which determine its onset."[47] A great deal occurred in the space of four years. Scientists now knew the anti-rachitic factor existed separately from vitamin A. They had also confirmed the effectiveness of heliotherapy in healing rickets. Both sides of this argument regarding etiology had proved correct. The environment and lack of a food supplement, and still something else, were involved in the onset of rickets. With vitamin D identified, researchers began looking for what Edwards Park called "the calcium depôt."[48] What controlled the level of calcium in the blood or the process of calcification? What happened to turn sunlight into the antirachitic factor?

Park was no longer a member of the research team at Johns Hopkins, having left the University in 1921 to become chair of the newly organized Department of Pediatrics at Yale. In a 1923 essay, titled "The Etiology of Rickets," he sought to summarize the advances in study and treatment, pointing clearly to the emergent fact that rickets was a deficiency disease. Coupled to the identification of vitamin D, John Howland's ongoing biochemical research at the Harriet Lane Home offered essential clues. "Rickets is a disturbance in the metabolism of the growing organism of such nature that the salt equilibrium, in particular as regards the calcium and phosphorus, in the circulating fluids is disturbed, and lime salts no longer deposit in the bones."[49] The proportion of calcium and phosphorus was as critical as the amount of the salts in blood and represented a factor equal in significance to a lack of the anti-rachitic factor in determining the onset of rickets.[50]

Such insights, examined in the light of the refined European research into human physiology, led to finer distinctions in the etiology of rickets, new definitions of the disease.[51] Park continued on to show how scientific investigation of cod liver oil had revealed the critical role of the substance in calcification and building of bones. Addressing the issue of heritability, Park was emphatically clear: "rickets cannot be inherited through the germ plasm."[52] Describing the origin of rickets, he observed that "the human organism is peculiarly dependent on the presence of radiant energy or its equivalent in the food and ... rickets may develop when the organism is deprived of them,"[53] noting that "pigmented skins apparently increase the susceptibility to rickets and a predisposition in that sense may be inherited."[54]

Pigmentation was not a topic widely considered. Benjamin Rush had theorized that skin pigmentation was the result of the environment, not biology. An individual with dark skin under proper circumstances could become white.[55] In the late 1890s, Doctor John Abel and assistant Walter Davis, working out of the pharmacological laboratory at Johns Hopkins, studied the chemical makeup of skin pigmentation, taking skin from an African American male cadaver. Conducting a variety of chemical treatments, Abel and Davis isolated the black pigment—"black sediment"—which fell to the bottom. Their research sought to connect skin pigmentation to a variety of diseases and conditions—rickets was not among them. The analysts undertook no exploration of function, but did briefly describe the findings of others, indicating that white skin absorbed far greater amounts of sunlight. Pigment absorbed the energy of the sun while protecting the vascular layers beneath.[56]

If exposure to ultraviolet radiation prevented or cured rickets, the ability to absorb sunlight was critical, as Park realized:

The negro and Italian children in American cities are especially susceptible to rickets because the pigment of their skin partially insulates them, so to speak, from the sun's rays, and makes them derive less benefit from that source than do fair skinned children. The diets of the negro and Italian child in our American cities are notoriously lacking in those foods which carry fat-soluble A and presumably X. The negro child in Africa does not develop rickets because he lives out of doors.[57]

Continuing the discussion, Park offered repeated examples of peoples across the globe free from rickets because of their ability to absorb sufficient sunlight in various fashions.[58]

Alfred Hess also recognized the potential effects of pigmentation on the ability to absorb ultraviolet radiation. In a series of experiments conducted on black and white Norway rats, Hess found that after measured exposure to ultraviolet light, the rats grew at the same rate, but the black rats developed rickets; the white did not. In his text, *Rickets, including Osteomalacia and Tetany*, published in 1929, Hess wrote, "This experiment has a direct application to the well-recognized susceptibility of negro infants to rickets." Hess was careful to insist that the greater degree of pigmentation was not the sole reason, but did say, "My personal opinion ... is that the negro, as well as some other southern races, evince a racial susceptibility to rickets when they migrate and live in a northern climate." Though Hess continued to perceive the epidemiology of rickets in terms of racial groups—the Italians, Greeks, and African Americans, he too eschewed the idea of rickets as a hereditary disorder.[59] Continued research convinced him beyond doubt that the disease derived from migration and extreme change of lifestyle.[60] Park and Hess both understood that the darker the pigmentation, the more sun was necessary to provide adequate presence of the anti-rachitic factor.

Hess and Park referred repeatedly to a widely heralded book published in 1922 by English physician J. Lawson Dick: *Rickets: a Study of Economic Conditions and Their Effects on the Health of the Nation*.[61] The work paralleled many of their own conclusions. Dick's perspective reiterated much David Paul von Hansemann had put forth, conditioned by the lessons of the First World War. Citing the demographics of accompanying industrialization, he wrote

> Rickets is almost wholly confined to a comparatively narrow belt running across America and Europe—a zone which is the wealthiest in the world and into which all the richest and choicest products of the earth are poured in their natural state. Today, the child and the wife of the collier live on a dietary much greater in food value and more extensive in variety than did even the wealthy of say three hundred or four hundred years ago. Notwithstanding, rickets is rampant among the colliers' children today while in these older times it was hardly known, if the evidence from the examination of the teeth, jaws and skeletons of ancient burials is to be believed.[62]

Rickets was everywhere in the industrializing world. The War had brought a sweeping epidemic of the disease; the victims were Caucasian. Simplistic racial explanations were unviable. Dick argued that the disease had compromised the manpower of the English military—though not killing outright, rickets weakened constitutions and made grown bodies vulnerable to debilities. Tuberculosis and syphilis came hand in hand with rachitic disease.[63] Edwards Park understood Dick's perspective perfectly. Recalling the Belgian orphans he had treated throughout the War, Park declared the severity of rickets cases equal only to that of the African American children in the United States.[64]

Lawson Dick was well aware of the disproportionate amount of rickets among African Americans. Noting a letter from Chicago pediatrician Clifford Grulee, he quoted, "in a large experience with negro babies in Chicago, I have never seen one between the ages of six and eighteen months, whether breast or artificially fed, that did not have very definite signs of rickets." Grulee ascribed the same conditions to babies of Greeks and Italians. He understood the phenomenon to be a result of migration from a tropical to a temperate climate.⁶⁵

Looking for rickets in America, Dick unsurprisingly found the disease in the East, in urban areas especially, but also in Chicago and in California. Associating the condition with African Americans, Italians and Greeks, Dick underlined the severity, believing rickets had overwhelmed these peoples—a subtle but important distinction from arguments maintaining racial susceptibility. Race was neither a sufficient nor a necessary explanation of rickets. Slowly but surely, perceptions were changing. Most physicians now recognized that children of all races had rickets in the United States.⁶⁶

Hess and Park each regarded David Paul von Hansemann's 1906 essay "On Rickets as a Folk Disease" one of the most important papers ever offered on the subject. Park translated a passage from von Hansemann's paper to conclude his own essay on the etiology of rickets: "Domestication does not relate merely to those things which pertain to the house ..., but refers to every effort on the part of man to further the survival of the race and of the individual by artificial means and to aid in the struggle against the forces of nature. By this definition it becomes at once apparent that not alone does man domesticate animals but has domesticated himself."⁶⁷ The answer to the problem of rickets lay in the conditions imposed by modern civilized life. A maddening conclusion, enlightening yet lacking the scientific precision necessary to actually combat the disease. Corresponding in later years, Park and Hess recognized their common ground, comprehending rickets as a pathological disease complicated by nutritional factors and a poorly understood, much misinterpreted racial component. Rickets defied simple explanation.⁶⁸

* * *

Edwards Park drew upon his experiences in post-war France to structure the Pediatrics Department at Yale University, shaping an emphasis on clinical medicine, balanced by a vision of the pediatrician as involved in "maternal-child health education."⁶⁹ Important among his decisions was the appointment of Doctor Martha May Eliot as Chief Resident and instructor in Pediatrics.

Eliot had worked with Park at Johns Hopkins, where she graduated from the Medical School in 1918. She was forced to intern elsewhere when John Howland refused to grant her an internship at the Harriet Lane Home.⁷⁰ Rejoining Park in New Haven, Eliot soon became associated with the Children's Bureau, serving as director of the Division of Child and Maternal Health, where she edited the pamphlet *Infant Care* for many years. Her work reflected a wholistic view of child health: "some Bureau in the Government should have all the interests of the child at heart."[71] Like Park, she believed social interaction with patients' families greatly improved the success of pediatric practice.[72]

Eliot explored the experiential aspect of her Children's Bureau work by directing the New Haven study of rickets. The survey of 216 babies born in New Haven began in 1923, lasting three years. Eliot titled the project "The Control of Rickets," focused on the idea that proper use of cod liver oil and sunbaths could bring mild chronic rickets under control. An important tool for the professional staff was the use of roentgen-rays. The instrument allowed physicians to look for lesions and deposits of cartilage and mineral salts in bones—the symptoms of rickets. Eliot and Park shared an enthusiasm for the new-found ability to diagnose rickets without complete reliance on clinical examination. X-rays appeared to offer a convenient replacement for what had come to seem ambiguous and untrustworthy reliance on symptoms such as enlarged epiphyses at the wrists, craniotabes, or beading of the ribs at the costochondral conjunctions (where cartilage met the bone in the sternum). Not knowing the dangers of radiation, staff enthusiastically pursued the use of the roentgenography, identifying rickets at early stages with monthly exposures. Sixty-five percent of patients were found to display signs of rickets before the age of four months; ninety percent before six months. The study concluded rickets was essentially universal among the New Haven population.[73]

Eliot and her staff set about educating mothers on how to recognize signs of rickets, give their children cod liver oil, expose the tads to adequate sun. In the winter months, the sun-bathing had to occur through an open window; plate glass blocked the ultraviolet rays. Some flexibility in the dosage of cod liver developed; the staff ultimately raised the dose to enhance effectiveness.[74]

Growth with breastfeeding was very rapid and led to large babies, a vulnerable category for rachitic disease among infants. The study found breastfed infants and premature babies to be especially at risk; virtually all the breastfed children had rickets. Analyzing breast milk, Eliot and her associates determined that no anti-rachitic factor was present. Judging by the results of the study, rickets could now be considered normal, while breastfeeding, long seen as natural, could be viewed as pathological. The conclusion added fuel to the long medical disagreement over the efficacy of breastfeeding, begun in the nineteenth century. Growing popularity of evaporated milk in the 1920s made infant formulas more attractive; by the 1950s, more than half of newborn infants in the United States were bottle fed. Though breastfeeding is today generally regarded as the healthiest nutritional option for infants, the American Academy of Pediatrics strongly recommends that vitamin D supplement the diet.[75]

Fourteen. Solving the Riddle of Rickets

Presenting a paper outlining the findings of the New Haven study at the American Medical Association meetings in 1925, Eliot declared "Our investigations have shown that a slight degree of early rickets is well nigh universal in our climate and in our state of society." Only a study of rickets in the tropics would answer the question of whether this was "normal."[76] In the discussion that followed Eliot's presentation, Park identified the key issue as whether "a mild degree of rickets is physiologic and means merely that the impetus of growth is greater than the power to calcify."[77] In other words, was a mild case of rickets simply normal for many children? Park agreed with Eliot that the disease persisted over many months with little visible change, sometimes undetected. Eliot called it "the extraordinary chronicity of rickets."[78]

Martha May Eliot continued her social approach to pediatric medicine at Yale, producing a film in 1925 presenting a clear message to parents: children need the sun. Titled *Sun Babies*, the film was funded in part by the Children's Bureau. There was no sound; subtitles were in English and Spanish. The introduction presents a romantic image of pale-skinned young children romping at a seashore. Further settings show children playing in the street with a hose, visiting the rickets clinic operated by Eliot and others. A nurse exhibits her authority by wearing a necktie. Different shades of skin represent varying ethnicities; Blacks and whites are pictured, but shown separately. Drawings illustrate bowed legs and the additional effects of rickets. Numerous scenes show babies sun bathing before an open window, or carefully placed in the sun outdoors—the mother is urged to remove her baby's coat and blanket, even in winter. Reflecting the recent discoveries in heliotherapy, the film was the one more effort on the part of the Children's Bureau to educate mothers.[79]

* * *

In his essay on the etiology of rickets, Edwards Park confessed "Knowledge concerning the metabolism of rickets is so confused that the wisdom of discussing it beyond the point of obtaining a general orientation seems doubtful."[80] He was not being gloomy. The next step in the unraveling of the mystery of rickets was very much a product of serendipity and coincidence. For all the care, the exactitude, the monotonous repetition necessary to the process, science remained a very human endeavor.

With the close of the rickets study in Vienna, members of the research team returned to the Lister Institute in London to further study the effects of ultraviolet radiation on the disease. Rats became the subjects, kept in individual lidded glass jars lined with sawdust. In 1923, researchers Harry Goldblatt and Katharine Marjorie Soames found that the livers of irradiated rats, fed to rachitic rats, promoted healing, while livers from non-irradiated rats did not.[81] Working in the same laboratory, Eleanor Margaret Hume (1887–1968) and Hannah Henderson Smith performed an experiment in which half the jars were irradiated with the rats inside; the rodents removed from the remainder to form a control group. To the surprise and consternation of the researchers, the two sets of rats exhibited almost identical healing. Perhaps air in the jars retained radiation, which the control rats absorbed on return. The experiment was repeated with an assistant blowing the air out of the jar after irradiation. The control rats no longer improved. Hume and Smith eventually realized the assistant was blowing out the sawdust, the rat feces, and the scraps of food with the air. The detritus in the jar had absorbed the radiation; when the rats consumed the food, the feces, and the sawdust on return to their jars, they imbibed the healing factor. The revelation was astonishing. Inert substances could absorb the second fat-soluble vitamin.[82]

Noting the uncorroborated work of Hume and Smith, Alfred Hess, assisted by Mildred Weinstock, undertook a series of experiments published in 1924, irradiating various fluids and foodstuffs. Working with rats, Hess ascertained that cottonseed oil and linseed oil absorbed antirachitic properties sufficient to offer protection from the disease. The oils retained the property for long periods; an "antirachitic factor therefore had been produced *in vitro* and outside the living organism."[83] Wheat grown in the dark had no effect on rickets; wheat grown in the light and irradiated proved successful. Fresh lettuce from the market was valueless; upon irradiation, the leaves became antirachitic. The accidental discovery of Hume and Smith was confirmed.[84]

The phenomenon was researched elsewhere at much the same time. Agricultural chemist Harry Steenbock (1886–1967) had assisted Elmer McCollum's fat-soluble vitamin research at the University of Wisconsin between 1912 and 1915, continued the work when his mentor departed for Johns Hopkins. Turning to studies of vitamin D, Steenbock found that "by irradiation with the quartz mercury vapor lamp, rat rations can be activated, making them growth-promoting and bone-calcifying, to the same degree as when the rats are irradiated directly."[85] Again, the discovery of Goldblatt and Soames was verified independently. Foodstuffs could absorb the anti-rachitic factor.

* * *

The history of rickets and vitamin D branches significantly at this point. Considered scientifically, the discovery of D was an essential step opening the door to further research. The nature of the vitamin remained unknown, the precise role in preventing rickets a mystery, the fact that the vitamin could be obtained through ingestion of certain foods, by exposure

Fourteen. Solving the Riddle of Rickets

to sunlight, or by consumption of irradiated foods a conundrum. Scientists addressed such questions over the next decade, shedding considerable light on the formation, composition, and behavior of D, though secrets remain to this day. From the standpoint of public health, such a comprehensive understanding of D was not critically important. While the scientists puzzled, the unassailable fact that society now possessed the practical means to eliminate rickets from the population had emerged.

* * *

Pursuing the scientific issue, Alfred Hess came to suspect that sterols—organic molecules comprising an essential component of cell membrane structure—could hold the answer. Chemical research on sterols was a new field; the term was not used until 1911.[86] Cholesterol, initially identified in the eighteenth century, was now found to comprise as much as 30 percent of animal cell membrane, while phytosterol provided the function in plants. Beginning in 1925, Hess, assisted by Mildred Weinstock and F. Dorothy Helman, produced no fewer than twenty-four papers over five years, reporting continued investigation into sterols and their relation to vitamin D. Offering an early hypothesis, Hess noted

> the epidermal portion of the skin contains a large amount of cholesterol situated in its deepest layers.... It would seem quite possible that the cholesterol in the skin is normally activated by ultraviolet radiation and rendered antirachitic—that the solar rays and similar artificial radiations are able to bring about this conversion. This point of view regards the superficial skin as an organ which reacts to particular light waves (the epidermal organ) rather than as a mere protective covering.[87]

Continued research cast doubt on the conjecture. The difficulty of isolating cholesterol in pure form posed an essential problem—very possibly the impurities remaining were in fact producing the antirachitic factor. Working at the National Institute for Medical Research in London, biochemists Otto Rosenheim (1871–1955) and T.A. Webster confirmed that some substance associated with cholesterol functioned as a precursor to the formation of vitamin D. Further papers from Hess agreed. By this point, Hess was in regular communication with researchers in Britain and Germany, sharing information, offering clues. Reaching out to Adolf Windaus (1876–1959), director of biochemical research at the University of Göttingen, Germany, Hess recommended in 1926 the investigation of ergosterol, an essential component in the cell membrane of fungi (of all things). Cooperating with Rosenheim and Webster in England as well as Hess, Windaus conducted a series of experiments with rats. In 1927, Windaus and Hess published a very brief article in the *Proceedings of the*

Society of Experimental Biology and Medicine announcing that ergosterol "was found to bring about a healing process of the bones when even as little as 0.003 mg. per capita was given."[88] Windaus was awarded the Nobel Prize for the discovery in 1928; many felt Alfred Hess should have been equally recognized. Windaus gave Hess credit for his part in the discovery, and shared the monetary award.[89]

What wanted explanation was how a sterol component of fungal cell structure could combat rickets in human beings. Continuing his research on the relationship between ergosterol and cholesterol over the next several years, Windaus soon identified variant forms of the antirachitic factor, designated D_1 and D_2. Hess continued his own research into the presence of sterols in foods. Researchers at London's National Institute of Medical Research defined the chemical structure of D_2, the form appearing in foods exposed to ultraviolet radiation. Ergosterol was the precursor. In 1937, Windaus isolated D_3, a compound labeled dehydrocholesterol, demonstrating that this sterol, found in animal skin, transformed into the vitamin with irradiation.[90]

In sum, by the mid–1930s, biochemical science had successfully demonstrated that chemical reactions triggered by irradiation converted sterols in food to forms of vitamin D. Animal bodies—including human bodies—manufactured D when sterols in the skin were exposed to sunlight. The full nature of the transformation, the manner in which the vitamin facilitated the absorption of calcium in the bones, would not be understood for decades, but the essence of the riddle was at last resolved. D was the answer. Most ironic of all, researchers eventually determined D was in fact not a vitamin, but a hormone—a chemical produced by an organ of the body, transferred via the bloodstream to another organ to regulate function.[91]

* * *

Though the ongoing scientific study of vitamin D and the behavior of the human body was and is vitally important, the more immediately critical impact of the discoveries surrounding the antirachitic factor was the practical application. Vitamin D prevented or cured rickets. That one crucial fact was enough; the issue thereafter was to make certain children of every clime imbibed their proper share, whether through direct exposure to ultraviolet radiation or as part of the diet. Public health campaigns such as the *Sun Babies* film played a role, but rickets was ultimately defeated by dietary efforts.

Cod liver oil was the most obvious remedy, but the stuff was not popular with children, for understandable reasons. The solution lay in the research of the mid–1920s, the experiments of Goldblatt and Soames,

Fourteen. Solving the Riddle of Rickets

Hess, and, most importantly, Harry Steenbock. The antirachitic factor could be imbedded in foods by irradiation. The fact had been confirmed in London, in New York, in Madison, Wisconsin. Steenbock, perfecting the technique in the biochemical laboratories at the University of Wisconsin, chose to act.[92]

Steenbock was motivated in part by a desire to see the public gain access to the benefits of his discoveries, in part to prevent charlatans from taking advantage. The news regarding vitamin D spread rapidly; snake oil salesmen seized the opportunity, pushing spurious products claiming to bestow the cure. Steenbock had previously tried to persuade the University's Board of Regents to patent his research on vitamin A, touching off an ugly controversy over the propriety of a public institution taking profits from research. In the end, the Board did nothing. Realizing the immense importance (and commercial significance) of vitamin D, Steenbock considered applying for patents on his own. In the end, administration officials assisted him in the formation of the Wisconsin Alumni Research Foundation (WARF). Steenbock would apply for the patents; the Foundation would regulate the licensing of the rights to interested corporations. The profits would fund further research. Vitamin D would become an essential component of the American diet.[93]

The Quaker Oats company was among the first to apply. Diets rich in oatmeal were known to promote rickets; Quaker Oats was determined to corner the cereal market. Oats fortified with vitamin D would certainly help. A deal was reached; the company would hold exclusive rights until 1940. Five major pharmaceutical companies followed, purchasing the right to manufacture supplements and concentrates.[94]

By far, the most obvious place for the vitamin was milk. Despite the statements of Edwards Park, Elmer McCollum and others insisting whole milk could not prevent rachitic disease, milk was an essential component in the process—vitamin D somehow facilitated the calcification of bones, but the bones had to have a supply of calcium to do the task. Milk was the essential source. By 1934, WARF was licensing the supplement to several large dairies throughout the United States. The problem was getting the D into the milk: irradiating cattle food proved ineffective, irradiating the milk directly altered the taste. Eventually, the milk was fortified with concentrates.

Technical problems resolved, the addition of vitamin D to milk proved an unparalleled success. By the 1940s, rickets had essentially disappeared from American homes.[95] This, despite the grim facts of the Great Depression—the grinding poverty, the malnutrition, the inadequate living arrangements, the spiritual despair—all the conditions once imputed to the spread of rickets. The disease was astonishingly simple to eradicate. Finding the cause had been the hard part.

The benefits were many. The vast majority of America's children would grow up healthy and strong; bowed legs would no longer be a fashion issue; the military needn't worry about flat feet. Surely contracted pelves—and the attendant difficulties in childbirth—would diminish significantly. The trajectory of American medical practice would in some ways change. In others, changes already in motion would persist.

Vitamin D rapidly became not only big business, but an essential part of the physician's prerogative. Utilizing the discovery, doctors exhorted mothers of infants and young children to surrender to the advances of a new age, fully acquiesce to the wisdom of medical authority. The necessity of maintaining sufficient levels of the vitamin became one more factor supporting the drive empowering "scientific motherhood." Only a doctor could adequately explain the importance. Like birth, motherhood was to be a domain shaped and directed by the physician, further establishing the dominance of modern medicine.[96]

Conclusion

The Sum of the Equation

The etiology of rickets defied analysis for a very long time. Looking back, what amazes is the number of analysts who offered what appeared to be highly unorthodox solutions to the problem, only to be proven correct, at least in part. Sunlight? Exercise? Fats in the diet? So much desperate theorizing, attempts to explain the inexplicable. Cod liver oil? German researcher D. Schütte reported the therapeutic benefits as early as 1824.[1] Few listened. Armand Trousseau of France advocated use of the nasty-tasting stuff in 1882, only to be largely ignored.[2] When John Bland-Sutton cured the rachitic lion cubs at the London Zoo employing a selection of foodstuffs including cod liver oil, he believed the essential ingredient was fat in the diet. He was nearly correct; D is a fat-soluble vitamin.[3]

An English missionary serving overseas, Theobald Palm carefully considered matters of diet and hygiene before concluding the reason the Japanese people suffered little rachitic disease was greater exposure to the direct rays of the sun. Arguing for a "Chemistry of Light," Palm prescribed careful research into the effects of sunlight on the human body in 1890.[4] His argument was heavily influenced by the work of German geographer August Hirsch, who demonstrated an apparent relationship between incidence of rickets and latitude in the 1880s.[5] But how to explain the dark-skinned peoples of the far north, who saw nothing of rickets despite an almost complete lack of sunlight for much of the year? Perhaps rickets was better explained as an industrial disease, inherent in the process of the urbanization gripping Europe and portions of the United States. The poor diet of so many in the cities was surely a factor; pediatricians did what they could to ensure a healthy supply of fresh milk—milk built strong bones. Developing Hirsch's hypothesis, German analyst David Paul van Hansemann in 1906 argued rickets was a product of modern civilization, a consequence of the domestication of the human species.[6] Rachitic disease was a weakening of the constitution. In Scotland, physician Leonard Findlay in 1908 supported the hypothesis, contending rickets was very much a product of the modern environment. Fresh air and exercise was the answer.[7]

Such a confusing welter of explanations; who could possibly anticipate that every last one of these theories offered a glimpse of the solution? Yet, with the discovery of vitamin D—not merely the identity, but the manner of its absorption—realization dawned. Cod liver oil was full of D, as were certain other fatty foods. Regular exposure to sunlight allowed the body to manufacture its own D. Industrialization and urbanization promoted rickets; smoggy atmospheres and darkened tenements blocked the sun. Fresh air and outdoor exercise brought children into the sunlight.

The extraordinary etiology does much to explain the curious historical incidence of rickets. Archaeological examination of bones recovered from the medieval cemetery near York, England revealed distinct signs of rickets, a finding unexpected at a pre-industrial site.[8] But industry itself was not the cause of rickets, rather, the lack of vitamin D. The people buried at Wharram Percy cemetery lived far from the sea, with little access to fatty fish oils. And, contrary to persistent rumor, people cannot get a tan standing in the English rain. A chilly, damp, relatively sunless climate was an apt location for rickets. When Britain did begin to industrialize in the eighteenth century, the resultant air pollution made a poor situation worse. Small wonder rickets was known as "the English disease."[9]

Rickets was known to occur among the slaves in the American South—the science of gynecology was constructed from experimentation on slave women afflicted with contracted pelves.[10] The disease may have been so commonplace among slaves that physicians overlooked the signs and dismissed its importance.[11] Yet, the incidence appears odd; slaves spent much of their lives out of doors in a climate redolent with sunlight; absorption of vitamin D should not have been a problem. But that is only half the equation: to avoid rickets, the body requires a supply of calcium. In 1981, Kenneth F. Kiple and Virginia Himmelsteib King argued persuasively that many of the enslaved—children especially—suffered rickets as a result of their mother's lactose intolerance, the inability to digest milk. "Sometime after weaning, a majority of the world's population loses the ability to digest milk, meaning the level of the lactose enzyme that metabolizes milk's lactose into absorbable sugars decreases." Because the slave diet offered little calcium a woman's body could absorb, prenatal diet was deficient.[12]

Free Blacks also suffered from rickets during America's antebellum period, as evidenced by the archaeological investigation at the cemetery of Philadelphia's First African Baptist Church, active between 1823 and 1848. Little is known of the lives of these African Americans; probably their diet was more rounded, and perhaps included alternate sources of calcium. But, unlike the Deep South, Philadelphia lies in the northern temperate zone, receiving the direct rays of the sun for a more limited portion of the year. As dark skin absorbs less sunlight, the acquisition of vitamin D may well have been insufficient.[13]

Rickets was a problem among Irish women emigrating to the New World during the Great Diaspora between 1845 and 1851. Some would suffer contracted pelves, becoming gynecologic experimental subjects at New York City's Woman's Hospital. Archaeological studies in Ireland have yielded evidence of rachitic disease in the teeth of young women dying during the famine. Again, the cause may not have been lack of sunlight, but insufficient calcium. Deprived of buttermilk in the 1820s, the Irish peasant diet lacked the necessary element. When the potato crop failed, young girls, already rachitic, emigrated to America.[14]

What of the peoples of the far north, the latitudes where human beings should have suffered most, were sunlight the whole answer? The infant children of the Inuit, or "Esquimaux," as Edwards Park discussed them, were breastfed by mothers consuming a steady diet rich in fatty fish oils carrying vitamin D. The long months of twilight, the small dark huts did not matter, provided there was an alternative source of the vitamin.[15]

The difficulty in unraveling the mystery of rickets lay in the natural disposition to focus on theories of mono-causation—there had to be a single root source of the disease: a germ, a genetic disposition, a nutritional deficiency, a bad habit. In the instance of rickets, there proved to be multiple causes—lack of vitamin D, lack of calcium—and multiple solutions, dependent on the cause. Once the disease was understood, virtual eradication became a possibility.

Rickets grew rampant with the advent of industrialization; overcrowded, polluted, ramshackle cities located in the temperate zone essentially shut out the sun, leaving foodstuffs as the only potential source of vitamin D. Unfortunately, very few foods actually contain D. Some fish, especially wild salmon or cod, some eggs—the yolk only, and some mushrooms, including the portabella variety, are the best food sources of D, but even these foods require a large amount to meet the body's needs. Most doctors and nutritionists currently agree it is difficult indeed to consume enough D to maintain the human body.[16] The working poor of the nineteenth and early twentieth century, doing their best on diets generally deficient, had essentially no chance at all.

* * *

The human species evolved in Africa, where there was endless sunlight. Short winter days were unknown. Living in relentless sun, natural selection among our earliest progenitors most probably favored a skin well-endowed with melanin, brown to black molecules found in the hair, the skin, and the iris of the eye. The darker pigment provided protection from overbearing sunshine. Early migrations took peoples into the neighboring tropics, but eventually human beings ventured into the temperate zones, where sunlight was more limited, seasonal variation marked. Absorption of ultraviolet light became increasingly critical to health.[17]

Darwin's theory of natural selection argues that evolutionary change derives from response to alterations in habitat. Moving into the temperate zones, peoples with skin rich in melanin would be placed at a disadvantage in survival—lighter skin absorbed more of the limited sunlight, bestowing an advantage. Rickets may well have become a factor. Over the long millennia, survival and sexual selection (on the whole, human beings choose partners in better physical condition) fostered growth of lighter-skinned populations. For much of human history, migration was a painfully slow process; dark-skinned peoples prevailed in tropical regions, lighter skinned in the temperate zones.[18]

This is delicate subject matter. Arguing that differences in skin color were products of evolutionary change opens the door to discussion of biological difference and racial definition. For centuries, Western science separated humankind into a hierarchically determined series of races, based largely on such superficial characteristics. The fact is, the human species exhibits a remarkable array of difference in matters such as skin and hair pigmentation, no essential variance at all in basic physiology or intelligence. We are a single species spread across an entire planet, manifesting differences in feature and habit that do not define us biologically. Not biology, but the shifting influence of social and cultural factors defines such race divisions as exist.[19] As Nina G. Jablonski, Professor of Anthropology at Penn State University clearly states, the evolution of skin color has no connection whatever to the evolution of other human traits.[20]

* * *

That obvious fact in no way discouraged the long, grim history of race-based analysis imbedded in the study of rickets, especially in America. Defining race by cultural interpretation of external physical traits was virtually universal in the United States, finding expression in persistent bias and stereotyping. Scientists and intellectuals believed rickets a degenerative disease characterizing the African American race, explained by heritage. On display was the defining element of a nation's entire existence: the metalanguage of race. Every intellectual discussion, scientific or otherwise, has been clouded by racial assumption.[21]

The inherent bias extended to the perception of immigrants. The

Conclusion: The Sum of the Equation

Irish, coming to America in the mid-nineteenth century, were almost universally perceived as a separate and inferior race. They came to be accepted only with the subsequent immigration of large numbers of southern and eastern European peoples. These human beings, regarded as inferior, met often humiliating treatment. The noted susceptibility to rickets was considered a defect of racial inheritance.[22]

The insistent prejudice was not merely harmful in itself; racial bias severely handicapped the study of rickets. Assuming different peoples suffered varying vulnerabilities, researchers too often categorized research subjects by race, seeking differentiation in results. The predisposition to invoke racial characteristics to explain away anomalous results was inherently destructive, the methodology deeply flawed. Most telling was the continued practice of applying results derived from treatment of Black and Irish patients to the ministration of protected whites, all the while insisting the groups were biologically different. The physiologies, the sensibilities were the same.[23]

* * *

Pelvimetric study in America developed in precisely this atmosphere. Researchers sought racial difference in pelvic diameter, measured cephalopelvic proportion based on perceived racial difference in the size and shape of an infant's skull, the birthing mother's hips. Such was the foundation for the emergence of obstetrical science as a medical specialty. The possibility of obstructed birth was a problem long recognized, though relatively rare until the advent of industrialization. Then came rickets, in colossal numbers. Surviving children grew to adulthood with weakened bodies, crooked limbs. And contracted pelves. Obstructed birth became a far more familiar eventuality, requiring an unusual degree of intervention. Birth, once the almost exclusive province of the midwife, increasingly required the assistance of a physician.

The growth of obstetrics was just one expression of a revolution in medical practice. Scientific investigation of human physiology and the etiology of disease resulted in essential breakthroughs, germ theory being the most essential. Antisepsis and anesthetics promoted surgical intervention. Innovative medical treatment demonstrably alleviated human suffering; the standing of the physician and the surgeon in society grew large.[24] Women were far more objectified than considered active participants, seldom treated as full human beings equal to men, regardless of education, professional ability, social standing, or racial origin. Throughout the nineteenth century and into the early years of the twentieth, American medical research was essentially guided by European practice; the foundations of modern American medicine were developed by physicians largely trained in Germany. This included the practice of what was disparagingly labeled "medical midwifery"—surgical intervention in childbirth.[25]

A key ingredient was the growing insistence on pelvimetrics—the measurement of an expectant woman's pelvis to determine whether she could give birth without surgical assistance. This can only be described as an invasive process, directed by a medical scientist, almost certainly male. Like any innovative scientific investigation, pelvimetry provoked contentious debate. What was the danger point? When was an obstructed birth likely to occur? Pelvic deformities appeared in a variety of forms, most associated with rickets. The lens of racial typing inevitably accompanied American studies, heavily influencing the designation of normal versus abnormal pelves, the incidence of contracted pelvis. Statistical estimates at Johns Hopkins University around the turn of the last century ranged from 10.25 to 15 percent; others reported incidence as high as 17.3 percent—more than one woman in six. The threshold measurement for contracted pelvis expanded from German researcher Carl Litzmann's designation of ten centimeters for the conjugata diagonalis in 1861 to an American estimate of thirteen centimeters—a full inch higher—determined in 1905. The larger the threshold, the greater the justification for medical intervention.[26]

By the early 1900s, contracted pelves had become a routine rationale for obstetric assistance. Interventions grew apace. Version remained the preferred technique—the physician maneuvering the fetus through the birth canal by hand. Forceps came into more frequent use. Ugly procedures such as craniotomy and symphysiotomy steadily gave way to Caesarean section, made possible by antisepsis and refinements of surgical technique. The use of anesthetics grew, even for women not requiring intervention. The parturient woman became an increasingly passive participant in the birth of her child.[27]

However invasive the intervention, a hospital or a clinic was the location preferred. Gaining power steadily, obstetricians came to view birth as an event entirely medical—even pathological. Obstetrical supervision became, in the minds of obstetricians, an absolute necessity. Writing in 1905, Joseph B. DeLee put the case perfectly:

> Careful study of existing conditions will convince any one that the safest place for the parturient woman is the special, well-equipped lying-in hospital. Here are all the facilities for the aseptic conduct of labor and the puerperium, here is the danger of child-bed infection properly evaluated, here only are the refinements of an operative technic possible.... Another benefit which is not so generally recognized is the effect on the physician. The maternity relieves him of a great deal of actual labor, it saves him many hours of tedious waiting, it lightens the burden of responsibility, and the knowledge that he is prepared for all

Conclusion: The Sum of the Equation   247

emergencies gives him a feeling of security which reflects itself in his work. The drudgery inherent in obstetric practice is thus largely eliminated.[28]

Removed from the comfortable surroundings of the home, separated from family, deprived of the soothing counsel of a midwife, required to lie flat on her back in an antiseptic labor area, lectured to be as quiet as possible, removed to a barren delivery room to be rigidly supervised by a team of nurses and a doctor draped in surgical white; surely it must have been a great comfort for the birthing woman to know the obstetrician felt secure.

* * *

Joseph B. DeLee and J. Whitridge Williams both served on the Advisory Council for Obstetrics Education at the White House Conference on Child Protection and Health called by President Hoover in 1930.[29] Unlike its predecessors, this meeting was fully dominated by the medical profession, as reflected in a confidential preliminary report issued to participants in 1930. The review fully encapsulated the obstetrical conjectures of the time. Contracted pelves were reckoned to occur in 8 to 24 percent of birthing women; "some are due to hereditary or germ defects."[30] Race was among the listed factors contributing to fetal, newly-born, and maternal mortality: 33.2 percent of Black obstetrical patients were said to exhibit contracted pelves. "It seems probable" the report contended, "that a large percentage of female pelvic deformities can be ascribed to rickets." In simple direct terms, for the ears of medical professionals only, obstetrics declared rickets likely to be the cause of deformity in pelvis and difficult birth, problems especially associated with African American women.[31]

Acknowledging that some states had introduced programs to educate midwives, the report nonetheless concluded, "The ultimate solution of the problem of good obstetrics lies not in the midwife, but in developing a sufficient number of doctors who are well trained in the fundamental principles of obstetrics."[32] Finally, "the practice of midwifery should always be under the supervision and control of direct medical authority."[33] The determination to do away with lay midwifery had reached the Federal level.

Even as obstetrical practice gained the formidable strength J. Whitridge Williams had long envisioned and fought to establish, he continued to express disquiet, arguing that the profession was going to extremes. Chief among his concerns was the growing tendency to view labor and birth as a pathological process, to respond accordingly. Anxious to hasten the birth, obstetricians were employing version before the end of labor's initial stage—far too soon. Forceps were often applied to the same purpose. Episiotomies were becoming commonplace. Artificial induction of

248   Conclusion: The Sum of the Equation

labor. Ready resort to Caesarean section. Physicians were far too eager to deploy the tools so recently molded in their profession. Deploring the state of matters, Williams concluded, "I consider the excessive tendencies of the present time as a result of, as well as an arraignment of our system of obstetrical education."[34]

* * *

The trends Williams so capably identified not only persisted; they became further entrenched. The experience of birth in America was well on the way to nearly complete transformation. By the 1930s, 50 percent of births in the United States occurred in hospitals; midwives assisted at just 15 percent, mainly in the South. By the 1950s, hospital births accounted for 95 percent of the total; mothers stayed in hospital for as long as ten days, forbidden to rise from bed. Episiotomies became routine, forceps delivery frequent. Use of Caesarean section grew steadily, accounting for more than twenty percent of births by the 1980s. Midwifery, surviving in Europe, very nearly disappeared throughout America. Hospital birth peaked in the 1980s at more than ninety-nine percent.[35]

A small rebellion began to gather strength. Birth to some had become a cold, clinical, cheerless, spiritless event. Surely there was more to this most elemental of all human experiences than the rigid mechanics defined and dictated by a male-dominated medical profession. By 2011, 2 percent of American births took place at home, assisted by a midwife. Interest continues to grow. The National Center for Disease Control and Prevention reports that the "risk profile" for out-of-hospital births is lower than hospital births.[36] At the same time, the incidence of Caesarean section has increased to more than 31 percent of American deliveries.[37]

Caesarean section developed as a surgical response to extreme obstruction in childbirth, a means of saving mother and child. As Williams noted, the procedure was embraced far too enthusiastically, becoming the preferred preventative when pelvimetric measurement indicated the slightest risk of obstruction. The definition of risk was highly elastic; obstetricians had inflated the danger point to justify surgical interventions.[38] Current definitions place the threshold for the conjugata diagonalis at 11.5 centimeters, a 1.5 centimeter reduction from the figure established little more than a century ago. Moreover, the Geneva Foundation for Medical Association and Research states that external pelvimetry (so diligently practiced at the Johns Hopkins Outdoor Obstetrical Service under Williams) is "of little value as it measures diameters of the false pelvis."[39] Pelvimetric measures are now the product magnetic resonance imaging (MRI) or computerized axial tomography (cat scans), but even these are called to question. The Cochrane Database of Systematic

Conclusion: The Sum of the Equation   249

Reviews reports there is too little evidence to decide whether pelvimetry is safe or beneficial.[40]

Cephalopelvic disproportion is now believed to occur in one pregnancy in two hundred-fifty—0.4 percent of births.[41] Certainly a much, much lower figure than the 8 to 24 percent described in 1930. Presumably the discovery of vitamin D and the subsequent near eradication of rickets explains much of the reduction. (Rickets has to some extent reappeared in the twenty-first century, due primarily to fear of skin cancers and the overuse of sunscreen.[42]) The impetus that drove research framing initial development of surgical obstetrics has largely disappeared. Yet the innovations of the late nineteenth and early twentieth centuries continue to dominate the culture of American birth. Few women now have Caesareans because they suffered rickets as a child.

* * *

Obstetrical science benefited essentially from the period in which the field developed, was in fact an integral expression of the era's values. The period from 1890 to 1920—and in some ways beyond—was the Age of Progressive Reform, a time when a restless America stood ready for change. The emergent ideal was a nation to be managed scientifically—every aspect of civilized life became a proving ground for empirical reform, to be guided by experts. Technicians trained in the social sciences—psychology, sociology, anthropology, economics—gained license to reorganize society, enhance efficiency, perhaps bring justice. A bureau for every purpose. Individual rights were to be subsumed in the good of the whole.[43]

Obstetrical aggression was another aspect of the general trend; physicians stood ready to remake the experience of birth in the name of science. The goal was not merely to make birth safer, but to gain absolute control, condemn and eliminate any competing vision, construct a model built on antisepsis, surgical intervention, rigid conformity, and drugs. Birth was one more target of America's reform impulse.

Accompanying and abetting that impulse was the fear of race suicide, the belief that America's ruling classes were doomed to be overwhelmed by hordes of immigrants, African Americans, and the genetically unfit.[44] Efforts to promote more effective birth procedures, diminish infant and maternal mortality, produce healthier babies, were consciously intended to make birth easier, more palatable, more attractive to white women of Anglo-Saxon heritage. Nowhere is the insistent thread of racially-defined analysis more visible. The surgical interventions offered at medical dispensaries for the poor—a clientele largely Black and immigrant—yielded knowledge and experience intended to assist their social betters. Most telling of all, obstetricians stood ready to assume a crucial role in the march of eugenics, offering permanent surgical solutions to eliminate the unfit.[45]

Very little of the Progressive Era is worthy of celebration. Certainly not the field of obstetrics. There is no denying the discoveries—the improvements in surgical technique, the gains in control of disease—were of enormous and everlasting value. The actual practice of obstetrical medicine was something else entirely. The pediatricians and the biochemists identified vitamin D, resolved the riddle of rickets. Obstetricians used rickets to gain control of birth.

Chapter Notes

Introduction

1. Irving Loudon, *Death in Childbirth: An International Study of Maternal Care and Maternal Mortality* (Oxford: Clarendon Press, 1993).

Chapter One

1. Joseph B. DeLee, M.D., "A Case of Flat Rachitic Pelvis; Prolapse of the Cord with the Head; Version and Extraction," *Journal of the American Medical Association* XXVIII, no. 7 (1897): 306–07.
2. Robert Tague and C. Owen Lovejoy, "The Obstetric Pelvis of A.L. 288–1 (Lucy)," *Journal of Human Evolution* 15, no. 1 (May 1986): 237–55.
3. Stephen Jay Gould, "The Most Compelling Pelvis Since Elvis," *Discover* 6, no. 12 (1985): 54–58.
4. Brian Handwerk, "An Evolutionary Timeline of Homo Sapiens," *Smithsonian Magazine*, last modified February 2, 2021, https://www.smithsonianmag.com/science-nature/essential-timeline-understanding-evolution-homo-homo-sapiens-180976807/.
5. Katharine Park, *Secrets of Women: Gender, Generation, and the Origins of Human Dissection* (New York: Zone Books, 2006), 90.
6. Karen Rosenberg and Wenda Trevathan, "Bipedalism and Human Birth: The Obstetrical Dilemma Revisited," *Evolutionary Anthropology* 4 (1996): 161–68; Jenny Carter and Thérèse Duriwz, *With Child: Birth Through the Ages* (Edinburgh: Mainstream, 1986), 13–56.
7. Park, *Secrets of Women*, 90.
8. Lewis Pyenson and Susan Sheets-Pyenson, *Servants of Nature: A History of Scientific Institutions, Enterprises and Sensibilities* (New York: W.W. Norton, 1999), 216.
9. Londa Schiebinger, *The Mind Has No Sex: Women in the Origins of Modern Science* (Cambridge: Harvard University Press, 1989), 191.
10. Ludmilla Jordanova, *Nature Displayed: Gender, Science and Medicine 1760–1820* (London: Addison Wesley Longman, 1999), 183–202.
11. Ibid.
12. Michel Foucault, *The Birth of the Clinic: An Archaeology of Medical Perception* (New York: Vintage, 1994), 124–48; Schiebinger, *The Mind Has No Sex*, 198–200.
13. Thomas LaQueur, *Making Sex: Body and Gender from the Greeks to Freud* (Cambridge: Harvard University Press, 1992).
14. Joan Wallach Scott, *Gender and the Politics of History* (New York: Columbia University Press, 1988), 28–50.
15. Schiebinger, *The Mind Has No Sex*, 1–6, 93, 158, 212.
16. Judith Walzer Leavitt, "Science Enters the Birthing Room: Obstetrics in America Since the Eighteenth Century," in *Childbirth: Changing Ideas and Practices in Britain and America 1600 to the Present*, ed. Philip K. Wilson (New York: Garland, 1996), 231–55.
17. Hendrick van Deventer, *The Art of Midwifery Improv'd*, translated from the Dutch and Latin (London: E. Curll et al., 1716). Originally published in Holland as *Manual Operations Which Are a New Light for Male and Female Midwives* in

1701; Adrian Wilson, *The Making of Man-Midwifery: Childbirth in England, 1660-1770* (Cambridge: Harvard University Press, 1995). Wilson offers key arguments concerning the significance of the introduction of forceps into obstetrics and considering Deventer and Elizabeth Nihell.

18. Wilson, *Making of Man-Midwifery*, 82.

19. Wendy Moore, "Keeping Mum," *British Medical Journal* 334, no. 7595 (March 31, 2007): 698; Jo Murphy Lawless, *Reading Birth and Death: A History of Obstetric Thinking* (Bloomington: Indiana University Press, 1999), 92-93; Charles D. Meigs, *Obstetrics: The Science and the Art*, 3rd ed., rev. (Philadelphia: Blanchard and Lea, 1856), 533.

20. Lawless, *Reading Birth and Death*, 37, 53, 74, 84.

21. Carter and Durier, *With Child*, 35, quoting from William Smellie, *Treatise on the Theory and Practice of Midwifery* (London, 1752); Wilson, *Making of Man-Midwifery*, 123-33.

22. Wilson, *Making of Man-Midwifery*, 123-33.

23. Nina Ratner Gilbart, *The King's Midwife: A History and Mystery of Madame du Coudray* (Berkeley: University of California Press, 1998), 60. In 1755 Parliament ruled that midwives could not use forceps.

24. Samuel Bard, *Compendium of the Theory and Practice of Midwifery* (New York: Collins, 1808); J. Whitridge Williams, *A Sketch of the History of Obstetrics in the United States up to 1860* (Baltimore, 1903), 29.

25. *Ibid.*, 529-64.

26. *Ibid.*, 533.

27. Robert P. Harris, "The Caesarean Operation of the United States," *American Journal of the Medical Sciences* 4 (Feb. 1871): 622-63 (chart, 663); "Remarks on the Cesarean Operation," *American Journal of the Medical Sciences* 11 (1878): 620-26; "A Study and Analysis of One Hundred Caesarean Operations Performed in the United States During the Present Century, and Prior to the Year 1878," *American Journal of the Medical Sciences* 12 (April 1879): 43-65.

28. Gabert and Bey, 597.

29. Meigs, *Obstetrics*, 571-99.

30. Deventer, *Art of Midwifery Improv'd*; Schiebinger, *The Mind Has No Sex*, 138-39; Chassar Moir, *Munro Kerr's Operative Obstetrics*, 6th ed. (1956), 310-11.

31. Jean-Louis Baudelocque, *L'Art des Accouchements* (Paris: Mequignon, 1781); Harold Speert, *Obstetric and Gynecological Milestones: Essays in Eponymy* (New York: Macmillan, 1858), 145.

32. Lawless, *Birth and Death*, 94-97.

33. Judith Leavitt, *Brought to Bed: Child-Bearing in America, 1750-1950*, expanded ed. (New Haven: Yale University Press, 1989) provides a strong history of the culture and specific historical context for birth in America.

34. Leavitt, *Brought to Bed*, 311-16; Theodore F. Riggs, "A Comparative Study of White and Negro Pelves: With a Consideration of the Size of the Child and Its Relation to Presentation and Character of the Races in the Two Races, 1891-1926," *Johns Hopkins Hospital Reports* 12 (1904): 422.

35. This is noted in many places, including Moir, *Kerr's Obstetrics*, 312.

36. Franz Carl Naegele, *Erfahrungeu. Abhandl. aud d. Gebiete der Krankh. des weibl. Geschlechtes nebst Grundzügen einer Methodenlehre der Geburtshülfe. Mit 4 Kupfertafeln* (Mannheim, 1812). Naegele, *The Obliquely Contracted Pelvis Containing Also an Appendix of the Most Important Defects of the Female Pelvis*, centennial ed., newly translated from the original German (New York, 1939).

37. Michael Sappol, *A Traffic of Dead Bodies: Anatomy and Embodied Social Identity in Nineteenth-Century America* (Princeton: Princeton University Press, 2002).

38. Lawrence Longo and Carl Theodor Litzmann, "Die Formen das Beckens, insbesondere des dengen weiblichen Beckens, nach eigenen Beobachtungen und Untersuchungen, hebst einem Anhange über die Osteomalacie," *American Journal of Obstetrics and Gynecology* 129 (Nov. 1, 1977): 571-72.

39. Joseph DeLee, *Principles and Practice of Obstetrics*, 6th ed. (Philadelphia: W.B. Saunders & Co., 1934), 779. Puerperal fever was a killer of women giving birth at this time. Simmelweis, a contemporary of Michaëlis, discovered its origins in the unwashed hands of physicians but very few heard his voice.

40. Michaëlis, *Das Enge Becken* (Leip-

zig: G. Wigand, 1851). Carl Litzmann, *Die Formen das Beckens, insbesondere des engen weiblichen Beckens, nach eigenen Beobactungen und Untersuchungen, hebst einem Anhange über die Osteomalacie* (Berlin: Georg Reimer, 1861).
41. Michaëlis, *Das Enge Becken.*
42. *Ibid.*, 3.
43. Longo, "Litzmann," 571–72.
44. Litzmann, *Die Formen das Beckens*, 50.
45. *Ibid.*, 50, 73. Julius Jarcho, *The Pelvis in Obstetrics* (New York: Paul B. Hoeber, 1933), 88. Litzmann organized chapters around defining each group of contracted pelves in *Die Formen des Beckens.*
46. Litzmann, *Die Formen das Beckens*, 7.
47. *Ibid.*, 13.
48. *Ibid.*, Chapter 2.
49. *Ibid.*, 95. An article in 1920 addresses the idea that the pelvis might change size during pregnancy and labor. The author identifies the disagreements actually as among physicians at the time who offered cases exemplifying changes of pelvic size. He used an X-ray to try to determine the truth but failed. He did acknowledge consensus for the most part that expansion was most likely in the sacrum. See Frank Lynch, "The Pelvic Articulation During Pregnancy, Labor and the Puerperium: An X-Ray Study," *Surgery, Gynecology and Obstetrics* 30 (1920): 575–80.
50. Jarcho, *Pelvis in Obstetrics*, 1. See 88 for a discussion of Litzmann's classification of pelves. Jarcho uses the word "abnormal," a word from the twentieth century, not from Litzmann.
51. William Smellie, *Philosophy of Natural History* (Edinburgh, 1790), vol. 1, 521–22, quoted in Schiebinger, *Nature's Body*, 145.
52. Philippe Rushton, *Race, Evolution and Behavior* (London: Charles Darwin Research Institution, 2000), 72.
53. Williams, "History of Obstetrics," 36; Herbert Thoms, *Chapters in American Obstetrics* (Springfield, IL: Charles C. Thomas, 1933), 45–53.
54. William DeWees, *A Compendius System of Midwifery* (Philadelphia: Blanchard and Lea, 1824).
55. Thomas F. Cock, *Manual of Obstetrics* (New York: Samuel S. and William Wood, 1853), 17.
56. *Ibid.*, 135.
57. *Ibid.*, 17–18.
58. *Ibid.*, 20.
59. *Ibid.*, 21.
60. *Ibid.*, 22.
61. Meigs, *Obstetrics*; Williams, *History of Obstetrics*; Irvine Loudon, *Death in Childbirth*, 166–71.
62. Meigs, *Obstetrics*, 583.
63. *Ibid.*, 519.
64. Hugh Hodge, *The Principles and Practice of Obstetrics* (Philadelphia: Henry Lea, 1866). Chapter 20 has a large portion on contracted pelves. Rambotham and Churchill were among several obstetricians from the British Isles who wrote texts and included contracted pelves as significant in the medical practice.
65. *Ibid.*, 386–408.
66. *Ibid.*, 386.
67. *Ibid.*
68. *Ibid.*
69. *Ibid.*, 395.
70. *Ibid.*, 404–07.
71. *Ibid.*, 394, Figure 96. Here Hodge cited precedent in Ramsbotham.
72. *Ibid.*, 398–400.
73. *Ibid.*, 399–400.
74. Deborah Kuhn McGregor, *From Midwives to Medicine: The Birth of American Gynecology* (New Brunswick: Rutgers University Press, 1998), 33–35.
75. Hodge, *Obstetrics*, 398–400.
76. *Ibid.*, 397.
77. H.R. Storer, "Report from the American Medical Association's Committee on Obstetrics," *Transactions of the American Medical Association* IV (1851): 349–407.

Chapter Two

1. Donald J. Ortner and Simon Hays, "Dry-Bone Manifestations of Rickets in Infancy and Early Childhood," *International Journal of Osteoarchaeology* 8 (1998): 45–55.
2. Mark Brown, "Evidence in the Bones Reveals Rickets in Roman Times," *The Guardian*, last modified August 20, 2018, https//www.theguardian.com/science/2018/20/roman-rickets-vitamin-d-deficiency.
3. Ortner and Mays, "Dry-Bone Manifestations of Rickets," 45–55.

4. *Ibid.*, 46.
5. *Ibid.*
6. Mary E. Lewis, "Impact of Industrialization: Comparative Study of Child Health in Four Sites from Medieval and Postmedieval England (A.D. 850–1859)," *American Journal of Physical Anthropology* 119, no. 3 (2002): 211–23.
7. *Ibid.*
8. *Ibid.*, 213.
9. *Ibid.*, 216.
10. *Ibid.*; Donald Ortner and Gretchen Theobald, "Paleopathological Evidence of Malnutrition," in *Cambridge World History of Food*, vol. 1, ed. Kenneth Kiple and Krimheld Conee Ornelas (Cambridge: Cambridge University Press, 2000), 36–37.
11. Glisson holds the title for the original treatise on rickets. Dispute lingers regarding Whistler's contribution since his career was later tainted by charges of moral corruption. For purposes of this study, details of early perceptions of the disease are most important. George Frederic Still, *The History of Paediatrics: The Progress of the Study of Diseases of Children Up to the End of the XVIIIth Century* (1931; Oxford: Oxford University Press, 1965). *The Compact Edition of the Oxford English Dictionary*, vol. II (Oxford: Oxford University Press, 1971), 2541. Richard Dunglison, *A Dictionary of Medical Science* (Philadelphia: Henry C. Lea, 1874), 883.
12. L. Paunier, "Rickets and Osteomalacia," in *Nutrition in Preventive Medicine: The Major Deficiency Syndromes, Epidemiology, and Approaches to Control*, ed. G.H. Beaton and J.M. Bengoa (Geneva: World Health Organization, 1976), 111.
13. Aaron Ihde, "Recognition of Rickets as a Deficiency Disease," *Pharmacy in History* 16 (1974): 83; Peter Dunn, "Francis Glisson (1597–1677) and the Discovery of Rickets," *Archives of Disease in Childhood* 78 (March 1998): 154–55.
14. "'The English Disease': Infantile Rickets and Scurvy in Pre-Industrial England," in *Childcare Through the Centuries*, ed. John Cule and Terry Turner (Cardiff: British Society for the History of Medicine, 1986), 121–35.
15. Ihde, "Studies on the History of Rickets, I," 84.
16. Anne Hardy, "Commentary: Bread and Alum, Syphilis and Sunlight: Rickets in the Nineteenth Century," *International Journal of Epidemiology* 32, no. 3 (July 2003): 337–40.
17. M.E. Lewis, "The Impact of Industrialisation: A Comparative Study of Child Health in Four Sites from Medieval and Post-Medieval England," *American Journal of Physical Anthropology* 119, no. 3 (2002): 221.
18. Alfred F. Hess, *Rickets: Including Osteomalacia and Tetany* (Philadelphia: Lea and Febiger, 1929), 22–37.
19. Sir William Jenner, *Clinical Lectures and Essays on Rickets, Tuberculosis, Abdominal Tumours* (London: Rivington, Percival & Co., 1895).
20. *Ibid.*, 45.
21. Abraham Jacobi, "Craniotabes," *American Journal of Obstetrics and Diseases of Women and Children* (Nov. 1870): 435–67.
22. W.F. Bynum, *The Science and Practice of Medicine in the Nineteenth Century* (Cambridge: Cambridge University Press, 1994), 100.
23. Rudolf Virchow, "Das Normale Knochenwachsthum und die Rachitische Störung Desselben," *Archiv für Pathologische Anatomie und Physiologie und für Klinische Medizin* 5 (1847): 409–507.
24. Rudolf Virchow, *Cellular Pathology as Based Upon Physiological and Pathological Histology*, translated from the second edition of the original by Frank Chance (Philadelphia: J.B. Lippincott, 1863), 432.
25. *Ibid.*, 434.
26. Erwin Ackeknecht, *Rudolf Virchow: The Development of Science* (New York: Arno Press, 1981), 78.
27. *Ibid.*, 387.
28. Hess, *Rickets*, 127–28.
29. Jenner, *Clinical Lectures*, 39–40.
30. Anne Hardy, "Rickets and the Rest: Child-Care, Diet and the Infectious Children's Diseases, 1850–1914," *Social History of Medicine* 5 (Dec. 1992): 389–412.
31. Jenner, *Clinical Lectures*, 39–40.
32. Hardy, "Rickets and the Rest."
33. Loudon, *Death in Childbirth*, 134–35.
34. *Ibid.*
35. Thomas Barlow, "On Cases Described as Acute Rickets Which Are Probably a Combination of Scurvy and Rickets," *Medico-Chirurgical Transactions* 66 (March 27, 1883): 159–220.

36. Hess, *Rickets*, 353–400.
37. Phillipe Hernigou, "Historical Overview of Rickets, Osteomalacia, and Vitamin D," *Revue du Rhumatisme* (English Edition) 62 (April 1995): 261–70.
38. Antoine Bernard Marfan, *Le Rachitism Etiologie, Pathogenie, Traitement, Prophylaxie* (Paris: Librairie J.-B. Baillièrre et Fils, 1942), 9.
39. Elizabeth Lomaz, "Infantile Syphilis as an Example of Nineteenth Century Belief in the Inheritance of Acquired Characteristics," in *Childbirth: Changing Ideas and Practices in Britain and America: 1600 to the Present*, vol. 5, ed. Philip Davis (New York: Garland, 1996), 328.
40. *Ibid*.
41. Roy Porter, *Blood and Guts: A Short History of Medicine* (New York: W.W. Norton, 2002), 1–20.
42. Gerald N. Grob, *The Deadly Truth: A History of Disease in America* (Cambridge: Harvard University Press, 2002), 164–65; William H. MacNeill, *Plagues and Peoples* (New York: Doubleday, 1977), 208–57.
43. Gregg Mitmann, Michelle Murphy, and Christopher Seller, "Landscapes of Exposure: Knowledge and Illness in Modern Environments," *Osiris* 19 (2004).
44. Mary Fulbrook, *A Concise History of Germany*, 2nd ed. (Cambridge: Cambridge University Press, 2004), 137. David Clay Large, *Berlin* (New York: Basic Books, 2000), 9.
45. August Hirsch, *Handbook of Geographical and Historical Pathology*, trans. Charles Creighton, M.D. (London: The New Sydenham Society, 1883).
46. August Hirsch, *Handbook of Geographical and Historical Pathology*, 3 vols., 2nd ed. (London: The New Sydenham Society, 1886), 3:738.
47. *Ibid.*, 3:740.
48. *Ibid.*, 3:734.
49. *Ibid.*, 3:734–35.
50. Isambard Owen, "Geographical Distribution of Rickets, Acute and Subacut Rhematism, Chorea, Cancer, and Urinary Calculus," *British Medical Journal* 1 (1889): 113–16.
51. *Ibid.*, 114; Loudon in *Death in Childbirth* notes the exceptionally high presence of rickets in Glasgow, 446–48.
52. Susan E. Klepp, "Seasoning and Society: Racial Differences in Mortality in Eighteenth-Century Philadelphia," *William and Mary Quarterly*, 3rd Series, vol. LI, no. 3 (July 1994): 473–506, 484, citing Andrew Maykuth, "Grave Injustice?" *Philadelphia Inquirer*, July 29, 1992, C4; David W. Dunlap, "A Black Cemetery Takes Its Place in History," *New York Times*, Feb. 28, 1993, E5; Spencer P. M. Harrington, "Stories the Bones Will Tell," *Archaeology* XLVI (March/April 1993): 36–37; Ira Berlin and Leslie M. Harris, "Uncovering, Discovering, and Recovering: Digging in New York's Slave Past Beyond the African Burial Ground," in *Slavery in New York*, ed. Ira Berlin and Leslie M. Harris (New York: New Press, 2005), 3, 7, 12.
53. J. Lawrence Angel, Jennifer Olsen Kelley, Michael Parrington and Stephanie Pinter, "Life Stresses of the Free Black Community as Represented by the First African Baptist Church, Philadelphia, 1823–1841," *American Journal of Physical Anthropology* 74 (1987): 213–29.
54. Ortner and Mays, "Dry-Bone Manifestations of Rickets in Infancy and Early Childhood," 45–55.
55. Angel, Kelley, Parrington and Pinter, "Life Stresses of the Free Black Community," 219, 221, 222; Charlotte Roberts and Keith Dorchester, *The Archeology of Disease*, 3rd ed. (Ithaca: Cornell University Press, 2005), 227, 228, 214.
56. Angel, Kelley, Parrington and Pinter, "Life Stresses of the Free Black Community," 213–29.
57. Todd Savitt, *Medicine and Slavery: The Diseases and Health Care of Blacks in Antebellum Virginia* (Urbana: University of Illinois Press, 1978), 137.
58. Letter from Edward Jarvis in J.B.D. De Bow, *Mortality Statistics of the 7th Census of the United States, 1850* (Washington, D.C.: Government Printing Office, 1855), 45.
59. J.B.D. De Bow, *Mortality Statistics*, 304.
60. *Ibid.*, 292–93.
61. *Ibid.*, 236–37.
62. Hess, *Rickets*, 22–37.
63. Aaron Ihde, "Studies on the History of Rickets, II: The Roles of Cod Liver Oil and Light," *Pharmacy in History* 17 (1974): 14. Elmer V. McCollum, *A History of Nutrition: The Sequence of Ideas in Nutrition Investigations* (Boston: Houghton Mifflin, 1957), 268.

64. McCollum, *History of Nutrition*; Hardy, "Commentary: Bread and Alum."
65. Roy Porter, *The Greatest Benefit to Mankind: A Medical History of Humanity* (New York: W.W. Norton, 1997), 322.
66. Rima Apple, *Mothers and Medicine: A Social History of Infant Feeding* (Madison: University of Wisconsin Press, 1987), 9.
67. Henry Thoreau, *Walden* (1854; Boston: Houghton Mifflin, 1995), 11.
68. Porter, *Greatest Benefit to Mankind*, 324.
69. Robert E. Kohler, *From Medical Education to Biochemistry: The Making of a Biomedical Discipline* (Cambridge: Cambridge University Press, 1982), 21.
70. John Snow, "On the Adulteration of Bread as a Cause of Rickets," *International Journal of Epidemiology* 32 (2003): 336–37; Hardy, "Commentary: Bread and Alum"; M. Dunnigan, "Commentary: John Snow and Alum-Induced Rickets from Adulterated London Bread: An Overlooked Contribution to Metabolic Bone Disease," *International Journal of Epidemiology* 32 (2003): 340–41; Nigel Paneth, "Commentary: Snow on Rickets," *International Journal of Epidemiology* 32 (2003): 341–43.
71. Jenner, *Clinical Lectures*, 45.
72. Ibid.
73. J. Henry Fruitnight, "The Treatment of Rachitis with the Lactophosphate of Lime," *Transactions of the American Pediatrics Society* 5 (1893): 168–74.
74. Apple, *Mothers and Medicine*, 13–62.
75. Hirsch, *Handbook of Geographical and Historical Pathology*, 736.
76. McNeill, *Something New Under the Sun*.
77. Gerald Grob, *The Deadly Truth*, 164–65.
78. Adolfo Murillo, "Historia de dos Operaciones Cesáreas en Chile," *Transactions of the Pan-American Medical Congress Held in the City of Washington, D.C., U.S.A., September 5, 6, 7, and 8 A.D. 1893*, 693–98.
79. Alfred F. Hess, "An Interpretation of the Seasonal Variation of Rickets," *Collected Writings*, 2 vols. (Springfield, IL: Charles C. Thomas, 1936), 1:669–75; reprinted from *American Journal of Diseases of the Child* (Aug. 1921).
80. Ihde, "Studies on the History of Rickets, II," 84.
81. William Buchan, "Advise to Mothers on the Subject of their Own Health," *Domestic Medicine* (Boston: Joseph Bumstead, 1809), 44.
82. Hardy, "Rickets and the Rest," 408.
83. Michael F. Holick, *The Vitamin D Solution* (New York: Hudson Street Press, 2010), 8–9; W. Mozozowski, "Letter," *Nature* 143, no. 3612 (Jan. 21, 1939): 121.
84. Antoine Bernard Marfan, *Maladies des Os* (Paris: Librairie J.-B. Baillière et Fils, 1912), 410.
85. Ruth A. Guy, "The History of Cod Liver Oil as a Remedy," *American Journal of Diseases of Children* 26 (1923): 112–16; D. Schutte, "Beobachtungen über den Nutzen des Berger Lebertrans (Oleum jecoris Aselli, von Gadus asellus L)," *Archiv fur Medizizinche Erfahrung im Gebiete der praktischen Medzin, Chirurgie, Geburtshülfe und Staatsarzneikunde* 2 (1824): 79.
86. A. Trousseau and H. Pidoux, *Treatise on Therapeutics*, trans. D.F. Lincoln, 9th ed. (New York: William Wood and Co., 1880), 161–67.
87. Trousseau, *Clinique Medical de l'Hôtel Dieu de Paris*, 4th ed. (Paris: Baillière, 1873), 529.
88. Marfan, *La Rachitisme Etiologie*, 112.
89. Ihde, "Studies on the History of Rickets, II," 15–16.
90. Fruitnight, "The Treatment of Rachiti," 174.
91. Ihde, "Studies on the History of Rickets, II," 16.
92. Ibid.
93. Hardy, "Rickets and the Rest"; Jenner, *Clinical Lectures*, 47.
94. Jenner, *Clinical Lectures*, 47.
95. Ibid., 48.
96. Ibid., 49.
97. Ibid.
98. John P. Jackson, Jr., and Nadine M. Weidman, *Race, Racism and Science: Social Impact and Interaction* (New Brunswick: Rutgers University Press, 2004), 9–12.

Chapter Three

1. Francis Bacon, "Novum Organum," *The Essays* (1635; New York: Penguin, 1986), 270.
2. Arthur O. Lovejoy, *The Great Chain*

of Being (Cambridge: Harvard University Press, 1936 and 1964); William Bynum, "The Great Chain of Being After Forty Years: An Appraisal," History of Science 13 (1975): 1–28.
 3. Lovejoy, Great Chain of Being, 227–41.
 4. Ibid., 233–35; Nell Irvin Painter, The History of White People (New York: W.W. Norton, 2010), 78; Rhodri Lewis, "William Petty's Anthropology: Religion, Colonialism, and the Problem of Human Diversity," Huntington Library Quarterly 74, no. 2 (June 2011): 261–88.
 5. Milford Woloff and Rachel Caspari, Race and Human Evolution (New York: Simon & Schuster, 1997).
 6. Leonard Lieberman and Fatimah Linda C. Jackson, "Race and Three Models of Human Origin," American Anthropology 97, no. 2 (June 1995): 233.
 7. Ibid., 79, 83, 85; Woloff and Caspari, Race and Human Evolution; Gould, Mismeasure of Man, 403, 412; Painter, History of White People, 72.
 8. Painter, History of White People, 91–101.
 9. J.M. Guardia, La Médicine a travers la Siècles Histoire Philosophe (Paris: J. B. Baillière et Fils, 1865), 524.
 10. Gerard Moran, The History of the Irish Famine: The Exodus (London: Routledge, 2018); Karen Sonnelitter, The Great Irish Famine: A History in Documents (Peterborough: Broadview Press, 2018); William R. Polk, The Birth of America: From Before Columbus to the Revolution (New York: Harper Perennial, 2006), 77.
 11. Percival Willoughby, Observations in Midwifery, ed. Henry Blenkinsop (Yorkshire: S.R. Publishers Limited, 1972), 16.
 12. Laura Briggs, "The Race of Hysteria: 'Overcivilization' and the 'Savage' Woman in Late Nineteenth-Century Obstetrics and Gynecology," American Quarterly 52 (June 2000): fn. 30.
 13. Ibid., 209.
 14. Rachel Holmes, The Hottentot Venus. The Life and Death of Saartjie Baartman: Born 1789—Buried 2002 (London: Bloomsbury, 2007), 13, 66–67.
 15. Gould, "The Hottentot Venus," The Flamingo's Smile: Reflections in Natural History (New York: W.W. Norton, 1985), 300–01.
 16. George Stocking, Race, Culture, and Evolution: Essays in the History of Anthropology (New York: Free Press, 1968), 39.
 17. Georg Cuvier, Recherches sur les ossemens fossiles, vol. 1 (Paris: Deterville, 1812), 105; Anne Fausto-Sterling, "Gender, Race, and Nation: The Comparative Anatomy of 'Hottentot' Women in Europe, 1815–1817," Deviant Bodies: Critical Perspectives on Difference in Science and Popular Culture ed. Jennifer Terry and Jacqueline Urla (Bloomington: Indiana University Press, 1995), 22–23; Schiebinger, Nature's Body, 160–83.
 18. Gould, "The Hottentot Venus," 294.
 19. Holmes, The Hottentot Venus, 153–69. Steven Jay Gould found the remains of Saartje Barrtman more than 150 years later when he toured the Museé de l'homme in the 1980s. Knowing her story, he recognized the jar as a public violation of her desired privacy. In 2002, after the end of apartheid in South Africa, the museum released her remains to be buried with honor on the Cape of Good Hope.
 20. Sander Gilman, "Black Bodies, White Bodies: Toward an Iconography of Female Sexuality in Late Nineteenth-Century Art, Medicine, and Literature," in Race, Writing and Difference (Chicago: University of Chicago Press, 1986), 223–21; Gould, "The Hottentot Venus," 155–66; Anne Fausto-Sterling, "Gender, Race, and Nation," 19–48; Laura Briggs, "The Race of Hysteria."
 21. Gould, "The Hottentot Venus."
 22. Gerardus Vrolik, "Observations of the Differences of Pelves of Various Races," quoted by Joseph Taber Johnson, "Apparent Peculiarities of Partutrition in the Negro Race," American Journal of Obstetrics and Diseases of Women and Children 8 (Jan. 1875): 105, 107.
 23. Johnson, "Apparent Peculiarities," 104.
 24. Schiebinger, Nature's Body, 158, 160.
 25. Anthony Fletcher, Gender, Sex, and Subordination in England 1500–1800 (New Haven: Yale University Press, 1999).
 26. Ibid.
 27. Johnson, "Peculiarities," 100.
 28. Robert Wald Sussman, The Myth of Race: The Troubling Persistence of an Unscientific Idea (Cambridge: Harvard University Press, 20014), 22–25, 172–73, 302–03.

29. Woloff and Casperi, *Race and Human Evolution*, 72; Gould, *Mismeasure of Man*, 105-41.
30. J.G. Gaison, "Pelvimetry," *Journal of Anatomy and Physiology* 16 (1881): 106. Renée Verneau, *Le Bassin dans les Sexes et les Races* (Paris: Librairie J.-B. Baillière et Fils, 1875); Lucille Hyme, "The Earliest Use of Indices for Sexing Pelves," *American Journal of Physical Anthropology* 15 (1957): 537-46.
31. Verneau, *Le Basins Dans Les Sexes*, 76.
32. Ibid., 127, 131.
33. Ibid.
34. Ibid.
35. William Greulich, Herbert Thoms, and Ruth Christian Twaddle, "A Study of Pelvic Type and Its Relationship to Body Build in White Women," *Journal of the American Medical Association* 112 (Feb. 11, 1939): 487; William Turner, "Index of the Pelvic Brim as a Basis of Classification," *Journal of Anatomy and Physiology* 20 (1885-1886): 125-43.
36. Turner, "Index of the Pelvic Brim."
37. Painter, *History of White People*, 151-89.
38. Reginald Horsman, *Race and Manifest Destiny: The Origins of American Racial Anglo-Saxonism* (Cambridge: Harvard University Press, 1981).
39. David A. Hollinger, "American Ethnoracial History and the Amalgamation Narrative," *Journal of American Ethnic History* 35, no. 4 (Summer 2006): 153-59.
40. Harriet Jacobs, *Incidents in the Life of a Slave Girl: Written by Herself* (Boston: Published for the author, Boston d'Eleotype Foundry, 1861); Frederick Douglass, *My Bondage and My Freedom* (New York: Miller, Orton and Mulligan, 1855).
41. Imaging in medicine has changed with technological innovation. Imaging as it was for Hodge but seemingly even more so, with little direct examination of the patient, stands at the heart of medical practice today. For imaging in birth see Alexander Tsiaras, *From Conception to Birth: A Life Unfolds* (New York: Doubleday, 2002).
42. McGregor, *From Midwives to Medicine*, 12, 22; Sussman, *Myth of Race*, 15-20.
43. Harriet A. Washington, *Medical Apartheid: The Dark History of Experimentation on Black Americans from Colonial Times to the Present* (New York: Doubleday, 2006), 34-35.
44. Gould, *Mismeasure of Man*, 82-101; Ann Fabian, *The Skull Collectors: Race, Science, and America's Unburied Dead* (Chicago: University of Chicago Press, 2010), 9-45.
45. Ibid.
46. Gould, *Mismeasure of Man*, 96-99.
47. Ibid., 100-01.
48. Meigs, *Obstetrics*, 518.
49. Meigs, *Obstetrics*, 58, figure 112. William Stanton, in *The Leopard's Spots: Scientific Attitudes Toward Race in America, 1815-1859* (Chicago: University of Chicago Press, 1960), 1-14.
50. Stanton, *The Leopard's Spots*, 1-14.
51. Ibid., 157.
52. Gould, *Mismeasure of Man*, 101-04.
53. Schiebinger, *The Mind Has No Sex*, 213.
54. Jennifer L. Morgan, *Laboring Women: Reproduction and Gender in New World Slavery* (Philadelphia: University of Pennsylvania Press, 2004), 35.
55. Klepp, "Seasoning and Society," 473-506; Dunlap, "A Black Cemetery Takes Its Place in History"; Harrington, "Stories the Bones Will Tell"; Berlin and Harris, eds., *Slavery in New York*, 3, 7, 12.
56. Robert Fogel and Stanley L. Engerman, *Time on the Cross: Evidence and Methods, A Supplement* (Boston: Little, Brown, 1974).
57. Richard H. Steckel, "The African American Population of the United States, 1790-1929," in *A Population History of North America*, ed. Michael Haines and Richard H. Steckel (Cambridge: Cambridge University Press, 2000), 449, 450. See also Richard H. Steckel, "A Peculiar Population: The Nutrition, Health, and Mortality of American Slaves from Childhood to Maturity," *Journal of Economic History* 46, no. 3 (Sept. 1986): 721-741.
58. Kiple points out that Steckel's comparative height study of slavery in the U.S. and Barbados show much greater health impact of slavery in the Barbados. Kenneth Kiple, "A Survey of Recent Literature on the Black Biological Past," *Social Science History* 10, no. 4 (Winter 1986): 349.
59. Kenneth F. Kiple and Virginia Himmelsteib King, *Another Dimension to the Black Diaspora: Diet, Disease, and Racism*

(Cambridge: Cambridge University Press, 1981), 106.
60. Todd Savitt, *Race and Medicine in Nineteenth- and Early Twentieth-Century America* (Kent: Kent State University Press, 2007), 80–84. Sappol, *A Traffic of Dead Bodies*, 5.
61. George N. Acker, "Rickets in Negroes," *Archives of Pediatrics* 11 (1894): 893.

Chapter Four

1. Charles Darwin, *On the Origin of Species: A Facsimile of the First Edition* (1859; Cambridge: Harvard University Press, 1961).
2. Stepan, *The Idea of Race in Science*, 1–19; Sussman, *The Myth of Race*, 19–25.
3. Introduction to Smith, *Essay on the Variety of Complexion and Figure*, ed. Winthrop Jordan, xxviii.
4. McGregor, *From Midwives to Medicine*, 12; Sussman, *The Myth of Race*, 36–47; Darwin, *Origin of Species*, 15–16.
5. Richard Hofstader, "The Vogue of Spencer," in *Darwin: Texts, Backgrounds, Contemporary Opinion, Critical Essays*, ed. Philip Appleman (New York: W.W. Norton, 1979), 389–99; Laura Briggs, "The Race of Hysteria: Overcivilization and the 'Savage' Woman in Late Nineteenth Century Obstetrics and Gynecology," *American Quarterly* 52, no. 2 (June 2000): 246–73, especially 248.
6. George Stocking, *Victorian Anthropology* (New York: Free Press, 1987) and *Race, Culture, and Evolution: Essays in the History of Anthropology* (1968; Chicago: University of Chicago Press, 1987).
7. Darwin, *The Descent of Man*, 2 vols. (London: John Murray, 1871); Stepan, *Idea of Race in Science*, 61–62.
8. *Ibid.*, 47–82; Gould, *Mismeasure of Man*, 416–19; Cynthia Russett, *Sexual Science: The Victorian Construction of Womanhood* (Cambridge: Harvard University Press, 1989).
9. Darwin, *Descent of Man*, 2:327.
10. *Ibid.*, 2:328–29.
11. Ernst Haeckel, *The History of Creation; or the Development of the Earth and Its Inhabitants by the Action of Natural Causes*, 5th ed., vol. 1 (New York: D. Appleton, 1911), 6 (emphasis Haeckel's) as quoted by Edward Larson, *Evolution: The Remarkable History of a Scientific Theory* (New York: Modern Library, 2006), 143.
12. Larson, *Evolution*, 144.
13. George Rosen, "Rudolf Virchow and Neanderthal Man," *American Journal of Surgical Pathology* 2 (June 1977): 183–88.
14. Carl C. Swisher, Garniss H. Curtis, and Roger Lewin, *Java Man: How Two Geologists Changed Our Understanding of Human Evolution* (Chicago: University of Chicago Press, 2000).
15. Stepan, *The Idea of Race in Science*, 173.
16. Darwin, *Origin of Species*, 10–14; Gould, *Structure of Evolutionary Theory*, 336, 622.
17. Edwin Black, *War Against the Weak: Eugenics and America's Campaign to Create a Master Race* (New York: Thunder's Mouth Press, 2003), 12–15; Harry Bruinius, *Better for All the World: The Secret History of Forced Sterilization and America's Quest for Racial Purity* (New York: Alfred A. Knopf, 2006), 11–12, 35–37.
18. Hofstader, "Vogue of Spencer"; David Duncan, *The Life and Times of Herbert Spencer* (Cambridge: Cambridge University Press, 2015).
19. Michael Bulmer, *Francis Galton: Pioneer of Heredity and Biometry* (Baltimore: Johns Hopkins University Press, 2003).
20. Stepan, *Idea of Race in Science*, 111–39; William Bynum, *Science and the Practice of Medicine in the Nineteenth Century* (Cambridge: Cambridge University Press, 1994); Gould, *Mismeasure of Man*, 107–09.
21. Porter, *Greatest Benefit to Mankind*, 304–96.
22. Paul De Kruif, *Microbe Hunters* (New York: Harcourt, Brace, 1926), 57–104; John Snow, "On the Adulteration of Bread as a Cause of Rickets," *International Journal of Epidemiology* 32 (2003): 336–337 (originally published 1857).
23. Thomas McKeown, *The Modern Rise of Population* (New York: Academic Press, 1976); Gerald Grob, *The Deadly Truth: A History of Disease in America* (Cambridge: Harvard University Press, 2002); Anne Hardy, "Rickets and the Rest: Child-Care, Diet and the Infectious Children's Diseases, 1850–1914," *Social History of Medicine* 5 (Dec. 1992): 389–412.

24. Ihde, "Recognition of Rickets as a Deficiency Disease," 85.
25. Leavitt, *Brought to Bed*, 116–41.
26. P.M. Dunn, "Sir James Young Simpson (1811–1870) and Obstetric Anaesthesia," *British Medical Journal* 86, no. 3 (May 2002): 207–09; Richard W. Wertz and Dorothy C. Wertz, *Lying-In: A History of Childbirth in America* (New York: Schocken Books, 1979), 117.
27. Amalie M. Kass, "Walter Channing: Brief Life of a Nineteenth-Century Obstetrician: 1786–1878," *Harvard Magazine* (March–April 2004): 44–45.
28. *The Compact Edition of the Oxford English Dictionary* (Oxford: Oxford University Press, 1971); McGregor, *From Midwives to Medicine*, 1–7.
29. McGregor, *From Midwives to Medicine*, 33–68.
30. Ibid., 69–166.
31. Thomas Addis Emmet, *Vesico-Vaginal Fistula from Parturition and Other Causes with Cases of Recto-Vaginal Fistula* (New York: Wm. Wood and Company, 1868).
32. Ibid.
33. Ibid.
34. Thomas A. Emmet, *Principles and Practice of Gynaecology* (Philadelphia: Henry C. Lea, 1879), 690–722.
35. Edward Laxton, *The Famine Ships: The Irish Exodus to America* (New York: Henry Holt, 1998), 1–18.
36. McGregor, *From Midwives to Medicine*, 100–03.
37. Deirdre Cooper Owens, *Medical Bondage: Race, Gender, and the Origins of American Gynecology* (Athens: University of Georgia Press, 2018), 73–107.
38. Emmet, *Principle and Practice of Gynaecology*.
39. J. Whitridge Williams, "The Frequency of Contracted Pelves in Baltimore," *Bulletin of the Johns Hopkins Hospital* 7 (1896): 165. See also George W. Dobbin, "The Frequency of Contracted Pelves in the Obstetrical Service of the Johns Hopkins Hospital," *The Journal of Obstetrics and Diseases of Women and Children* 36 (Aug. 1897): 148.
40. William Thompson Lusk, *The Science and Art of Midwifery* (New York: D. Appleton, 1882), 433.
41. Loudon, *Death in Childbirth*, 132–37.

42. Emmet, *Principles and Practice of Gynaecology*, 21.
43. Thomas Addis Emmet, *Principles and Practice of Gynecology* (handwritten first draft).
44. George J. Engelmann, *Labor Among Primitive Peoples Showing the Development of the Obstetric Science of Today from the Natural and Instinctive Customs of All Races, Civilized and Savage, Past and Present* (St. Louis: J.H. Chambers and Co., 1884).
45. Ibid., 9–10.
46. Alice B. Stockham, *Tokology: A Book for Every Woman* (Chicago: Sanitary Publishing Co. 1883), Chapter 1. See also Ann Marie Plane, "Childbirth Practices Among Native American Women of New England and Canada, 1600–1800," in *Women and Health in America*, 2nd ed., ed. Judith R. Leavitt (Madison: University of Wisconsin Press, 1999), 38–64.
47. Armand Corre, *La Mère et l'Enfant dans les Races Humaines* (Paris, 1882), 16.
48. Ibid., 74–75.
49. Samuel Gache, "Le Rachitisme en Amérique et Son Influence Obstétricale," *Annales de Gynecologie et Obstetrique* 60 (1903): 175–95.
50. Ibid.
51. Janet Golden, ed., *Infant Asylums and Children's Hospitals: Medical Dilemmas and Developments, 1850–1920: An Anthology of Sources* (New York: Garland, 1989), Introduction.
52. Richard Meckel, *Save the Babies: American Public Health Reform and the Prevention of Infant Mortality* (Ann Arbor: University of Michigan Press, 1998).
53. Edwards A. Park, "A Model and A Gem," in *The Harriet Lane Home: A Model and A Gem*, ed. Edwards A. Park (Baltimore: Department of Pediatrics, School of Medicine, Johns Hopkins University, 2006), 52.
54. McNeill, *Plagues and Peoples*, 197.
55. LeRoy Ashby, *Endangered Children: Dependency, Neglect and Abuse in American History* (New York: Twayne, 1997), 101–78.

Chapter Five

1. Evelyn Brooks Higginbotham, "African American Women's History and the

Metalanguage of Race," in *We Specialize in the Wholley Impossible: Essays in Black Women's History*, ed. Darlene Clark Hine, Wilma King, and Linda Reed (Brooklyn: Carlson, 1995), 3-24.
2. David Blight, *Race and Reunion: The Civil War in American History* (Cambridge: Harvard University Press, 2001), 300-37.
3. Keith Wailoo, *Dying in the City of the Blues: Sickle Cell Anemia and the Politics of Race and Health* (Chapel Hill: University of North Carolina Press, 2001), 26.
4. W.E.B. DuBois, *The Souls of Black Folk: Essays and Sketches* (Chicago: A.C. McClurg, 1904), vii.
5. Peggy Pascoe, *What Comes Naturally: Miscegenation Law and the Making of Race in America* (New York: Oxford University Press, 2010).
6. Steckel, "The African American Population of the United States," 453.
7. *Ibid.*, 462.
8. *Ibid.*, 456-57.
9. Isabel Wilkerson, *The Warmth of Other Suns: The Epic Story of America's Great Migration* (New York: Random House, 2009).
10. Ronald Takaki, *A Different Mirror: A History of Multicultural America* (Boston: Little, Brown, 1993), 246-310; Roger Daniels, *Coming to America: A History of Immigration and Ethnicity in American Life* (New York: Harper Perennial, 2002), 185-286.
11. Hirsch, *Handbook of Geographical and Historical Pathology*, 3:732-42.
12. Christian Warren, "Northern Chills, Southern Fevers: Race-Specific Mortality in American Cities," *Journal of Southern History* 63 (Feb. 1997): 51-52, footnotes 73, 53, 54.
13. *Ibid.*, 14.
14. Acker, "Rickets in Negroes," 893-94.
15. Charles West, *Diseases of Children* (Philadelphia: Longmans, Green and Company, 1874), 588; Hirsch, *Handbook of Geographical and Historical Pathology*, 3:732-42.
16. Joseph Taber Johnson, "Apparent Peculiarities of Parturition in the Negro Race with Remarks on Race Pelves," *American Journal of Obstetrics and Diseases of Women and Children* 8 (1875): 88-123.
17. *Ibid.*, 108.

18. *Ibid.*, 88.
19. Briggs, "The Race of Hysteria." Diane Price Herndl, "The Invisible (Invalid) Woman: African American Women, Illness, and Nineteenth-Century Narrative," in *Women and Health in America*, 2nd ed., ed. Judith Walzer Leavitt (Madison: University of Wisconsin Press, 1999), 131.
20. Johnson, "Apparent Peculiarities of Parturition in the Negro Race," 88-123.
21. *Ibid.*, 99, 111.
22. *Ibid.*, 88, 122.
23. *Ibid.*, 100.
24. Hirsch, *Handbook of Geographical and Historical Pathology*, 3:332-42.
25. Parry, "Observations on the Frequency and Symptoms of Rachitis, with the Results of the Author's Clinical Experience," *American Journal of the Medical Sciences* 63 (1872): 18.
26. *Ibid.*, 45.
27. *Ibid.*, 40-41.
28. *Ibid.*
29. *Ibid.*, 41.
30. *Ibid.*, 17-52.
31. J. Forsyth Meigs and William Pepper, *A Practical Treatise on the Diseases of Children*, 7th ed. (Philadelphia: Blakiston, Son and Co., 1883), 694.
32. Parry, "Observations on the Symptoms of Rachitis," 17-52, 305-29.
33. W.H. Parrish, "A Case of Craniotomy," *Transactions of the Philadelphia Obstetrics Society* (Nov. 1874): 39; John Parry, "The Comparative Merits of Craniotomy and the Caesarean Section in Pelves with a Conjugate Diameter of Two and a Half Inches or Less," *American Journal of the Medical Sciences* 5 (1873): 646.
34. Parrish, "A Case of Craniotomy," 38-39.
35. *Ibid.*
36. *Ibid.*
37. *Ibid.*, 40.
38. Parry, "Comparative Merits of Craniotomy and Caesarean Section," 646.
39. *Ibid.*, 651.
40. Johnson, "Parturition in the Negro Race," 88.
41. Parry, "Comparative Merits of Craniotomy and Caesarean Section," 646-51, 664.
42. *Ibid.*, 644-45.
43. *Ibid.* Briggs, "The Race of Hysteria."
44. Parry, "Comparative Merits of

Craniotomy and Caesarean Section," 646-51, 664; Robert P. Harris, "The Caesarean Operation in the United States," *American Journal of Obstetrics* 4 (Feb. 1872): 622-63.

45. Parry, "Comparative Merits of Craniotomy and Caesarean Section," 61-62, citing Robert Harris.

46. Harris, "The Caesarean Operation in the United States," 622-663; Cooper Owens, *Medical Bondage*, 78-83.

47. Harris, "The Caesarean Operation in the United States," 623, 639-40.

48. Acker, "Rickets in Negroes," 893-94.

49. *Ibid.*

50. *Ibid.*, 894.

51. *Ibid.*

52. Phillip Cutright and Edward Shorter, "The Effects of Health on the Completed Fertility of Nonwhite and White U.S. Women Born Between 1867 and 1935," *Journal of Social History* 13 (1979): 191-209.

53. Steckel, "African American Population of the United States," 473.

54. Stanley Engerman, "Changes in Black Fertility, 1890-1940," in *Family and Population in Nineteenth-Century America*, ed. Tamare Hareven and Maris Vinovskis (Princeton: Princeton University Press, 1978), 126-53.

55. Joseph McFalls and George Masnick, "Birth Control and the Fertility of the U.S. Black Population," *Journal of Family History* 6 (Spring 1981): 89-106; Carole R. McCann, *Birth Control Politics in the United States, 1916-1945* (Ithaca: Cornell University Press, 1994), 136-39.

56. John Haller, "The Physician Versus the Negro: Medical and Anthropological Concepts of Race in the Late Nineteenth Century," *Bulletin of the History of Medicine* 44, no. 2 (March-April 1970): 154-67, especially 155.

57. Acker, "Rickets in Negroes," 898.

58. See for instance, Daniel Immerwahr, "American Blacks and Birth Control," in *Population Reference Bureau* 2 (Washington, D.C.: PRB, 1976), 6-7; Joseph McFalls, Jr., and Marguerite H. McFalls, *Disease and Fertility* (Orlando: Academic Press, 1984). McCann, *Birth Control Politics in the United States, 1916-1945*.

59. Vanessa Gamble, *Making a Place for Ourselves: The Black Hospital Movement 1920-1945* (Oxford: Oxford University Press, 1987), 15-19.

60. *Ibid.*

61. *Ibid.*, 19-23. See also David McBride, *Integrating the City of Medicine: Blacks in Philadelphia Health Care, 1910-1965* (Philadelphia: Temple University Press, 1989).

62. Gladys-Marie Fry, *Night Riders in Black Folk History* (Chapel Hill: University of North Carolina Press, 1975), Chapter 6. Vanessa Northington Gamble, "Under the Shadow of Tuskegee: African Americans and Health Care," in *Tuskegee's Truths: Rethinking the Tuskegee Syphilis Study*, ed. Susan Reverby (Chapel Hill: University of North Carolina Press, 2000), 431-442.

63. Williams, *Ovarian Cysts*, 1246.

64. *Ibid.*

65. Higginbotham, "Metalanguage of Race," 3-24.

66. Susan L. Smith, *Sick and Tired of Being Sick and Tired* (Philadelphia: University of Pennsylvania Press, 1995), 39-40.

67. Edward H. Beardsley, *A History of Neglect: Health Care for Blacks and Mill Workers in the Twentieth Century South* (Knoxville: University of Tennessee Press, 1990), 102.

68. Irving M. Snow, "An Explanation of the Great Frequency of Rickets Among Neapolitan Children in American Cities," *Archives of Pediatrics* 12 (1895): 18-34. Snow alternated the terms "race" and "nationality."

69. *Ibid.*

70. *Ibid.*, 20.

71. *Ibid.*, 23.

72. *Ibid.*

73. *Ibid.*, 27.

74. *Ibid.*, 28-29.

75. J.P. Crozer Griffith, discussant, in Snow, "Explanation of the Great Frequency of Rickets," 29.

76. *Ibid.*; Griffith, *The Care of Baby* (Philadelphia: W.B. Saunders, 1911).

77. L. Emmett Holt, discussant, in Snow, "Explanation of the Great Frequency of Rickets," 29-30.

78. *Ibid.*

79. George Acker, discussant, in Snow, "Explanation of the Great Frequency of Rickets," 34.

80. S.S. Adams, discussant, in Snow, "Explanation of the Great Frequency of Rickets," 31.

81. Nancy Tomes, *The Gospel of Germs:*

Men, Women, and the Microbe in American Life (Cambridge: Harvard University Press, 1998).
82. Jacqueline Wolf, *Don't Kill Your Baby: Public Health and the Decline of Breast Feeding* (Athens: Ohio University Press, 2001).
83. Snow, "Explanation of the Great Frequency of Rickets," 30.

Chapter Six

1. Russell Chesney and Gail Hedberg, "Rickets in Lion Cubs at the London Zoo in 1889," *Pediatrics* 123, no. 5 (May 2009): 948–49. W.B. Cheadle, "Rickets," in *A System of Medicine*, ed. T. Clifford Allbutt and John S. Billings (New York: Macmillan, 1901), 129.
2. Ihde, "Studies on the History of Rickets, II," 14.
3. Cheadle, "Rickets."
4. *Ibid.*, 113.
5. *Ibid.*, 111.
6. *Ibid.*
7. Mitmann, Murphy, and Seller, *Landscapes of Exposure*; McNeill, *Something New Under the Sun*.
8. Florence Nightingale quoted in Mike Davis, *Late Victorian Holocausts: El Niño-Famines and the Making of the Third World* (London: Verso, 2002), 25.
9. Davis, *Late Victorian Holocausts*, 26.
10. *Ibid.*, 173.
11. Hirsch, *Handbook of Geographical and Historical Pathology*, 3:732; Frank R. Barrett, *Disease and Geography: The History of an Idea* (Toronto: Atkinson College, Department of Geography, 2000), 106, 109.
12. Hirsch, *Handbook of Geographical and Historical Pathology*, 3:788.
13. *Ibid.*, 3:336, 3:366–67.
14. Brian Fagan, *Floods, Famines, and Emperors: El Niño and the Fate of Civilizations* (New York: Basic Books, 1999), 45–64.
15. Hirsch, *Handbook of Geographical and Historical Pathology*, 3:736.
16. *Ibid.* 3:732–42.
17. Owen, "Geographical Distribution of Rickets," 113–16.
18. *Ibid.*, 114; Theobald A. Palm, "The Geographical Distribution and Aetiology of Rickets," *The Practitioner* 45 (Nov. 1890): 273.
19. Palm, "Geographical Distribution of Rickets," 321–29.
20. Cited by Palm as William Huntly, *Habits and Diet of the Natives of Rajputana, with Reference to the Etiology and Treatment of Rickets*, Palm, "Geographical Distribution of Rickets," 324–28.
21. Palm, "Geographical Distribution of Rickets," 324–28.
22. *Ibid.*, 332.
23. *Ibid.*, 336.
24. Hardy, "Rickets and the Rest," 408.
25. Palm, "Geographical Distribution of Rickets," 335.
26. *Ibid.*, 334.
27. *Ibid.*, 270–79, 321–42.
28. *Ibid.*, 340.
29. *Ibid.*, 270–79, 321–42.
30. *Ibid.*
31. David Smith and Malcolm Nicolson, "The 'Glasgow School' of Paton, Findlay and Cathcart: Conservative Thought in Chemical Physiology, Nutrition and Public Health," *Social Studies of Science* 19 (1989): 195–238.
32. Leonard Findlay, "The Underlying Cause in the Pathogenesis of Rickets," *Journal of the American Medical Association* 83 (Nov. 8, 1924): 1474. Findlay, "The Etiology of Rickets; A Clinical and Experimental Study," *The British Medical Journal* 18 (July 4, 1908): 13–17.
33. Findlay, "Underlying Cause in the Pathogenesis of Rickets," 1473.
34. McNeill, *Under the Sun*, 66; Hardy, "Bread and Alum," 338.
35. Findlay, "Etiology of Rickets," 16.
36. *Ibid.*, 17.
37. *Ibid.*, 13.
38. *Ibid.*
39. Hess, *Rickets*, 205.
40. Edwards A. Park, "The Etiology of Rickets," *Physiological Reviews* 3 (1923): 154.
41. David Paul von Hansemann, "Ueber Rachitis als Volkskrankheit" ["On Rickets as a Folk-Disease"], *Berliner Klinische Wochenschrift: Organ für praktische Aerzte* 9 (Feb. 26, 1906): 248–54, trans. Blueberry Morningsnow.
42. Park, "The Etiology of Rickets," 154.
43. von Hansemann, "Ueber Rachitis."
44. *Ibid.*
45. *Ibid.*
46. *Ibid.* Thanks to Professor Peter Shapinsky for his expertise in Japanese history.

On Japanese architecture see K. Tada, G. Mehta and N. Murata, *Japanese Style: Architecture and Interiors and Design* (North Clarendon, VT: Tuttle, 2005).

47. von Hansemann, "Ueber Rachitis."
48. *Ibid.*
49. John Lovett Morse, "The Frequency of Rickets in Infancy in Boston and Vicinity," *Journal of the American Medical Association* 34 (1900): 724.
50. "Obituary: John Lovett Morse," *American Journal of Diseases of Children*, found in *Archives of Pediatrics* 59, no. 6 (1942): 1328.
51. Morse, "Frequency of Rickets in Infancy in Boston," 724.
52. Hess, *Rickets*, 214–15.
53. Morse, "Frequency of Rickets in Infancy in Boston," 724.
54. *Ibid.*
55. *Ibid.*, 725.
56. *Ibid.*
57. *Ibid.*, 726.
58. John Lovett Morse and Fritz B. Talbot, *Diseases of Nutrition and Infant Feeding* (New York: Macmillan, 1915), 316.
59. Morse, "Rickets in Infancy," 726.
60. *Ibid.*
61. L. Emmett Holt, discussant, in Snow, "Neopolitan Children," 29–30.
62. Morse, "Rickets in Infancy," 725, 726.
63. Apple, *Mothers and Medicine*, 32; John Lovett Morse, *The Care and Feeding of Children* (Cambridge: Harvard University Press, 1914); Borden S. Veeder, *Pediatric Profiles* (St. Louis: C.V. Mosby Company, 1957), 99.
64. Fruitnight, "The Treatment of Rachitis," 168–74. See Hess, *Rickets*, 350.
65. Thomas Southworth, "The Importance of the Early Recognition and Treatment of Rachitis," *Journal of the American Medical Association* 50 (1908): 89–93.
66. *Ibid.*, 93.
67. J.C. Cook, discussant in Southworth, "Importance of Early Recognition," 92.
68. L.T. Royster, discussant in Southworth, "Importance of Early Recognition," 93.
69. *Ibid.*
70. Leonard Findlay, "Introduction," Medical Research Committee, *A Study of Social and Economic Factors in the Causation of Rickets*, Special Report Series, No. 20 (London: Published by His Majesty's Stationery Office, 1918), 16–17.
71. Findlay, "Etiology of Rickets."
72. "What a Woman Should Be," *The New York Times*, Jan. 24, 1897.
73. Antoinette Donnelly, "Are We a Bowlegged Sex?" *The Chicago Tribune*, July 2, 1916.
74. Dr. W.A. Evans, "How to Keep Well," *The Chicago Tribune*, Jan. 20, 1918: 18, C5.
75. Dr. A. Wilberforce Williams, "Talks on Preventive Measures, First Aid Remedies, Hygienics and Sanitation," *The Chicago Defender*, Sept. 8, 1917, 12.

Part Two

1. Robert H. Wiebe, *The Search for Order 1877–1920* (New York: Hill and Wang, 1966); Thomas C. Leonard, *Illiberal Reformers: Race, Eugenics, and American Economics in the Progressive Era* (Princeton: Princeton University Press, 2016).
2. *Ibid.*
3. The quote is from Mark Twain, *Puddn'Head Wilson* (Hartford, CT: American Publishing Company, 1894).

Chapter Seven

1. William Osler, *The Principles and Practice of Medicine* (New York: D. Appleton, 1899), 434.
2. Regina Morantz-Sanchez, *Sympathy and Science: Women Physicians in American Medicine* (Oxford: Oxford University Press, 1985), 115–16.
3. Kenneth M. Ludmerer, *Learning to Heal: The Development of American Medical Education* (Baltimore: Johns Hopkins University Press, 1985), 34.
4. Harvey Cushing, *The Life of William Osler*, vol. 1 (Birmingham: Special Edition, Classics of Modern Medicine, 1982), quoting from William Osler's letter to *Canada Medical and Surgical Journal* 2 (1873–1874): 308.
5. Harvey et al., *A Model of Its Kind*, 6–12.
6. *Sixth Report of the Superintendent of the Johns Hopkins Hospital. For the Year ending January 31, 1895* (Baltimore: Johns Hopkins University Press, 1895), 17–18.
7. *Ibid.*

8. *Sixth Report of the Superintendent of The Johns Hopkins Hospital*, 18–19.
9. *Ibid.*, 136.
10. William Travis Howard, *Public Health Administration and the Natural History of Disease in Baltimore, Maryland, 1797-1920* (Washington, D.C.: Carnegie Institute of Washington, 1924), 183, from U.S. Census data. See also Department of Commerce, Bureau of the Census, *Negro Population: 1790-1840* (Washington, D.C.: Government Printing Office, 1918), 98. The federal government statistics distinguish Baltimore from Baltimore City, p. 113. Howard does not.
11. Karen Olson, "Old West Baltimore: Segregation, African-American Culture, and the Struggle for Equality," *The Baltimore Book*, 57–61.
12. Argersinger, "The City That Tries to Suit Everybody," 82.
13. Washington, *Medical Apartheid*, 153.
14. Harry Dowling, *City Hospitals: The Undercare of the Underprivileged* (Cambridge: Harvard University Press, 1982), 32; Alan Mason Chesney, *Johns Hopkins Hospital and the Johns Hopkins University School of Medicine: A Chronicle* (Baltimore: Johns Hopkins University Press, 1943), 1:164–65.
15. Gamble, *Making a Place*, 28.
16. Chesney, *Johns Hopkins Hospital*, 1:164–165.
17. Charles E. Rosenberg, "Social Class and Medical Care in 19th Century America: The Rise and Fall of the Dispensary," in *Sickness and Health: Readings in the History of Medicine and Public Health*, ed. Judith Walzer Leavitt and Ronald Numbers (Madison: University of Wisconsin Press, 1978), 309–22. Originally published in 1974.
18. George Rosen, "The Efficiency Criterion in Medical Care, 1900–1920," *Bulletin of the History of Medicine* 50 (1976): 28–44.
19. J. Whitridge Williams, "Dispensary Abuse and Certain Problems of Medical Practice," *Journal of the American Medical Association* 66 (1916): 1902–908; F.S. Newell, "The Ideal Obstetric Outpatient Clinic," and Discussion, from J. Whitridge Williams and others, *Transactions of the American Association for the Study and Prevention of Infant Mortality* 4 (1913): 191–207.
20. Irving Loudon, "The Origin and Growth of the Dispensary Movement in England," *Bulletin of the History of Medicine* 55 (1981): 341.
21. Chesney, *Johns Hopkins Hospital*, 1:291.
22. *Ibid.*, 68–69.
23. *Ibid.*, 2:150.
24. *Ibid.*, 2:114.
25. *Ibid.*, 2:211–13.
26. A. McGehee Harvey, *Adventures in Medical Research: A Century of Discovery at Johns Hopkins* (Baltimore: Johns Hopkins University Press, 1976), 188.
27. Williams, "Dispensary Abuse," 1903.
28. *Ibid.*, 1902–08.
29. Alan Frank Guttmacher, "Recollections of John Whitridge Williams," *Johns Hopkins Alumni Bulletin* 23 (1935): 233–43.
30. *Ibid.*
31. McGregor, *Midwives to Medicine*, 203–19.
32. J. Whitridge Williams, "Carcinoma of the Cervix Uteri in the Negress," *Johns Hopkins Hospital Reports* 2 (1890): 224–26; Williams, "Tuberculosis of the Generative Organs," *Transactions of the American Gynecological Society* 17 (1892): 409–80.
33. Harvey, Brieger, Abrams and McKusick, *A Model of Its Kind*; Harvey, *Adventures in Medical Research*, Chapter 16; Chesney, *Johns Hopkins Hospital*, vols. 1 and 2.
34. Judith Walzer Leavitt, "The Growth of Medical Authority: Technology and Morals in Turn-of-the-Century Obstetrics," *Women and Health in America*, 636–58; Susan E. Lederer, *Subjected to Science: Human Experimentation in America Before the Second World War* (Baltimore: Johns Hopkins University Press, 1995), 1–26; Cooper Owens, *Medical Bondage*, 78–83; Barbara Duden, *Disembodying Women: Perspectives on Pregnancy and the Unborn* (Cambridge: Harvard University Press, 1993).
35. James Cassedy, *American Medicine and Statistical Thinking, 1800-1860* (Cambridge: Harvard University Press, 1984), 4, 17, 19, 181–82.
36. J. Whitridge Williams, "Pelvimetry for the General Practitioner," *The Medical News* 58 (1891): 322–23.
37. *Ibid.*

38. Howard A. Kelly, Discussion of J. Whitridge Williams, "Pelvimetry," 363–64.
39. Chesney, *Johns Hopkins Hospital*, 2:232.
40. Ibid., 2:165, 2:210.
41. Ibid., 2:461.
42. J. Whitridge Williams, Letter to Superintendent Dr. Winford H. Smith, Johns Hopkins Hospital, April 10, 1916, "J. Whitridge Williams Collection," 1903–1936 inclusive, Alan Mason Chesney Medical Archives, Johns Hopkins University.
43. Guttmacher, "Recollections of John Whitridge Williams."
44. Ibid.
45. Gail Bederman, *Manliness and Civilization: A Cultural History of Gender and Race in the United States, 1880–1917* (Chicago: University of Chicago Press, 1995), 170–216.
46. Outstanding, in the TR lexicon.
47. William Cronon, *Nature's Metropolis: Chicago and the Great West* (New York: W.W. Norton, 1992).
48. Gould, *Mismeasure of Man*, 109–14.
49. Rockefeller Archives, Collection RF, group 1.1, series 200L, box 185, folder 2220, "Conference on Public Health," University of Pennsylvania, Philadelphia, Pennsylvania (Nov. 8, 1915), 183. See also Fee, *Disease and Discovery*, 49.
50. J. Whitridge Williams, "The Frequency of Contracted Pelvis in the First Thousand Women Delivered in the Obstetrical Department of the Johns Hopkins Hospital," *Obstetrics* 1, no. 5 (May 1899): 245, repeated in subsequent analyses; list of books sent to Welch Library, "J. Whitridge Williams Collection," Chesney Medical Archives.
51. Hodge, *Principles and Practice of Obstetrics*.
52. Thomas P. Duffy, "The Flexner Report—100 Years Later," *Yale Journal of Biology and Medicine* 84, no. 3 (Sept. 1984): 269–76; Abraham Flexner, *Medical Education in the United States and Canada: A Report to the Carnegie Foundation for the Advancement of Teaching* (New York: Carnegie Foundation, 1910), Arno reprint edition, 1972, 180–81.
53. Flexner, *Medical Education in the United States and Canada*, 180–81.
54. Higginbotham, "Metalanguage of Race," 3–24.
55. Gamble, *Making a Place*, 29.
56. Flexner, *Medical Education in the United States and Canada*, 180–81.
57. Savitt, *Race and Medicine in Nineteenth and Early Twentieth Century America*, 121–268.
58. J. Whitridge Williams, *Obstetrics: A Textbook for the Use of Students and Practitioners* (New York: D. Appleton, 1903).

Chapter Eight

1. William Carlos Williams, "A Face of Stone," *The Doctor Stories*, comp. Robert Coles (New York: New Directions, 1984), 78–87; T. Hugh Crawford, *Modernism, Medicine and William Carlos Williams* (Norman: University of Oklahoma Press, 1993).
2. Wolf, *Deliver Me from Pain*, 1–73; Wertz and Wertz, *Lying In*, 132–35; Leavitt, *Brought to Bed*, 116–41.
3. Paul Findley, "The Lost Art of Obstetrics," *Northeast Medicine* 17 (1918): 67–70, quoted in Irving Loudon, "The Transformation of Maternal Mortality," 1558.
4. Katharine Park, *Secrets of Women: Gender, Generation and the Origins of Human Dissection* (Princeton: Princeton University Press, 2010), 121–60.
5. Discussion of C.A. Von Ramdohr, "The Difference in Treatment, in Hospital and Private Practice, of Dystocia Due to Contracted Pelvis," *Transactions of the Obstetrical Society of New York* 23 (1890): 180–85.
6. Williams, "Frequency of Contracted Pelves in Baltimore," 165; Dobbin, "Frequency of Contracted Pelves in the Obstetrical Service," 148.
7. Edward Reynolds, "On the Frequency of Contract Pelvis among American Women, as Deduced from 2227 Cases of Labor," *Transactions of the American Gynecological Society* 15 (1890): 367.
8. Ibid., 369.
9. Ibid., 371.
10. Williams, "Frequency of Contracted Pelves in Baltimore," 166.
11. J. Whitridge Williams, Working Copy, *Obstetrics*, 2nd ed. (1908), 681.
12. George W. Dobbin, "The Frequency of Contracted Pelvis in the Obstetrical Service of the Johns Hopkins Hospital,"

American Journal of Obstetrics and diseases of women and children 36, no. 2 (Aug. 1897): 145–63, see 149.

13. George W. Dobbin, "The Use of Pelvimetry in Gynecology, Illustrated by a Case of Vesico-Vaginal Fistula," *American Journal of Obstetrics* XXXII (1895): 201–07.

14. Ibid.

15. Dobbin, "Frequency of Contracted Pelves in the Obstetrical Service," 151.

16. *Ibid.*, 153.

17. Dobbin, "The Operative Treatment of Labor, Complicated by Pelvic Deformities; Based upon a Critical Review of the First Thousand Patients Delivered in the Obstetrical Department of the Johns Hopkins Hospital," *Obstetrics* 1, no. 7 (July 1899): 353–418, esp. 354.

18. Bederman, *Manliness and Civilization*, 1–44, 170–216; Briggs, "The Race of Hysteria."

19. J. Whitridge Williams, "A Further Contribution Concerning the Frequency and Clinical Significance of Funnel Pelves," *Surgery, Gynecology and Obstetrics* 13 (1911): 95, discussion, 96.

20. Edward Davis, "The Frequency and Mortality of Abnormal Pelves," *American Journal of Obstetrics and Diseases of Children* XI (1901): 15.

21. Ibid. 11–15, 66–78.

22. James Clifton Edgar, "Pelvic Deformity in New York," *Transactions, American Gynecological Society* 27 (1902): 329.

23. *Ibid.*, 325.

24. Ibid.

25. *Ibid.*, 324–37.

26. Dobbin, "Operative Treatment of Labor," 353–418.

27. Effa V. Davis, "A Study of the Bony Pelvis in One Hundred and Fifty Cases," *Journal of the American Medical Association* 45 (Dec. 1905): 1709–710.

28. Ibid.

29. *Ibid.*, 1710.

30. Ibid.

31. A.F.A. King, "Uniformity in Pelvic and Cranial Measurements," *Transactions of the American Gynecological Society* 29 (1904): 233–46.

32. Ibid.

33. *Ibid.*, 245–46.

34. Harvey A. Gabert and Mohammed Bey, "History and Development of Cesarean Operation," *Obstetrics and Gynecology Clinics of North America* 15 (1988): 597.

35. *Ibid.*; Meckel, *Save the Babies*, 159–61.

36. Adophe Pinard, "Indication del'Operation Césarienne, Considérée en Rapport avec celle de la Symphyséotomie, de la Craniotomie de l'"Accouchement Prématore Artificiel," *Annales de Gynecologie* 52 (Aug. 1899): 98–99.

37. Klaus, *Every Child a Lion*, 32–33.

38. Judith Walzer Leavitt, "The Growth of Medical Authority: Technology and Morals in Turn-of-the-Century Obstetrics," in *Women and Health in America*, ed. Leavitt, 636–58.

39. Henry Bettmann, "Premature Labor and the Newborn Child," *American Journal of Obstetrics and Diseases of Women and Children* 25 (1892): 315–28.

40. Joseph B. DeLee, "Progress Toward Ideal Obstetrics," *American Association for the Study and Prevention of Infant Mortality* 6 (1915): 116.

41. Joseph B. DeLee, "The Prophylactic Forceps Operation," *American Journal of Obstetrics and Gynecology* 1 (Oct. 1920): 77–80.

42. Ibid.

43. Joseph B. DeLee, "The Technique of the Chicago Lying-In Hospital and Dispensary," *Surgery, Gynecology and Obstetrics* 3 (1906): 805–15; J.P. Greenhill, "Joseph B. DeLee (1859–1942)," *Yearbook of Obstetrics and Gynecology* (Chicago: Yearbook Publishers, 1942); Judith Walzer Leavitt, "Joseph B. DeLee and the Practice of Preventive Obstetrics," *American Journal of Public Health* 78, no. 10 (Oct. 1988): 1353–360.

44. Joseph B. DeLee, *The Principles and Practice of Obstetrics* (Philadelphia: W.B. Saunders, 1913), 272.

45. Greenhill, "Joseph B. DeLee"; Leavitt, "DeLee and the Practice of Preventive Obstetrics."

46. Timothy Johnson, "John Whitridge Williams," in *The First One Hundred Years: Department of Gynecology and Obstetrics, The Johns Hopkins University School of Medicine*, ed. John Rock, Timothy Johnson and J. Donald Woodruff (Baltimore: Johns Hopkins University Press, 1991), 135.

47. Greenhill, "Joseph B. DeLee (1859–1942)."

48. Wertz and Wertz, *Lying In*, 132–77; Leavitt, *Brought to Bed*, 171–95.

49. Tina Cassidy, *Birth: The Surprising History of How We are Born* (New York: Atlantic Monthly Press, 2006); Wertz and Wertz, *Lying In*, 132–77; Leavitt, *Brought to Bed*, 171–212.

50. Gabert and Bey, "History and Development of Cesarean Section," 591–605.

51. Loudon, *Death in Childbirth*, 258–66.

52. Ibid., 599; Jane Eliot Sewell, *Caesarean Section—A Brief History, a Brochure to Accompany an Exhibition on the History of Caesarean Section at the National Library of Medicine* (April 30, 1993–August 31, 1993) Washington, D.C., American College of Obstetricians and Gynecologists, 1993.

53. Gabert and Bey, "History and Development of Cesarean Section," 600.

54. J. Morris Slemons, "Progress in Obstetrics: 1890–1940," *American Journal of Surgery* 51 (1941): 89–90.

55. William Diekmann, "Cesarean Section Mortality," *American Journal of Obstetrics and Gynecology* 50 (1945): 41–42.

56. Sewell, *Caesarean Section—A Brief History*.

57. Barton Cooke Hirst, "Symphysiotomy," *The Medical News* 63 (Dec. 2, 1893): 627.

58. Leavitt, "Growth of Medical Authority," 639–40; J. W. Williams, "Is Pubiotomy a Justifiable Operation? A Second Communication," *American Journal of Obstetrics and Diseases of Children* 61 (1910): 721–52.

59. Leavitt, *Brought to Bed*, 87–170.

60. A.F.A. King, Edward Davis and J. Whitridge Williams, "Report of the Committee Appointed at the Previous Meeting to Consider 'Uniformity in Pelvic and Cranial Measurements,'" *Transactions of the American Gynecological Society* 30 (1905): 80–82.

61. DeLee, *Principles and Practice of Obstetrics*, 657.

62. Laurel Thatcher Ulrich, *A Midwife's Tale: The Life of Martha Ballard, Based on Her Diary, 1785–1812* (New York: Oxford University Press, 1990).

63. Arnold Van Gennep, *Rites of Passage*, trans. Monika Vizedom and Gabrielle Caffee (Chicago: University of Chicago Press, 1960).

64. Bederman, *Manliness and Civilization*, 23–25.

65. Munro Kerr, "Diagnosis and Treatment of Contracted Pelves," *Transactions of the American Gynecological Society* XXXVI (1911): 156–85.

66. Ibid., 178–80.

67. Ibid., 183.

68. Ibid., 183–85.

69. Leavitt, *Brought to Bed*, 25.

70. Loudon, *Death in Childbirth*, 549–50; Loudon, "The Transformation of Maternal Mortality," 1558–560.

71. Robert Morse Woodbury, "The Trend of Maternal-Mortality Rates in the United States Death-Registration Area, 1900–1921," *American Journal of Public Health* 14, no. 9 (Sept. 1, 1924): 738–43; Loudon, *Death in Childbirth*, 569–95.

72. Loudon, *Death in Childbirth*, 569–95; Ransom Hooker, *Maternal Mortality in New York City: A Study of All Puerperal Deaths, 1930–1932* (New York: The Commonwealth Fund, 1933); Charles R. King, "The New York Maternal Mortality Study: A Conflict of Professionalization," *Bulletin of the History of Medicine* 65 (1991): 476–502.

73. Loudon, "Transformation of Maternal Mortality," 1559.

74. Joseph B. DeLee, "The Maternity Ward of the General Hospital," *The Modern Hospital Yearbook* 6 (1926): 67–72; DeLee, "What Are the Special Needs of the Modern Maternity?" *The Modern Hospital* 28 (March 1927): 59–69; DeLee, "How Should the Maternity Be Isolated?" *The Modern Hospital* 29 (Sept. 1927): 65–72; DeLee and Heinz Siendentopf, "The Maternity Ward of the General Hospital," *Journal of the American Medical Association* 100 (Jan. 7, 1933): 6–14. See also Leavitt, *Brought to Bed*, 183–86.

75. J. Whitridge Williams, "Is an Architecturally Isolated Building Essential for a Lying-In Hospital," *Modern Hospital* 28 (April 1927) 58, quoted by Joseph DeLee, "Facing the Facts," *Journal of American Medical Association* 100 (Jan. 1933): 12.

Chapter Nine

1. Fielding H. Garrison, "A History of Pediatrics," in *Abt-Garrison History of Pediatrics*, ed. A.F. Abt (Philadelphia:

W.B. Saunders, 1925), as cited in Alexandra Minna Stern and Harold Merkel, eds., *The Formative Years: Children's Health in the United States,1880-2000* (Ann Arbor: University of Michigan Press, 2005), 48.

2. Janet Golden, Introduction, *Infant Asylums and Children's Hospitals: Medical Dilemmas and Developments, 1850-1920, An Anthology of Sources,* ed. Janet Golden (New York: Garland, 1989), introduction; Russell Viner, "Abraham Jacobi and the Origins of Scientific Pediatrics in America," *The Formative Years,* ed. Stern and Markel, 23-46.

3. Abraham Jacobi, "Foundlings and Foundling Institutions," *Infant Asylums,* 33-136.

4. Viner, "Jacobi and the Origins of Scientific Pediatrics."

5. Quoted in Jerome S. Leopold, "Abraham Jacobi (1830-1919)," *Pediatric Profiles,* ed. Borden S. Veeder (St. Louis: The C.V. Mosby Company, 1957), 15.

6. Jacobi, "Foundlings and Foundling Institutions," 33-136.

7. Rima Apple, *Perfect Motherhood: Science and Childrearing in America* (New Brunswick: Rutgers University Press, 2006), 37.

8. Abraham Jacobi, "Craniotabes," *American Journal of Obstetrics and Diseases of Women and Children* (Nov. 1870): 435-67.

9. Abraham Jacobi, "Why Hospitals for Children are Needed," ca., 1880 reprint, *Collectanea Jacobi,* ed. William Robinson (New York, 1908) in Robert Bremner, ed., *Children and Youth in America: A Documentary History,* 2 vols. (Cambridge: Harvard University Press, 1971), 2:831-836.

10. J. Whitridge Williams, "Vulvo-Vaginitis in Children," *Maryland Medical Journal* XXVII, no. 7 (June 11, 1892): 705-12.

11. Holt alluded to the great growth in membership of the American Pediatrics Society; there were forty-four physicians present at the first meeting in 1888. Holt, "The Scope and Limitations of Hospitals for Infants," *Transactions for the American Pediatric Society* 10 (1898): 147-60.

12. George Rosen, "The Efficiency Criterion in Medical Care, 1900-1920: An Early Approach to an Evaluation of Health Service," *Bulletin of the History of Medicine* 50 (1976): 28-44.

13. L. Emmett Holt, "The Children's Hospital, the Medical School and the Public," *Johns Hopkins Hospital Bulletin* 25 (1913): 89-92. Jacobi, "Why Hospitals for Children Are Needed," in *Children and Youth in America,* 2:831.

14. Ashby, *Endangered Children,* 55-101.

15. John Holt, Jr., quoted in *The Harriet Lane Home: A Model and a Gem* (Baltimore: Department of Pediatrics, School of Medicine, Johns Hopkins University, 2006), 90.

16. Jacobi, "Why Hospitals for Children Are Needed," 2:831-36.

17. Barbara Ehrenreich and Deirdre English, *For Her Own Good: 150 Years of the Experts' Advice to Women* (Garden City, NY: Anchor Books, 1979), 69-98.

18. Edwards A. Park and Howard H. Mason, "Luther Emmett Holt," *Pediatric Profiles,* 33-60.

19. *Ibid.*

20. Apple, *Perfect Motherhood,* 36.

21. Park and Mason, "Luther Emmett Holt," 33-60.

22. *Ibid.*

23. Philip Van Ingen, "Infant Mortality in Institutions," *Proceedings of the National Conference of Charities and Correction* (1915): 126-29.

24. Hammonds, *Childhood's Deadly Scourge,* 17-87.

25. Holt, "Scope and Limitations of Hospitals," 147-60.

26. Meckel, *Save the Babies,* 40-51.

27. Apple, *Mothers and Medicine*; Jacqueline H. Wolf, "Discarding Nature's Plan: A Social History of Infant Feeding in Chicago, 1892-1938," Ph.D. diss. University of Illinois at Chicago, 1998; Wolf, *Don't Kill Your Baby*; Janet Golden, "From Wet Nurse Directory to Milk Bank: The Delivery of Human Milk in Boston, 1909-1927," *Bulletin of the History of Medicine* 62 (1988): 589-605.

28. Park and Mason, "Luther Emmett Holt," 39.

29. John M. Barry, *The Great Influenza: The Epic Story of the Deadliest Plague in History* (New York: Viking, 2004), 72; Harvey, Brieger, Abrams, and McKusick, *Model of Its Kind,* 1:22.

30. Letters exchanged between Simon Flexner and Alfred Hess; Simon Flexner and Edwards A. Park; Simon Flexner

Papers, American Philosophical Society Library, Philadelphia, Pennsylvania.
31. Park et al., *Harriet Lane Home*, 47-70.
32. Harvey et al., *A Model of Its Kind*, 55.
33. "Agreements between the Harriet Lane Home for Invalid Children of Baltimore City and the Johns Hopkins Hospital," September 1, 1906. Collection HLH, Series 4D, folder 1, Chesney Medical Archives.
34. Edwards A. Park, "The One Man We Desire above All Others: Clemens von Pirquet, 1908-1911," *Harriet Lane Home* 43, fn.1.
35. Report to the Trustees on the Occasion of the Twentieth Anniversary, "The Harriet Lane Home for Invalid Children," Collection HLH, folder 1, Chesney Archives; Harvey et al., *A Model of Its Own Kind*, 1:56-57; Chesney, *Johns Hopkins Hospital and School of Medicine*, 3:78.
36. Park, "One Man," 26.
37. *Ibid.*, 30-32.
38. *Ibid.*, 20.
39. Chesney, *Johns Hopkins Hospital and School of Medicine*, 3:220.
40. Helen Taussig et al., "Final Meeting in the Harriet Lane Home Amphitheater," *Johns Hopkins Medical Journal* 137 (1975): 20-25.
41. Wilburt C. Davison, "John Howland," *Pediatric Profiles*, 161-63.
42. Harvey, *Adventures in Medical Research*, 200; Park, "Model and a Gem," 57.
43. Harvey et al., *Model of Its Kind*, 56.
44. "New Hospital Opens," copy for the *Evening Sun*, Baltimore, Nov. 20, 1912, Collection HLH, folder 1, Chesney Archives.
45. Holt, "The Children's Hospital, the Medical School and the Public," 89.
46. *Ibid.*, 91.
47. *Ibid.*, 92.
48. Sappol, *A Traffic of Dead Bodies*, 98-135.
49. Davison, "John Howland," 169.
50. Henry M. Seidel, "Larger than Life: Edwards A. Park, 1927-1946," *Harriet Lane Home*, 119-62.
51. Apple, *Mothers and Medicine*; Park et al., *The Harriet Lane Home*, 56.
52. Saul Benison, *Tom Rivers: Reflections on a Life in Medicine and Science* (Cambridge: MIT Press, 1967), 48.

53. *Ibid.*
54. Alfred Hess saw Howland in this same light. He respected him greatly but disliked his military style. Abraham Flexner, "Alfred Fabian Hess, 1875-1933," Hess, *Collected Writings*, 1:xxiii.
55. Edwards A. Park, "A Lush Meadow of Opportunity," *Harriet Lane Home*, 72.
56. Edwards A. Park, "A Most Companionable Man: Howland's Persona," *The Harriet Lane Home*, 103-18.
57. Park, "Lush Meadow of Opportunity," 90; John Howland and W. McKim Marriot, "Acidosis Occurring in Diarrhea," *American Journal of the Disabled Child* XI, no. 5 (1916): 309-25.
58. John Howland and W. McKim Marriot, "The Calcium Content of the Blood in Rachitis and Tetany," *Transactions of the American Pediatrics Society* 28 (1916): 202. Letter from Edwards A. Park to Alan Mason Chesney, March 20, 1939, Baltimore. Collection HLH, folder 1, Chesney Archives.
59. Benjamin Kramer and John Howland, "Calcium and Phosphorus in the Serum in Relation to Rickets," *American Journal of the Diseases of the Child* 22 (1921): 105. The citation puts Howland's name first. Park contended that Kramer was the real innovator in this and several other instances. Letter from Edwards A. Park to Alan Mason Chesney, March 20, 1939. Letter from Edwards A. Park to Alan Mason Chesney, March 22, 1929, Baltimore. Collection HLH, folder 1, Chesney Archives.
60. L. Emmett Holt and John Howland, *The Diseases of Infancy and Childhood*, 7th ed., fully rev. (New York: D. Appleton, 1916), 243.
61. *Ibid.*, 242.
62. L. Emmett Holt and John Howland, *The Diseases of Infancy and Childhood*, 8th ed., fully rev. (New York: D. Appleton, 1922), 241.
63. Holt and Howland, *Diseases of Infancy and Childhood*, 7th ed., 243-44.
64. *Ibid.*
65. Holt and Howland, *Diseases of Infancy and Childhood*, 8th ed., 242-43.

Chapter Ten

1. Outdoor Obstetrical Service Records, Medical Records Division, Alan Mason

Chesney Medical Archives, Johns Hopkins Medical Institutions, Baltimore, Maryland. The records are on microfilm. Unless otherwise noted, the discussion of the OOS Case records derives entirely from this source. The request for waiver of HIPAA (Health Insurance and Accountability Act) authorization for research use or disclosure of protected health information (Application # 2004-15) was approved on 11 October 2004, conditional on nondisclosure of protected health information of individuals in the requested materials without authorization of the descendants. In accordance with this condition, the patient records discussed cannot be individually identified.
2. Cassedy, *American Medicine and Statistical Thinking*, 60-64.
3. Nancy M. Theriot, "Negotiating Illness: Doctors, Patients, and Families in the Nineteenth Century," *Journal of the History of the Behavioral Sciences* 37 (Fall 2001): 349-68; Jonathan Gillis, "The History of the Patient History since 1850," *Bulletin of the History of Medicine* 80 (Fall 2006): 490-512.
4. J. Whitridge Williams, "Frequency of Contracted Pelves in the First Thousand Women Delivered in the Obstetrical Department of the Johns Hopkins Hospital," *Obstetrics* 1, no. 5 (May 1899): 245.
5. Dobbin, "Operative Treatment of Labor," 353-418.
6. J. Whitridge Williams, "Pelvimetry for the General Practitioner," *The Medical News* 58, no. 12 (March 21, 1891): 321-24; George W. Dobbin, "The Use of Pelvimetry in Gynecology, Illustrated by a Case of Vesico-Vaginal Fistula," *American Journal of Obstetrics and Diseases of Women and Children* 33 (1895): 204; Moir, ed., *Munro Kerr's Operative Obstetrics*, 316.
7. Williams, "Pelvimetry," 323.
8. Leavitt, *Brought to Bed*, 116-41.
9. Williams, "Pelvimetry," 322-24.
10. Williams, "History of Obstetrics," 29-36.
11. Jennifer Block, *Pushed: The Painful Truth about Childbirth and Modern Maternity Care* (Cambridge: DaCapo, 2007), 19-21, 109-12.
12. Williams, "Frequency of Contracted Pelves in Baltimore," 164.
13. Williams, *Obstetrics*, 1st ed., 1-23, 580-675.

14. Edgar, "Pelvic Deformity in New York," 324-37; King, "Uniformity in Pelvic and Cranial Measurements," 233-46.
15. Loudon, *Death in Childbirth*, 142.
16. Ibid., 130; Litzmann, *Die Formen des Beckens*, chapter eleven.
17. Dobbin, "Frequency of Contracted Pelvis," 145-63; Dobbin, "The Operative Treatment of Labor," 353-418.
18. Williams, "Frequency of Contracted Pelves in the First Thousand Women," 241-53.
19. Williams, *Obstetrics*, 1st ed., 581.
20. Ibid., 283-91.
21. Susan Bordo, *Unbearable Weight: Feminism, Western Culture, and the Body* (Berkeley: University of California Press, 1993), 175-78.
22. Robbie E. Davis-Floyd, *Birth as an American Rite of Passage* (Berkeley: University of California Press, 1992), 187-240.
23. Laura Briggs, "The Race of Hysteria," 247.
24. Judith Walzer Leavitt, "Under the Shadow of Maternity: American Women's Responses to Death and Debility Fears in Nineteenth-Century Childbirth," *Women and Health in America*, 328-46.
25. J. Whitridge Williams, "The Funnel Pelvis," *Transactions of the American Gynecological Society* 64 (July 1911): 106-24.
26. J. Whitridge Williams "Frequency, Etiology and Practical Significance of Contractions of the Pelvic Outlet," *Surgery, Gynecology, and Obstetrics* 8 (June 1909): 619-38, esp. 620.
27. Emmet, *Vesico-Vaginal Fistula*.
28. Turner, "Index of the Pelvic Brim," 125-43.
29. C. Breus and A. Kolisko, *Die pathologischen Beckenformen* (Leipzig: F. Deuticke, 1902-1912).
30. Michaela Klien, *Die Geburtsilfliche Bedeutung der Verengerungen des Beckenausgangs, insbesondere des Trichterbeckens* Volkmann's Sammlung klin (1896, #196). Williams, "Frequency, Etiology, and Practical Significance of Contractions," 620-21.
31. Williams, *Obstetrics*, 4th ed. (New York: D. Appleton, 1917), 902.
32. Ibid.
33. Ibid., 624.
34. Williams, "The Funnel Pelvis," 106-24.

35. J. Morris Slemons, *John Whitridge Williams: Academic Aspects and Bibliography* (Baltimore: Johns Hopkins University Press, 1935), 27–36.
36. Williams, "Further Contribution Concerning Funnel Pelves," 95.
37. Williams, "Frequency, Etiology and Practical Significance of Contractions," 622.
38. J. Whitridge Williams, "Is Pubiotomy a Justifiable Operation?" *American Journal of Obstetrics and the Diseases of the Child* 58 (1908): 202–31; J. Whitridge Williams, "The Effect of Pubiotomy upon the Course of Subsequent Labors," *American Journal of Obstetrics and the Diseases of the Child* 72, no. 1 (July 1915): 1–25.
39. Judith Walzer Leavitt, "The Growth of Medical Authority," 640; Williams, "Is Pubiotomy a Justifiable Operation?" 721–52.
40. Williams, "The Funnel Pelvis," 106–24.
41. Ibid.
42. J. Whitridge Williams, "Indications for Therapeutic Sterilization in Obstetrics," *Journal of the American Medical Association* 91, no. 17 (Oct. 27, 1928), 1240; Black, *War Against the Weak*.
43. Frances Goldsborough, "The Maternal Mortality in the First 5000 Obstetrical Cases at the Johns Hopkins Hospital," *Bulletin of the Johns Hopkins Hospital* 19 (1908): 13.
44. Robert Woods, "Lying-In and Laying-Out: Fetal Health and the Contribution of Midwifery," *Bulletin of the History of Medicine*, 81 (Winter 2007): 730–59.
45. J. Whitridge Williams, "Pelvic Indications for the Performance of Cesarean Section," *Transactions of the American Gynecological Society* 26 (1901): 260–76.

Chapter Eleven

1. J. Whitridge Williams, "A Case of Spondylolisthesis, with Description of the Pelvis," *American Journal of Obstetrics and Diseases of Women and Children* 40, no. 2 (Aug. 1899): 145–71.
2. Ibid., 150.
3. Ibid.
4. Ibid., 150–57.
5. Ibid., 163.
6. Holmes, *The Hottentot Venus*, 169–90.
7. Williams, "A Case of Spondylolisthesis," 163–69.
8. Leavitt, "Growth of Medical Authority," 636–58; Susan E. Lederer, *Subjected to Science*, 1–26; Cooper Owens, *Medical Bondage*, 78–83.
9. Harvey et al., *A Model of Its Kind*, 38.
10. Williams, "Frequency of Contracted Pelves in Baltimore," 164.
11. Ibid., 243; Williams, *Obstetrics*, 2nd ed., 582.
12. Williams, "Pelvic Indications for Cesarean Section," 261.
13. Ibid., 263.
14. Ibid., 250.
15. Beardsley, *A History of Neglect*, 15–17.
16. J.W. Williams, *Obstetrics*, 3rd rev. ed. (New York: D. Appleton, 1912), 789.
17. Williams, "Pelvic Indications for Cesarean Section," 260–76; Cassedy, *American Medicine and Statistical Thinking*, 80–91.
18. Williams, *Obstetrics* (handwritten copy), 262–63.
19. Williams, *Obstetrics*, 1st ed., 640.
20. Dobbin, "Operative Treatment of Labor," 357.
21. Williams, "Frequency of Contracted Pelvis in the First 1000 Women," 249–51.
22. Williams, "Pelvic Indications for the Performance of Cesarean Section," 263.
23. Ibid., 264–65.
24. Ibid., 261–63.
25. Theodore F. Riggs, "A Comparative Study of White and Negro Pelves," *The Johns Hopkins Hospital Reports* 12 (1904): 421.
26. Ibid.
27. Riggs, "Comparative Study of White and Negro Pelves," 421–54.
28. Clayton Arbuthnot Lane, "A Clinical Comparison of the Maternal Pelvis and of the Foetus in Europeans, Eurasians, and Bengalis: And the Enunciation of a New Law in Accordance with Which the Size of the Child at Birth Is Determined," *Lancet* (Sept. 26, 1903): 885–89; Vrolik, "Observations of the Differences of Pelves"; Shiebinger, *Nature's Body*, 158, 160.
29. Lane, "Clinical Comparison of the Maternal Pelvis and of the Foetus in

Europeans, Eurasians, and Bengalis," 885-89.
30. Riggs, "Comparative Study of White and Negro Pelves," 423.
31. Ibid., 422.
32. Ibid. 422-23.
33. Ibid., 438.
34. Ibid., 446.
35. Ibid., 437.
36. Ibid., 430-36.
37. Ibid., 447-50, 453.
38. Ibid., 438.
39. Ibid., 444, 446.
40. Ibid., 446.
41. Ibid., 443.
42. Ibid., 453.
43. Elizabeth Fee, "Nineteenth-Century Craniology: The Study of the Female Skull," *Bulletin of the History of Medicine* 53 (1979): 415-33; Gould, *Mismeasure of Man*, 140; Franz Boas, "Changes in the Bodily Form of Descendants of Immigrants," *American Anthropologist*, New Series, vol. 14, no. 3 (July-Sept. 1912): 530-62.
44. Riggs, "Comparative Study of White and Negro Pelves," 452-53.

Chapter Twelve

1. Murray H. Bass, "Albert Fabian Hess," *Pediatric Profiles*, 175-81; Abraham Flexner, "Albert Fabian Hess, 1975-1933," *Collected Writings: Alfred F. Hess*, 2 vols. (Springfield, IL: Charles C. Thomas, 1936), 1:ix-xxviii.
2. Wade Oliver, *The Man Who Lived for Tomorrow: A Biography of William Hallock Park, M.S.* (New York: E.P. Dutton, 1941); Evelyn Hammonds, *Childhood's Deadly Scourge: The Campaign to Control Diphtheria in New York City, 1880-1930* (Baltimore: Johns Hopkins University Press, 1999).
3. Bass, "Albert Fabian Hess," 175-81; Flexner, "Albert Fabian Hess," 1:ix-xviii.
4. Quoted from the handbook of the Federation for the Support of Jewish Philanthropic Societies of New York City in Konrad Bercovici, "Orphans as Guinea Pigs," *The Nation* 112 (1921): 912-13.
5. Lederer, *Subjected to Science*, 106.
6. Flexner, "Albert Fabian Hess," *Collected Writings*, 1:xvii-xxii.
7. Alfred F. Hess, "Infantile Scurvy: The Blood, the Blood-Vessels and the Diet," *American Journal of Diseases of Children* 8 (1914): 386-405; Hess, *Collected Writings*, 1:294-315.
8. Roger K French, "Scurvy," *The Cambridge World History of Human Disease*, ed. Kenneth F. Kiple (Cambridge: Cambridge University Press, 1993), pp. 1001-005.
9. Hess, "Infantile Scurvy," 400.
10. Ibid., 386-405.
11. Ibid., 404.
12. Ibid., 404-05.
13. Ibid.
14. Albert von Haller, *The Vitamin Hunters*, trans. Hella Freud Bernays (Philadelphia: Chilton, 1962), 55-56; Lee R. McDowell, *Vitamin History: The Early Years* (Sarasota: Design, 2013), 9-10, 62.
15. Hess, "Infantile Scurvy," 404.
16. Ibid., 403-05.
17. Hess, *Collected Writings*, 1:316-635; Hess, *Scurvy: Past and Present*.
18. Alfred Hess and Lester Unger, "Prophylactic Therapy for Rickets in a Negro Community," *Journal of the American Medical Association* (Nov. 30, 1917): 1583-586, reprinted in Hess, *Collected Writings*, 1:487-99.
19. Ibid. See also George Rosen, "The First Neighborhood Health Care Movement, Its Rise and Fall," *American Journal of Public Health* 61, no. 8 (Aug. 1971): 1620-637.
20. George Rosen, "The Case of the Consumptive Conductor, or Public Health on a Street Car: A Centennial Tribute to Alfred Hess, M.D.," *American Journal of Public Health* 65, no. 9 (Sept. 1975): 977-78.
21. Hess and Unger, "Prophylactic Therapy for Rickets," 487.
22. Ibid.
23. Ibid.
24. Ibid.
25. Ibid., 488.
26. Ibid.
27. Ibid.
28. Ibid., 487-89; Alfred F. Hess and Lester J. Unger, "The Diet of the Negro Mother in New York City," *Journal of the American Medical Association* (March 30, 1918): 900-02; Hess, *Collected Writings*, 1:500-09.
29. Hess and Unger, "Prophylactic Therapy for Rickets," 494.

30. Ibid.; Discussion following Alfred F. Hess, "Rickets as Influenced by the Diet of the Mother During Pregnancy and Lactation," *Journal of the American Medical Association* 83, no. 20 (Nov. 15, 1924): 1563-566.
31. Hess and Unger, "The Diet of the Negro Mother in New York City," Hess, *Collected Writings*, 1:500-09. This is the more complete reprint version of the original article in *The Journal of the American Medical Association* (March 30, 1918).
32. See Jane Ziegelman, *97 Orchard: An Edible History of Five Immigrant Families in One New York Tenement* (New York: Harper, 2010).
33. Hess and Unger, "Diet of the Negro Mother in New York City," Hess, *Collected Writings*, 1:507-09.
34. Discussion following Hess, "Rickets as Influenced by the Diet of the Mother," 1563-566.
35. Franz Boas, "Changes in the Bodily Form of Descendants of Immigrants," *Senate Document 208, 61st Congress, Second Session* (Washington, D.C.: Government Printing Office, 1911), 530-562.
36. R. Fred Wacker, *Ethnicity, Pluralism and Race: Race Relations Theory in America Before Myrdal* (Westport, CT: Greenwood Press, 1983).
37. Franz Boas to Alfred Hess, April 8, 1919. American Philosophical Society, Franz Boas Papers, Alfred Hess Folder #1 B: B61.
38. Alfred Hess to Franz Boas, October 15, 1923, Franz Boas to Alfred Hess, October 23, 1923, American Philosophical Society, Boas Papers, Hess Folder #1 B: B61.
39. Franz Boas, *The Mind of Primitive Man* (New York: Macmillan, 1911), 274.
40. Robert Woodbury, *Statures and Weights of Children Under Six Years of Age*, Children's Bureau Publication #87 (Washington, D.C.: Government Printing Office, 1921), 63-64. Woodbury analyzed the effect of rickets on white children only, perhaps limited by data, showing less growth for those affected.
41. Franz Boas, "Remarks on the Anthropological Study of Children," *Transactions of the 15th International Congress on Hygiene and Demography* (Washington, 1913), reprinted in Boas, *Race, Language and Culture* (Chicago: University of Chicago, 1940), 94-102; Boas, "Growth," in the same volume, 103-30.
42. Hess, *Rickets: Including Osteomalacia and Tetany*, 89.
43. Ibid., 92.
44. Ibid. 278.
45. Hess and Unger, "Prophylactic Therapy"; Hess and Unger, "The Diet of the Negro Mother."
46. Holt and Howland, *Diseases of Infancy and Childhood*, 7th ed., 242.
47. Ibid.
48. Albert Love and Charles Davenport, "Defects Found in Drafted Men," *The Scientific Monthly* 10, no. 1 (Jan. 1920): 5-25.
49. Ibid., 8.
50. Beth Linker, "Feet for Fighting: Locating Disability and Social Medicine in First World War America," *Social History of Medicine* 20, no. 1 (April 2007): 91-109.
51. Davenport and Love, "Defects Found in Drafted Men," 22.
52. Ibid., 22-24.
53. Hess, *Rickets*, 308.

Chapter Thirteen

1. Grace Meigs, "Maternal Mortality from All Conditions Connected with Child Birth, in the United States and Certain Other Countries," U.S. Department of Labor, Children's Bureau, Miscellaneous Series No. 6, Bureau Publication No. 19 (Washington, D.C.: Government Printing Office, 1917). Quotation, 7.
2. Woodbury, "Trend of Maternal-Mortality Rates," 739.
3. See James Young, "Maternal Mortality and Maternal Mortality Rates," *American Journal of Obstetrics and Gynecology* 31 (1936): 198-212 for an analysis of the pitfalls of comparative maternal mortality rates.
4. Leslie Reagan, *When Abortion Was a Crime: Women, Medicine, and Law in the United States, 1867-1973* (Berkeley: University of California Press, 1997), 39, 77, 91, 95, 109-11; Leavitt, *Brought to Bed*, 18, 174.
5. Loudon, "Transformation of Maternal Mortality," 1558.
6. DeLee, "Progress Toward Ideal Obstetrics," 114.
7. Leavitt, *Brought to Bed*, 36-63; Char-

lotte Borst, *Catching Babies: The Professionalization of Childbirth, 1870-1920* (Cambridge: Harvard University Press, 1995).

8. Gertrude Jacinta Fraser, *African American Midwifery in the South: Dialogues of Birth, Race, and Memory* (Cambridge: Harvard University Press, 1998), 103.

9. Schwartz, *Birthing a Slave*, 291-319.

10. Valerie Lee, *Granny Midwives and Black Women Writers: Double-Dutched Readings* (New York: Routledge, 1996); Fraser, *African American Midwifery in the South*.

11. Lee, *Granny Midwives and Black Women Writers*, 6.

12. Ibid.; Fraser, *African American Midwifery in the South*.

13. Meckel, *Save the Babies*, 108-18.

14. J.H. Mason Knox, "Address by the President," *Transactions of the American Association for the Study and Prevention of Infant Mortality* (1910): 29.

15. Ibid., 30.

16. Black, *War Against the Weak*, 4-73; Klaus, *Every Child a Lion*, 35-38.

17. Daniel Kevles, *In the Name of Eugenics: Genetics and the Uses of Human Heredity* (New York: Alfred A. Knopf, 1985), 44-45.

18. Black, *War Against the Weak*, 32-37.

19. Ibid., 116-18, quotation, 117; Black, *War Against the Weak*, 57, 89.

20. Meckel, *Save the Babies*, 116-18.

21. L. Emmett Holt, "Infant Mortality, Ancient and Modern: An Historical Sketch," *Transactions of the American Association for Study and Prevention of Infant Mortality, Archives of Pediatrics* 30 (1913): 25.

22. Gordon, *Woman's Body, Woman's Right*, 136-58; Bederman, *Manliness and Civilization*, 199-206.

23. John W. Harris, "Biographical Sketch of J. Whitridge Williams," Alan Mason Chesney Archives, J. Whitridge Williams Papers, Folder J, Whitridge Williams Death

24. J. Whitridge Williams, "What the Obstetrician Can Do to Prevent Infant Mortality," *Transactions of the American Association for the Study and Prevention of Infant Mortality* 1 (1910): 190-203. Stanley A. Halpern, *American Pediatrics: The Social Dynamics of Professionalism* (Berkeley: University of California Press, 1988); Lindenmeyer, *A Right to Childhood*, 36.

25. Lawrence D. Longo and Christina M. Thomson, "Prenatal Care and Its Evolution," *Proceedings of the Second Motherhood Symposium of the Women's Studies Research* (University of Wisconsin-Madison, 1981), reprinted in Philip K. Wilson, ed., *Childbirth: Changing Ideas and Practices in Britain and America, 1600 to the Present*, vol. 2: *The Medicalization of Obstetrics: Personnel, Practice, and Instruments* (New York: Garland, 1996), 157.

26. Williams, "What the Obstetrician Can Do to Prevent Infant Mortality," 196.

27. J. Whitridge Williams, "The Midwife Problem and Medical Education," *Transactions of the American Association for the Study and Prevention of Infant Mortality* 2 (1911): 189.

28. Ibid.

29. Judy Barrett Litoff, "Forgotten Women: American Midwives at the Turn of the Twentieth Century," *The Historian* 40, no. 2 (Feb. 1978): 235-51.

30. Guy Steele, "The Midwife Problem and Its Legal Control," *Maryland Medical Journal* 48 (Jan. 1905): 1-6.

31. Lilian Welsh, *Reminiscences of Thirty Years in Baltimore* (Baltimore: The Norman, Remington Co., 1925), 31-61.

32. Robin Muncy, *Creating a Female Dominion in American Reform, 1890-1935* (New York: Oxford University Press, 1991), 142.

33. Morantz-Sanchez, *Sympathy and Science*, 133, 160, 173; Welsh, *Reminiscences of Thirty Years in Baltimore*, 93.

34. F. Elisabeth Crowell, "The Midwives of New York," *Charities and the Commons* 17 (Jan. 1907) in *The American Midwife Debate: A Sourcebook on Its Modern Origins*, ed. Judy Barrett Litoff (Westport, CT: Greenwood Press, 1986), 42-43.

35. Reagan, *When Abortion Was a Crime*, 90.

36. Ibid., 31-61.

37. Mary Sherwood, "The Midwives of Baltimore," *Journal of the American Medical Association* 52, no. 25 (1909): 2009-010.

38. Ibid.

39. Ibid., 2010.

40. Ibid., 2009.

41. Ibid.

42. *Ibid.*, 2009-010.
43. Helmina Jeidell and Willa Fricke, "The Midwives of Anne Arundel County, Maryland," *Johns Hopkins Hospital Bulletin* XXIII, no. 29 (Sept. 1912): 279-81.
44. Anna Rochester, *Infant Mortality: Results of a Field Study in Baltimore, Maryland Based on Births in One Year* (Washington, D.C.: Government Printing Office, 1923), Bureau Publication #119. Quotation, p. 19.
45. *Ibid.*
46. *Ibid.*, 77.
47. *Ibid.*, 43.
48. *Ibid.*, 65.
49. *Ibid.*, 68.
50. *Ibid.*, 85, 106.
51. *Ibid.*, 58.
52. *Ibid.*, 101.
53. *Ibid.*, 130.
54. Lindenmeyer, *A Right to Childhood*, 52-75; Robyn Muncy, *Creating a Female Dominion in American Reform 1890-1935* (Oxford: Oxford University Press, 1991), 38-65; Ladd-Taylor, *Mother-Work*, 104-27.
55. Ladd-Taylor, *Motherwork*, 104-27; Muncy, *Creating a Female Dominion*, 38-65.
56. *Standards of Child Welfare: A Report of Children's Bureau Conferences, Many and June 1919*, U.S. Department of Labor, Children's Bureau Publication no. 60 (Washington, D.C.: Government Printing Office, 1919), 67-70.
57. Julia C. Lathrop, "Standards of Child Welfare," *Annals of the American Academy of Political and Social Science* 98 (1921): 1-8.
58. *Ibid.*
59. *Ibid.*, 8.
60. Lindenmeyer, 87.
61. *Ibid.*, 88-89.
62. Halpern, *American Pediatrics*, 86-87.
63. Barbara Katz Rothman, *Recreating Motherhood*, 2nd ed. (New Brunswick: Rutgers University Press, 2000), 145.
64. Skocpol, *Protecting Soldiers and Mothers*, 520.
65. Sonya Michel, *Children's Interests, Mothers' Rights: The Shaping of America's Child Care Policy* (New Haven: Yale University Press, 1999), 7.
66. J. Whitridge Williams, "The Significance of Syphilis in Prenatal Care and in the Causation of Fetal Deaths," *Bulletin of the Johns Hopkins Hospital* 31, no. 351 (May 1920): 142.
67. *Ibid.*
68. *Ibid.*, 99.
69. Meckel, *Save the Babies*, 114, 202.
70. Harvey et al., *A Model of Its Kind*, 105-06.
71. Lauren P. Morton, "Baltimore's First Birth Control Clinic: The Bureau for Contraceptive Advice, 1927-1932," *Maryland Historical Magazine* 102, no. 4 (2007): 300-19.
72. "To the Physicians of Maryland," October 17, 1927, in "Fourth Report for the Bureau for Contraceptive Advise" (1932), Alan Mason Chesney Medical Archives Folder: Baltimore Birth Control Clinic, Box #III/62/4.
73. Barry Alan Mehler, "History of the American Eugenics Society, 1921-1940," Ph.D. Dissertation in History, University of Illinois at Champaign-Urbana, 1988, 402. See also the Adolf Meyer Papers at the Alan Mason Chesney Medical Archives.
74. Elizabeth Fee, *Disease and Discovery: A History of the Johns Hopkins School of Hygiene and Public Health 1916-1939* (Baltimore: Johns Hopkins University Press, 1987), 204-10.
75. Adolf Meyer, "The Right to Marry," *The Survey* 36 (June 3, 1916): 243-46.
76. J. Whitridge Williams, "Comments on Curtis, Watson et al: Discussion of Genital Warts," *Transactions of the American Gynecological Society* 53 (1928): 43.
77. Kenneth Blackfan, "Growth and Development of the Child," *White House Conference on Child Health and Protection*, Part IV (New York: Century Co., 1932); Gould, *Mismeasure of Man*, 40-49.
78. Philip R. Reilly, M.D., J.D., *The Surgical Solution: A History of Involuntary Sterilization in the United States* (Baltimore: Johns Hopkins University Press, 1991), 45; Harry Bruinius, *Better for All the World: The Secret History of Forced Sterilization and America's Quest for Racial Purity* (New York: Alfred A. Knopf, 2006).
79. Williams, "Indications for Therapeutic Sterilization in Obstetrics," 1240.
80. *Ibid.*
81. *Ibid.*, 1241.
82. *Ibid.*, 1238.
83. *Ibid.*, 1240.
84. *Ibid.*
85. John W. Harris, "A Study of the

Results Obtained in Sixty-Four Caesarean Sections Terminated by Supravaginal Hysterectomy," *Bulletin of the Johns Hopkins Hospital* 33 (Sept.1922): 318–19.
86. *Ibid.*
87. J. Whitridge Williams, "A Histological Study of Fifty Uteri Removed at Cesarean Section," *Transactions of the American Gynecological Society* 42 (1920): 350–51.
88. *Ibid.*; Lutz Kuelber, "Eugenics: Compulsory Sterilization in 50 American States," www.uvm.edu/lkuelber/eugenics.
89. J. Whitridge Williams and Ko Chi Sun, "A Statistical Study of the Incidence and Treatment of Labor Complicated by Contracted Pelvis in the Obstetric Service of the Johns Hopkins Hospital from 1896 to 1924," *American Journal of Obstetrics and Gynecology* 11 (June 1926): 735–55.
90. *Ibid.*, 741.
91. *Ibid.*, 741–42.
92. *Ibid.*, 755.
93. Haller, "The Physician versus the Negro," 154–167.
94. Williams, "Statistical Study," 735.
95. *Ibid.*, 745.
96. J. Whitridge Williams, "A Critical Analysis of Twenty-One Years' Experience with Caesarean Section," *Bulletin of the Johns Hopkins Hospital* 32 (June 1921): 173–84.
97. J.H. Mason Knox and Paul Zantai, "The Health Problem of the American Negro," *American Journal of Public Health* 6 (1926): 809.
98. *Ibid.*, 808; J. H. Mason Knox, "The Preschool Child in Rural Maryland," *Transactions of the Medical and Chiriurgical Faculty of the State of Maryland* 126 (1924): 45.
99. *Ibid.*

Chapter Fourteen

1. C. Breus and A. Kolisko, *Die pathologische Beckenform* (Leipzig: F. Deuticke, 1904). Alfred F. Hess, *Rickets*, 224.
2. Edwards A. Park, "Rickets in Baltimore Since the Advent of Vitamin D Treatment," in *Symposium on Nutrition: The Physiological Role of Certain Vitamins and Trace Elements*, ed. Roger M. Herriott (Baltimore: Johns Hopkins University Press, 1953), 126; Barrie Vernon-Roberts, "Christian Georg Schmorl: Pioneer of Spinal Pathology and Radiology," *Spine* 19 no. 23 (1994): 2724–727.
3. *Ibid.* G. Schmorl, "Die pathologische Anatomie der rachitischen Knochenerkrankung mit besonderer Berücksichtigung ihrer Histologie und Pathogenese," *Erbn. d. inn. Med. u. Kinder* iv (1909), as cited in Edwards A. Park, "The Etiology of Rickets," *American Physiological Society* 3 (1923): 133.
4. C.G. Schmorl, "Die pathologische Anatomiie der rrachitischen Knochenerkrankung mit besonderer Berucksichtigung ihrer Histologie und Pathogenese," *Ergebn. d. inn. Med. u. Kinder* iv. (1909): 403; Hess, "Infantile Rickets," 37, 39.
5. George Sarton, "The Discovery of X-Rays," *Isis* 26 (March 1937): 358; Daniel Server, "The Rise of Radiation Protection: Science, Medicine and Technology in Society, 1895–1935," Ph.D. Diss., Princeton University, 1976.
6. Server, viii.
7. Herbert Thoms, "The Clinical Significance of X-Ray Pelvimetry," *American Journal of Obstetrics and Gynecology* 12, no. 4 (Jan. 1926): 543–50.
8. Amand Routh, "On Caesarean Section in the United Kingdom with Tables of 1282 Cases of Caesarean Section by Over 100 Obstetricians and Gynaecologists of the United Kingdom, Who Were Living on June 1, 1910," *Journal of Obstetrics and Gynaecology of the British Empire* XIX (Jan. 1911): 1–233.
9. *Ibid.*
10. Leonard Findlay, "Introductory Historical Survey," in Margaret Ferguson, *A Study of Social and Economic Factors in the Causation of Rickets*, written under D. Noël Paton and Leonard Findley (London: Medical Research Committee, 1918), 18.
11. *Ibid.*
12. Ferguson, *Study of Social and Economic Factors in the Causation of Rickets*, 94–95.
13. David F. Smith and Malcolm Nicholson, "Chemical Physiology Versus Biochemistry, the Clinic Versus the Laboratory. The Glasegian Opposition to Edward Mellanby's Theory of Rickets," *Proceedings of the Royal College of Physicians of Edinburgh* 19 (1989): 51–60.
14. Alfred Hess and Lester J. Unger, "The Clinical Role of the Fat Soluble Vitamin: Its Relation to Rickets," *Journal of*

the *American Medical Association* 74 (Jan. 24, 1920), 223; Hess, *Collected Writings*, 1:605-22.
15. von Haller, *The Vitamin Hunters*, 52.
16. F.G. Hopkins, "The Effect of Heat and Aeration upon the Fat-Soluble Vitamine," *Biochemistry Journal* 14 (1920): 725-33.
17. John Paranscandola and Aaron M. Ihde, "Edward Mellanby and the Antirachitic Factor," *Bulletin of the History of Medicine* 51 (Winter 1977): 507-15.
18. Edward Mellanby, "An Experimental Investigation on Rickets," *Lancet* 1, no. 196 (March 15, 1919): 407-12; Edward Mellanby, "Experimental Rickets: The Effects of Cereals and Their Interaction with Other Factors of Diet and Environment in Producing Rickets," Medical Research Council Special Report No. 93 (London: His Majesty's Stationery Office, 1925); Ihde, "Recognition of Rickets as a Deficiency Disease," 83-88.
19. Park, "Etiology of Rickets," 115.
20. K. Huldschinsky, "Heilung von Rachitis durch künstliche Hohensonne," *Detsch. Med. Wochenscht* 45 (1919): 712-13.
21. Privy Council: Medical Research Council, *Studies of Rickets in Vienna, 1919-1922* (London: His Majesty's Stationary Office, 1923).
22. *Ibid.*
23. H.S. Hutchison, "The Aetiology of Rickets, Early and Late," *Quarterly Journal of Medicine* XV (1921-1922): 167-95, with two plates.
24. *Ibid.*
25. *Ibid.*, 184.
26. *Ibid.*, 194.
27. Elmer F. McCullom and M. Davis, "Observations on the Isolation of the Substance in Butter Fat Which Exerts a Stimulating Effect on Growth," *Journal of Biological Chemistry* 19 (1914): 245-50; Fee, *Disease and Discovery*, 62-63.
28. Park et al., *The Harriet Lane Home*, 91.
29. Hess and Unger, "The Fat Soluble Vitamin"; Hess, *Collected Writings*, 1:619.
30. *Ibid.*, 1:619-20.
31. *Ibid.*, 1:605.
32. *Ibid.*, 1:611-17.
33. *Ibid.*, 1:621.
34. Alfred F. Hess and Lester J. Unger,

"Use of the Carbon Arc Light in the Prevention and Cure of Rickets," *Journal of the American Medical Association* (May 27, 1922); Hess, *Collected Writings*, 1:713-719.
35. Alfred. F. Hess and M.G. Gutman, "The Cure of Infantile Rickets by Sunlight," *Journal of the American Medical Association* (Jan. 7, 1922); Hess, *Collected Writings* 1:676-681.
36. *Ibid.*
37. P.G. Shipley, E.A. Park, E.V. McCullom, N. Simmonds and H.T. Parsons, "Studies on Experimental Rickets: The Production of Rachitis and Similar Diseases in the Rat by Deficient Diets," *Journal of Biological Chemistry* XLV (July 1921): 333-41; Alfred F. Hess, "Experimental Rickets in Rats: II. The Failure of Rats to Develop Rickets On a Diet Deficient in Vitamin A," *Journal of Biological Chemistry* (July 1921); Hess, *Collected Writings*, 1:656.
38. Hess, "Clinical Role of the Fat Soluble Vitamin," 611.
39. G.F. Powers, E.A. Park and Nina Simmonds, "The Influence of Radiant Energy upon the Development of Xerophthalmia in Rats: A Remarkable Demonstration of the Beneficial Influence of Sunlight and Out-of-Door Air Upon the Organism," *Journal of Biological Chemistry* LVII (Jan. 29, 1923): 576.
40. Elmer V. McCullom, Nina Simmonds, J.E. Becker, and P.G. Shipley, "Studies on Experimental Rickets XXI. An Experimental Demonstration of the Existence of a Vitamin Which Promotes Calcium Deposition," *Journal of Biological Chemistry* 53 (1922): 293-312.
41. G.F. Powers, E.A. Park, P. Shipley, et al., "The Prevention of Rickets in the Rat by Means of Radiation with the Mercury Vapor Quartz Lamp," *Proceedings of the Society for Experimental Biology and Medicine* 19 (1921): 293-312.
42. P.G. Shipley, E.A. Park, E.V. McCollum and Nina Simmonds, "The Function of the Organic Factor as Exemplified by Cod Liver Oil," *Transactions of the American Pediatrics Society*, 33rd Session (June 1921): 1-7, Discussion: Alfred Hess, 5.
43. *Ibid.*, Discussion: Edwards A. Park, 6-7.
44. McCullom, Simmonds, Becker, and Shipley, "Studies on Experimental Rickets XXI," 304.

45. "Finds New Vitamin is Bone Protector," *New York Times*, June 19, 1922, 1.
46. Elmer McCollum and Nina Simmonds, *Food, Nutrition and Health* (Baltimore: Published by the Authors, 1925), iii.
47. Findlay, "Historical Survey," 43.
48. Park, "Etiology of Rickets," 133.
49. *Ibid.*, 153.
50. Elmer V. McCullom, Nina Simmonds, J.E. Becker, and P.G. Shipley, "Studies on Experimental Rickets XXI. An Experimental Demonstration of the Existence of a Vitamin Which Promotes Calcium Deposition," *Journal of Biological Chemistry* 53 (1922): 293-312.
51. Harold Harrison and Helen Harrison, *Disorders of Calcium and Phosphate Metabolism in Childhood and Adolescence* (Philadelphia: W.B. Saunders Co., 1979).
52. Park, "Etiology of Rickets," 112.
53. *Ibid.*, 149.
54. *Ibid.*
55. Takaki, *Iron Cages*, 32; Smith, *Variety of Complexion and Figure in the Human Species*, 59.
56. John J. Abel and Walter S. Davis, "On the Pigment of Negro's Skin and Hair," *Journal of Experimental Medicine* I (July 1896): 369.
57. Park, "Etiology of Rickets," 150.
58. *Ibid.*, 150-51.
59. Hess, *Rickets*, 92.
60. Hess and Unger, "Prophylactic Therapy" and "The Diet of the Negro Mother."
61. J. Lawson Dick, *Rickets: A Study of Economic Conditions and Their Effects on the Health of the Nation, in Two Parts Combined in One Volume* (London: William Heinemann, 1922).
62. *Ibid.* 85-86.
63. *Ibid.*, 29.
64. Helen Taussig, "Pediatric Profile, Edwards A. Park, 1878-1969," *The Journal of Pediatrics* 77 (Oct. 1970): 724-25; Edwards A. Park, "Memoires Originaux: Un Dispensaire do La Croix-Rouge Americaine en France,"*Archives de Médicine des Enfants* 22 (1919): 393-413. Edwards A. Park and Co-Workers, "The Organization of a Children's Dispensary on the Basis of Appointments for Patients," *The Modern Hospital* 13 (1919): 101-08, 185-89.
65. Dick, *Rickets* 58.
66. *Ibid.*, 66.
67. Park, "Etiology of Rickets,"154.

68. Edwards A. Park Papers, Alfred Hess Folder, 1931-1933, Chesney Archives.
69. Ellen More, *Restoring the Balance: Women Physicians and the Profession of Medicine, 1850-1995* (Cambridge: Harvard University Press, 1995), 172.
70. *Ibid.*, 172-74.
71. Letter from Martha Eliot to E.A. Park, Nov. 29, 1930, Schlesinger Library, Martha M. Eliot Collection, Folder 250.
72. Oral History with Pauline Stitt, in Regina Markell Morantz, Cynthia Stodola Pomerleau and Carol Hansen Fenichel, eds., *In Her Own Words: Oral Histories of Women Physicians* (New Haven: Yale University Press, 1982), 117-18.
73. Martha May Eliot, "The Control of Rickets: Preliminary Discussion of the Demonstration in New Haven" *Journal of the American Medical Association* 85, no. 9 (1925): 656-63; Martha May Eliot, M.D., "The New Haven Demonstration of Community Control of Rickets," *The Public Health Journal* 17, no. 3 (March 1926): 114-16.
74. Eliot, "New Haven Demonstration."
75. Thanks to Molly Jean-Mary, N.P., M.Ph., at the Boston Children's Hospital. See "Vitamin D Deficiency May Lurk in Babies," *New York Times*, Aug. 26, 2008.
76. Eliot, "Control of Rickets: Preliminary Discussion," 656-60.
77. *Ibid.*, 661.
78. *Ibid.*
79. *Sun Babies*, produced by the Children's Bureau, 1926. Information provided by the National Archives, Washington, D.C. The local ID number for the film is 102.2, the Archive ID 13608.
80. Park, "Etiology of Rickets," 139.
81. Harry Goldblatt and Katharine Marjorie Soames, "The Supplementary Value of Light Rays to a Diet Graded in Its Content of Fat-Soluble Organic Factor," *Biochemical Journal* 17 (1923): 622-29.
82. E.M. Hume and H.H. Smith, "The Effect of the Radiation of the Environment with Ultra-Violet Light upon the Growth and Calcification of Rats, Fed on a Diet Deficient in Fat-Soluble Vitamins: The Part Played by Irradiated Sawdust," *Biochemistry Journal* 18 (1924): 1334-345; Kenneth J. Carpenter and Ling Zhao, "Forgotten Mysteries in the Early History of Vitamin D," *Journal of Nutrition* 129 (Feb. 1999): 923-27.

83. Alfred Hess and Mildred Weinstock, "Antirachitic Properties Imparted to Inert Fluids by Ultraviolet Radiation," *Proceedings of the Society of Biology and Medicine* 22 (1924): 6–7; Hess, *Collected Writings*, 2:136–46.

84. Alfred Hess and Mildred Weinstock, "Antirachitic Properties Imparted to Lettuce and to Growing Wheat by Ultraviolet Irradiation," *American Journal of the Disabled Child* (1924): 5; Hess, *Collected Writings*, 2:114; Hess and Weinstock, "Antirachitic Properties Imparted to Inert Fluids," 2:136–46.

85. Harry Steenbock and Archie Black, "Fat-Soluble Vitamins. XVII. The Induction of Growth-Promoting and Calcifying Properties in a Ration by Exposure to Ultra-Violet Light," *Journal of Biological Chemistry* 61 (April 1924): 405–22; Rima D. Apple, *Vitamania: Vitamins in American Culture* (New Brunswick: Rutgers University Press, 1996).

86. Charles E. Bills, "Physiology of the Sterols, Including Vitamin D," *Physiological Reviews* 15, no. 1 (Jan. 1935): 1–12.

87. Alfred A. Hess and Mildred Weinstock, "The Antirachitic Value of Irradiated Phytosterol and Cholesterol," *Journal of Biological Chemistry* 63 (1925): 305–09; Hess, *Collected Writings*, 2:157–59, esp. 159.

88. Alfred F. Hess and Adolf Windaus, "The Development of Marked Activity in Ergosterol Following Ultraviolet Irradiation," *Proceedings of the Society for Experimental Biology and Medicine* 24 (1927); Hess, *Collected Writings*, 2:272.

89. George Wolf, "The Discovery of Vitamin D: The Contribution of Adolf Windaus," *The Journal of Nutrition*, 34, no. 6 (June 2004): 1299–302. This essay was very helpful in sorting out the steps in the discovery of Vitamin D, as was Bills, "Physiology of the Sterols," 1, and McDowell, *Vitamin History*, 116–21, Flexner, "Alfred Fabian Hess," xvi.

90. Wolf, "Discovery of Vitamin D."

91. Holick, *Vitamin D Solution*, 3–24.

92. Rima D. Apple, "Patenting University Research: Harry Steenbock and the Wisconsin Alumni Research Association," *Isis* 80, no. 3 (Sept. 1989): 374–94.

93. Ibid., 380–85.

94. Ibid.

95. Harold E. Harrison, "The Disappearance of Rickets," *American Journal of Public Health* 56, no. 5 (May 1966): 734–37; Holick, *The Vitamin D Solution*, 69–70.

96. Apple, *Mothers and Medicine*, 110. Her book *Vitamania* details the commerce in cod liver oil and Vitamin D.

Conclusion

1. Schütte, *Archiv fur Medizinche Erfahrung*, 79.

2. Trousseau and Pidoux, *Treatise on Therapeutics*, 161–67; Trousseau, *Clinique Medical de l'Hôtel Dieu de Paris*, 529.

3. Chesney and Hedberg, "Rickets in Lion Cubs at the London Zoo in 1889," 948–49; Cheadle, "Rickets," 129.

4. Palm, "The Geographical Distribution and Aetiology of Rickets," 273.

5. Hirsch, *Handbook of Geographical and Historical Pathology*, vol. 3, 734.

6. Von Hansemann, "On Rickets as a Folk-Disease," 249.

7. Findlay, "The Underlying Cause in the Pathogenesis of Rickets," 1474.

8. Ortner and Mays, "Dry-Bone Manifestations of Rickets in Infancy and Early Childhood," 45–55.

9. Lewis, "The Impact of Industrialisation: A Comparative Study of Child Health in Four Sites from Medieval and Post-Medieval England," 221.

10. McGregor, *From Midwives to Medicine*.

11. Kenneth F. Kiple, *The Caribbean Slave: A Biological History* (Cambridge: Cambridge University Press, 2002), 76–103.

12. Kiple and King, *Another Dimension to the Black Diaspora*, 79–95, 195, esp. 84; Nicholas Cardell and Mark Hopkins, "The Effect of Milk Intolerance on the Consumption of Milk by Slaves in 1960," *Journal of Interdisciplinary History* 8, no. 3 (Winter 1978): 507–10.

13. Angel et al., "Life Stresses of the Free Black Community," 213–29.

14. Polk, *The Birth of America*, 77; Laxton, *The Famine Ships*, 1–18; Dick Ahlstrom, "Teeth of Children Who Died in Famine Carry Hidden History," *The Irish Times*, Sept. 9, 2015, 35.

15. Park, "Etiology of Rickets," 151.

16. U.S. Department of Health and Human Services, National Institute of

Health, Office of Dietary Supplements, "Vitamin D: Fact Sheet for Health Professionals," last modified August 17, 2021, www/ods.od.nih.gov/factsheets/VitaminD-HealthProfessional/.

17. Leonard Lieberman and Fatimah Linda C. Jackson, "Race and Three Models of Human Origin," *American Anthropologist* 97, no. 3 (June 1995): 231–38.

18. Nina G. Jablonski, *Living Color: The Biological and Social Meaning of Skin Color* (Berkeley: University of California Press, 2014), 9–71.

19. American Association of Physical Anthropologists, "AAPA Statement on Race and Racism," *American Journal of Physical Anthropology* 101 (1996): 569–70.

20. Ibid.

21. Higginbotham, "African-American Women's History and the Metalanguage of Race," 3–24.

22. Polk, *Birth of America*, 77; Laxton, *Famine Ships*, 1–18; Noel Ignatiev, *How the Irish Became White* (London: Routledge, 1995).

23. Cooper Owens, *Medical Bondage*, 73–107.

24. Porter, *Greatest Benefit to Mankind*, 428–61.

25. Ludmerer, *Learning to Heal*, 34.

26. King, Davis and Williams, "Report of the Committee Appointed to Consider 'Uniformity,'" 80–82.

27. Cassedy, *American Medicine and Statistical Thinking*, 4, 17, 19, 181–82; Williams, "Pelvimetry for the General Practitioner," 322–23.

28. DeLee, *Obstetrics*, 272.

29. Fred Lyman Adair, "The White House Conference," *American Journal of Obstetrics and Gynecology* 21, no. 3 (1931): 442–44.

30. *Preliminary Committee Reports of the White House Conference on Child Health and Protection* (New York: Century, 1930), 42.

31. Ibid.

32. Ibid., 29.

33. Ibid., 30.

34. J. Whitridge Williams, "A Criticism of Certain Tendencies in American Obstetrics," *New York State Journal of Medicine* 22, no. 11 (Nov. 1922): 493–99, esp. 499.

35. Leavitt, *Brought to Bed*, 171–95; Wertz and Wertz, *Lying In*, 132–77.

36. Marian F. MacDorman, T.J. Mathews and Eugene Declercq, "Trends in Out-of-Hospital Births in the United States, 1990–2012," NCHS Data Brief No. 144, March 2014, last modified November 6, 2015, www.cdc.gov/nchs/products/databriefs/db144.

37. Centers for Disease Control and Prevention, National Center for Health Statistics, last modified May 21, 2020, www.cdc.gov/nchs/fastats.

38. King, Davis and Williams, "Report of the Committee Appointed to Consider Uniformity,'" 80–82.

39. Diaa M. El-Mowafi, "Obstetrics Simplified: Contracted Pelvis," Geneva Foundation for Medical Association Research, last modified July 16, 2021, www.gfmer.ch/Obstetrics simplified/contracted pelvis htm.

40. R.C. Pattinson, A. Cuthbert, and V. Vannevel, "Pelvimetry for Fetal Presentations at or Near Term for Deciding on Mode of Delivery," *Cochrane Database of Systematic Reviews*, Issue 3, article no. CD000161, last modified March 30, 2017, https://www.cochrane.org/CD000161/PREG pelvimetry-fetalcephalic-presentations-ornear-term-deciding-mode-delivery.

41. Lori Smith, "The Common Labor Complications: Cephalopelvic Disproportion," *Medical News Today*, www.medicalnewstoday.com. The figure is cited at several websites, attributed to the American College of Nurse-Midwives. Several additional sites state only that the condition is "very rare."

42. Holick, *Vitamin D. Solution*, 10–11, 70.

43. Wiebe, *Search for Order*; Leonard, *Illiberal Reformers*.

44. Ladd-Taylor, "When the Birds Have Flown the Nest," 444–74.

45. Brunius, *Better for All the World*; Black, *War Against the Weak*.

Bibliography

Primary Sources

Journal Articles and Essays

Abel, John J., and Walter S. Davis. "On the Pigment of Negro's Skin and Hair." *Journal of Experimental Medicine* I (July 1896): 369.

Acker, George N. "Rickets in Negroes." *Archives of Pediatrics* 11 (1894): 893-98.

Adair, Fred Lyman. "The White House Conference." *American Journal of Obstetrics and Gynecology* 21, no. 3 (1931): 442-44.

Barlow, Thomas. "On Cases Described as Acute Rickets Which Are Probably a Combination of Scurvy and Rickets." *Medico-Chirurgical Transactions* 66 (March 27, 1883): 159-220.

Bettman, Henry. "Premature Labor and the Newborn Child." *American Journal of Obstetrics and Diseases of Women and Children* 25 (1892): 315-28.

Bills, Charles E. "Physiology of the Sterols, Including Vitamin D." *Physiological Reviews* 15, no. 1 (Jan. 1935): 1-12.

Boas, Franz. "Changes in the Bodily Form of Descendants of Immigrants." *American Anthropologist*, New Series, vol. 14, no. 3 (July-Sept. 1912): 530-62.

Davis, Edward. "The Frequency and Mortality of Abnormal Pelves." *American Journal of Obstetrics and Diseases of Children* XI (1901): 15.

Davis, Effa. "A Study of the Bony Pelvis in One Hundred and Fifty Cases." *Journal of the American Medical Association* 45 (Dec. 1905): 1709-710.

DeLee, Joseph B., M.D. "A Case of Flat Rachitic Pelvis; Prolapse of the Cord with the Head; Version and Extraction." *Journal of the American Medical Association* XXVIII, no. 7 (1897): 306-07.

Dunn, Peter. "Francis Glisson (1597-1677) and the Discovery of Rickets." *Archives of Disease in Childhood* 78 (March 1998): 154-55.

Edgar, James Clifton. "Pelvic Deformity in New York." *Transactions, American Gynecological Society* 27 (1902): 324-37.

Eliot, Martha May, M.D. "The New Haven Demonstration of Community Control of Rickets." *The Public Health Journal* 17, no. 3 (March 1926): 114-16.

Gaison, J.G. "Pelvimetry." *Journal of Anatomy and Physiology* 16 (1881): 106.

Goldblatt, Harry, and Katharine Marjorie Soames. "The Supplementary Value of Light Rays to a Diet Graded in Its Content of Fat-Soluble Organic Factor." *Biochemical Journal* 17 (1923): 622-29.

Goldsborough, Frances. "The Maternal Mortality in the First 5000 Obstetrical Cases at the Johns Hopkins Hospital." *Bulletin of the Johns Hopkins Hospital* 19 (1908): 13.

Greulich, William, Herbert Thoms, and Ruth Christian Twaddle. "A Study of Pelvic Type and Its Relationship to Body Build in White Women." *Journal of the American Medical Association* 112 (Feb. 11, 1939).

Guy, Ruth A. "The History of Cod Liver Oil as a Remedy." *American Journal of Diseases of Children* 26 (1923): 112-16.

Hansemann, David Paul von. "Ueber Rachitis als Volkskrankheit" ["On Rickets as a Folk-Disease"]. *Berliner Klinische Wochenschrift: Organ für praktische Aerzte* 9 (Feb. 26, 1906): 248-54.

Harris, Robert P. "The Caesarean Operation in the United States." *American*

Journal of Obstetrics 4 (Feb. 1872): 622–63.
Hirst, Barton Cooke. "Symphysiotomy." *The Medical News* 63 (Dec. 2, 1893): 627.
Hopkins, F.G. "The Effect of Heat and Aeration upon the Fat-Soluble Vitamine." *Biochemistry Journal* 14 (1920): 725–33.
Howland, John, and W. McKim Marriot. "The Calcium Content of the Blood in Rachitis and Tetany." *Transactions of the American Pediatrics Society* 28 (1916): 202.
Huldschinsky, K. "Heilung von Rachitis durch künstliche Hohensonne." *Detsch. Med. Wochenscht* 45 (1919): 712–13.
Hume, E.M., and H.H. Smith. "The Effect of the Radiation of the Environment with Ultra-Violet Light upon the Growth and Calcification of Rats, Fed on a Diet Deficient in Fat-Soluble Vitamins: The Part Played by Irradiated Sawdust." *Biochemistry Journal* 18 (1924): 1334–345.
Hutchinson, H.S. "The Aetiology of Rickets, Early and Late." *Quarterly Journal of Medicine* XV (1921–1922): 167–95.
Jacobi, Abraham. "Craniotabes." *American Journal of Obstetrics and Diseases of Women and Children* (Nov. 1870): 435–67.
Jeidell, Helmina, and Willa Fricke. "The Midwives of Anne Arundel County, Maryland." *Johns Hopkins Hospital Bulletin* XXIII, no. 29 (Sept. 1912): 279–81.
Johnson, Joseph Taber. "Apparent Peculiarities of Parturition in the Negro Race with Remarks on Race Pelves." *American Journal of Obstetrics and Diseases of Women and Children* 8 (Jan. 1875): 88–123.
Kerr, Munro. "Diagnosis and Treatment of Contracted Pelves." *Transactions of the American Gynecological Society* XXXVI (1911): 156–85.
King, A.F.A., Edward Davis, and J. Whitridge Williams. "Report of the Committee Appointed at the Previous Meeting to Consider 'Uniformity in Pelvic and Cranial Measurements.'" *Transactions of the American Gynecological Society* 30 (1905): 80–82.
King, Charles R. "The New York Maternal Mortality Study: A Conflict of Professionalization." *Bulletin of the History of Medicine* 65 (1991): 476–502.
Knox, J.H. Mason. "Address by the President." *Transactions of the American Association for the Study and Prevention of Infant Mortality* (1910): 29.
Knox, J.H. Mason, and Paul Zantai. "The Health Problem of the American Negro." *American Journal of Public Health* 6 (1926): 809.
Kramer, Benjamin, and John Howland. "Calcium and Phosphorus in the Serum in Relation to Rickets." *American Journal of the Diseases of the Child* 22 (1921): 105.
Lane, Clayton Arbuthnot. "A Clinical Comparison of the Maternal Pelvis and of the Foetus in Europeans, Eurasians, and Bengalis: And the Enunciation of a New Law in Accordance with which the size of the Child at Birth Is Determined," *Lancet* (Sept. 26, 1903): 885–89.
Lathrop, Julia C. "Standards of Child Welfare." *Annals of the American Academy of Political and Social Science* 98 (1921): 1–8.
Linker, Beth. "Feet for Fighting: Locating Disability and Social Medicine in First World War America." *Social History of Medicine* 20, no. 1 (April 2007): 91–109.
Love, Albert, and Charles Davenport. "Defects Found in Drafted Men." *The Scientific Monthly* 10, no. 1 (Jan. 1920): 5–25.
McCullom, Elmer F., and M. Davis. "Observations on the Isolation of the Substance in Butter Fat Which Exerts a Stimulating Effect on Growth." *Journal of Biological Chemistry* 19 (1914): 245–50.
McCullom, Elmer V., Nina Simmonds, J.E. Becker, and P.G. Shipley. "Studies on Experimental Rickets XXI. An Experimental Demonstration of the Existence of a Vitamin Which Promotes Calcium Deposition." *Journal of Biological Chemistry* 53 (1922): 293–312.
Meigs, Grace. "Maternal Mortality from All Conditions Connected with Child Birth, in the United States and Certain Other Countries." U.S. Department of Labor, Children's Bureau, Miscellaneous Series No. 6, Bureau Publication No. 19 (Washington, D.C.: Government Printing Office, 1917).
Mellanby, Edward. "Experimental Rickets: The Effects of Cereals and their Interaction with Other Factors of Diet and Environment in Producing Rickets." Medical Research Council Special

Report No. 93. London: His Majesty's Stationery Office, 1925.

Meyer, Adolf. "The Right to Marry." *The Survey* 36 (June 3, 1916): 243–46.

Morton, Lauren P. "Baltimore's First Birth Control Clinic: The Bureau for Contraceptive Advice, 1927–1932." *Maryland Historical Magazine* 102, no. 4 (2007): 300–19.

Owen, Isambard. "Geographical Distribution of Rickets, Acute and Subacute Rheumatism, Chorea, Cancer, and Urinary Calculus." *British Medical Journal* 1 (1889): 113–16.

Palm, Theobald A. "The Geographical Distribution and Aetiology of Rickets." *The Practitioner* 45 (Nov. 1890): 273.

Parascandola, John, and Aaron M. Ihde. "Edward Mellanby and the Antirachitic Factor." *Bulletin of the History of Medicine* 51 (Winter 1977): 507–15.

Park, Edwards A. "The Etiology of Rickets." *Physiological Reviews* 3 (1923).

Parrish, W.H. "A Case of Craniotomy." *Transactions of the Philadelphia Obstetrics Society* (Nov. 1874): 39.

Powers, G.F., E.A. Park, and Nina Simmonds. "The Influence of Radiant Energy upon the Development of Xerophthalmia in Rats: A Remarkable Demonstration of the Beneficial Influence of Sunlight and Out-of-Door Air Upon the Organism." *Journal of Biological Chemistry* LVII (Jan. 29, 1923): 576.

Reynolds, Edward. "On the Frequency of Contract Pelvis Among American Women, as Deduced from 2227 Cases of Labor." *Transactions of the American Gynecological Society* 15 (1890): 367.

Riggs, Theodore F. "A Comparative Study of White and Negro Pelves: With a Consideration of the Size of the Child and Its Relation to Presentation and Character of the Races in the Two Races, 1891–1926." *Johns Hopkins Hospital Reports* 12 (1904): 421–22.

Routh, Amand. "On Caesarean Section in the United Kingdom with Tables of 1282 Cases of Caesarean Section by over 100 Obstericians and Gynaecologists of the United Kingdom, Who Were Living on June 1, 1910." *Journal of Obstetrics and Gynaecology of the British Empire* XIX (Jan. 1911): 1–233.

Sarton, George. "The Discovery of X-Rays." *Isis* 26 (March 1937): 358.

Sherwood, Mary. "The Midwives of Baltimore." *Journal of the American Medical Association* 52, no. 25 (1909): 2009–2010.

Shipley, P.G., E.A. Park, E.V. McCollum, and Nina Simmonds. "The Function of the Organic Factor as Exemplified by Cod Liver Oil. "*Transactions of the American Pediatrics Society*, 33rd Session (June 1921).

Smith, David F., and Malcolm Nicholson. "Chemical Physiology Versus Biochemistry, the Clinic Versus the Laboratory. The Glasegian Opposition to Edward Mellanby's Theory of Rickets." *Proceedings of the Royal College of Physicians of Edinburgh* 19 (1989): 51–60.

Snow, Irving M. "An Explanation of the Great Frequency of Rickets Among Neapolitan Children in American Cities," *Archives of Pediatrics* 12 (1895): 18–34.

Southworth, Thomas. "The Importance of the Early Recognition and Treatment of Rachitis." *Journal of the American Medical Association* 50 (1908): 89–93.

Steele, Guy. "The Midwife Problem and Its Legal Control." *Maryland Medical Journal* 48 (Jan. 1905): 1–6.

Steenbock, Harry, and Archie Black. "Fat-Soluble Vitamins. XVII. The Induction of Growth-Promoting and Calcifying Properties in a Ration by Exposure to Ultra-Violet Light." *Journal of Biological Chemistry* 61 (April 1924): 405–22.

Storer, H.R. "Report from the American Medical Association's Committee on Obstetrics." *Transactions of the American Medical Association* IV (1851): 349–407.

Thoms, Herbert. "The Clinical Significance of X-Ray Pelvimetry." *American Journal of Obstetrics and Gynecology* 12, no. 4 (Jan. 1926): 543–50.

Turner, William. "Index of the Pelvic Brim as a Basis of Classification." *Journal of Anatomy and Physiology* 20 (1885–1886): 125–43.

Van Ingen, Philip. "Infant Mortality in Institutions." *Proceedings of the National Conference of Charities and Correction* (1915): 126–29.

Woodbury, Robert Morse. "The Trend of Maternal-Mortality Rates in the United States Death-Registration Area, 1900–1921." *American Journal of Public Health* 14, no. 9 (Sept. 1, 1924): 738–43.

Bibliography

Books

Bard, Samuel. *Compendium of the Theory and Practice of Midwifery*. New York: Collins, 1808.

Cock, Thomas F. *Manual of Obstetrics*. New York: Samuel S. and William Wood, 1853.

Darwin, Charles. *The Descent of Man*, 2 vols. London: John Murray, 1871.

———. *On the Origin of Species: A Facsimile of the First Edition*. 1859. Cambridge: Harvard University Press, 1961.

De Kruf, Paul. *Microbe Hunters*. New York: Harcourt, Brace, 1926.

DeLee, Joseph. *Principles and Practice of Obstetrics*, 6th ed. Philadelphia: W.B. Saunders & Co., 1934.

DeWees, William. *A Compendius System of Midwifery*. Philadelphia: Blanchard and Lea, 1824.

Dick, J. Lawson. *Rickets: A Study of Economic Conditions and Their Effects on the Health of the Nation, in two parts combined in one volume*. London: William Heinemann, 1922.

DuBois, W.E.B. *The Souls of Black Folk: Essays and Sketches*. Chicago: A.C. McClurg, 1904.

Emmet, Thomas A. *Principles and Practice of Gynaecology*. Philadelphia: Henry C. Lea 1879.

Ferguson, Margaret. *A Study of Social and Economic Factors in the Causation of Rickets*. Written under D. Noël Paton and Leonard Findley. London: Medical Research Committee, 1918.

Findlay, Leonard. "Introduction." Medical Research Committee, *A Study of Social and Economic Factors in the Causation of Rickets*. Special Report Series, No. 20. London: Published by His Majesty's Stationery Office, 1918.

Flexner, Abraham. *Medical Education in the United States and Canada: A Report to the Carnegie Foundation for the Advancement of Teaching*. New York: Carnegie Foundation, 1910.

Haeckel, Ernst. *The History of Creation; or the Development of the Earth and Its Inhabitants by the Action of Natural Causes*, 5th ed., vol. 1. New York: Appleton, 1911.

Haller, Albert von. *The Vitamin Hunters*. Trans. Hella Freud Bernays. Philadelphia: Chilton, 1962.

Hess, Alfred F. *Collected Writings*, 2 vols. Springfield, IL: Charles C. Thomas, 1936.

Hirsch, August. *Handbook of Geographical and Historical Pathology*, 3 vols., 2nd ed. London: The New Sydenham Society, 1886.

Hodge, Hugh. *The Principles and Practice of Obstetrics*. Philadelphia: Henry Lea, 1866.

Holt, L. Emmett, and John Howland. *The Diseases of Infancy and Childhood*, 8th ed, fully rev. New York: D. Appleton, 1922.

Hooker, Ransom. *Maternal Mortality in New York City: A Study of All Puerperal Deaths, 1930–1932*. New York: The Commonwealth Fund, 1933.

Jenner, Sir William. *Clinical Lectures and Essays on Rickets, Tuberculosis, Abdominal Tumours*. London: Rivington, Percival & Co., 1895.

Litzmann, Carl. *Die Formen das Beckens, insbesondere des engen weiblichen Beckens, nach eigenen Beobactungen und Untersuchungen,hebst einem Anhange über die Osteomalacie*. Berlin: Georg Reimer, 1861.

Lusk, William Thompson. *The Science and Art of Midwifery*. New York: D. Appleton, 1882.

Marfan, Antoine Bernard. *Le Rachitism Etiologie, Pathogenie, Traitement, Prophylaxie*. Paris: Librairie J.-B. Baillièrre et Fils, 1942.

McCollum, Elmer V. *A History of Nutrition: The Sequence of Ideas in Nutrition Investigations*. Boston: Houghton Mifflin, 1957.

McCollum, Elmer, and Nina Simmonds. *Food, Nutrition and Health*. Baltimore: Published by the Authors, 1925.

Meigs, Charles. *Obstetrics: The Science and the Art. Treatise on Obstetrics*, 3rd ed., rev. Philadelphia: Blanchard and Lea, 1856.

Meigs, J. Forsyth, and William Pepper. *A Practical Treatise on the Diseases of Children*, 7th ed. Philadelphia: Blakiston, Son and Co., 1883.

Morse, John Lovett, and Fritz B. Talbot. *Diseases of Nutrition and Infant Feeding*. New York: Macmillan, 1915.

Naegele, Franz Carl. *The Obliquely Contracted Pelvis Containing Also an Appendix of the Most Important Defects of*

Bibliography

the *Female Pelvis*, centennial ed., newly translated from the original German. New York, 1939.

Osler, William. *The Principles and Practice of Medicine.* New York: D. Appleton, 1899.

Privy Council: Medical Research Council, *Studies of Rickets in Vienna, 1919–1922.* London: His Majesty's Stationary Office, 1923.

Rochester, Anna. *Infant Mortality: Results of a Field Study in Baltimore, Maryland Based on Births in One Year.* Washington, D.C.: Washington Government Printing Offices, 1923, Bureau Publication #119.

Speert, Harold. *Obstetric and Gynecological Milestones: Essays in Eponymy.* New York: Macmillan, 1858.

Trousseau, A., and H. Pidoux. *Treatise on Therapeutics*, 9th ed. Trans. D.F. Lincoln. New York: William Wood and Co., 1880.

Virchow, Rudolf. *Cellular Pathology as Based Upon Physiological and Pathological Histology.* Translated from the second edition of the original by Frank Chance. Philadelphia: J.B. Lippincott, 1863.

Welsh, Lilian. *Reminiscences of Thirty Years in Baltimore.* Baltimore: The Norman, Remington Co., 1925.

West, Charles. *Diseases of Children.* Philadelphia: Longmans, Green and Company, 1874.

Williams, J. Whitridge. *Obstetrics: A Textbook for the Use of Students and Practitioners.* New York: D. Appleton, 1903.

Williams, William Carlos. *The Doctor Stories.* Comp. Robert Coles. New York: New Directions, 1984.

Woodbury, Robert. *Statures and Weights of Children Under Six Years of Age.* Children's Bureau Publication #87. Washington, D.C.: Government Printing Office, 1921.

Secondary Sources

Journal Articles and Essays

Angel, J. Lawrence, Jennifer Olsen Kelley, Michael Parrington, and Stephanie Pinter. "Life Stresses of the Free Black Community as Represented by the First African Baptist Church, Philadelphia, 1823–1841," *American Journal of Physical Anthropology* 74 (1987): 213–29.

Apple, Rima D. "Patenting University Research: Harry Steenbock and the Wisconsin Alumni Research Association." *Isis* 80, no. 3 (Sept. 1989): 374–94.

Briggs, Laura. "The Race of Hysteria: 'Overcivilization' and the 'Savage' Woman in Late Nineteenth-Century Obstetrics and Gynecology." *American Quarterly* 52 (June 2000): 246–73.

Carpenter, Kenneth J., and Ling Zhao. "Forgotten Mysteries in the Early History of Vitamin D." *Journal of Nutrition* 129 (Feb. 1999): 923–27.

Chesney, Russell, and Gail Hedberg. "Rickets in Lion Cubs at the London Zoo in 1889." *Pediatrics* 123, no. 5 (May 2009): 948–49.

Cutright, Phillip, and Edward Shorter. "The Effects of Health on the Completed Fertility of Nonwhite and White U.S. Women Born between 1867 and 1935." *Journal of Social History* 13 (1979).

Duffy, Thomas P. "The Flexner Report—100 Years Later." *Yale Journal of Biology and Medicine* 84, no. 3 (Sept. 1984): 269–76.

Dunn, P.M. "Sir James Young Simpson (1811–1870) and Obstetric Anaesthesia." *British Medical Journal* 86, no. 3 (May 2002): 207–09.

Fee, Elizabeth. "Nineteenth-Century Craniology: The Study of the Female Skull." *Bulletin of the History of Medicine* 53 (1979): 415–33.

Gabert, Harvey A., and Mohammed Bey. "History and Development of Cesarean Operation." *Obstetrics and Gynecology Clinics of North America* 15 (1988): 597.

Gillis, Jonathan. "The History of the Patient History since 1850." *Bulletin of the History of Medicine* 80 (Fall 2006): 490–512.

Golden, Janet. "From Wet Nurse Directory to Milk Bank: The Delivery of Human Milk in Boston, 1909–1927." *Bulletin of the History of Medicine* 62 (1988): 589–605.

Haller, John. "The Physician versus the Negro: Medical and Anthropological Concepts of Race in the Late Nineteenth Century." *Bulletin of the History of Medicine* 44, no. 2 (March–April 1970): 154–67.

Hardy, Anne. "Commentary: Bread and Alum, Syphilis and Sunlight: Rickets in the Nineteenth Century." *International Journal of Epidemiology* 32, no. 3 (July 2003): 337–40.

Hardy, Anne. "Rickets and the Rest: Child-care, Diet and the Infectious Children's Diseases, 1850–1914," *Social History of Medicine* 5 (December 1992), 389–412.

Harrison, Harold E. "The Disappearance of Rickets." *American Journal of Public Health* 56, no. 5 (May 1966).

Higginbotham, Evelyn Brooks. "African American Women's History and the Metalanguage of Race." *We Specialize in the Wholley Impossible: Essays in Black Women's History*, ed. Darlene Clark Hine, Wilma King, and Linda Reed. Brooklyn: Carlson, 1995, 3–24.

Hollinger, David A. "American Ethnoracial History and the Amalgamation Narrative." *Journal of American Ethnic History* 35, no. 4 (Summer 2006): 153–59.

Hyme, Lucille. "The Earliest Use of Indices for Sexing Pelves." *American Journal of Physical Anthropology* 15 (1957): 537–46.

Ihde, Aaron. "Studies on the History of Rickets, I: Recognition of Rickets as a Deficiency Disease." *Pharmacy in History* 16 (1974).

Ihde, Aaron. "Studies on the History of Rickets, II: The Roles of Cod Liver Oil and Light." *Pharmacy in History* 17 (1974).

Immerwahr, Daniel. "American Blacks and Birth Control." *Population Reference Bureau* 2. Washington, D.C.: PRB, 1976.

Klepp, Susan E. "Seasoning and Society: Racial Differences in Mortality in Eighteenth-Century Philadelphia." *William and Mary Quarterly*, 3rd Series, vol. LI, no. 3 (July 1994): 473–506.

Leavitt, Judith Walzer, "Joseph B. DeLee and the Practice of Preventive Obstetrics." *American Journal of Public Health* 78, no. 10 (Oct. 1988): 1353–360.

Lewis, Mary E. "Impact of Industrialization: Comparative Study of Child Health in Four Sites from Medieval and Postmedieval England (A.D. 850–1859)." *American Journal of Physical Anthropology* 119, no. 3 (2002): 211–23.

Lieberman, Leonard, and Fatimah Linda C. Jackson. "Race and Three Models of Human Origin." *American Anthropologist* 97, no. 3 (June 1995): 231–38.

Litoff, Judy Barrett. "Forgotten Women: American Midwives at the Turn of the Twentieth Century." *The Historian* 40, no. 2 (Feb. 1978): 235–51.

Loudon, Irvine. "The Origin and Growth of the Dispensary Movement in England." *Bulletin of the History of Medicine* 55 (1981): 341.

McFalls, Joseph, and George Masnick. "Birth Control and the Fertility of the U.S. Black Population." *Journal of Family History* 6 (Spring 1981): 89–106.

Ortner, Donald J., and Simon Hays. "Dry-Bone Manifestations of Rickets in Infancy and Early Childhood." *International Journal of Osteoarchaeology* 8 (1998): 45–55.

Rosen, George. "The Efficiency Criterion in Medical Care, 1900–1920: An Early Approach to an Evaluation of Health Service." *Bulletin of the History of Medicine* 50 (1976): 28–44.

Slemons, J. Morris. "Progress in Obstetrics: 1890–1940." *American Journal of Surgery* 51 (1941): 89–90.

Smith, David, and Malcolm Nicolson. "The 'Glasgow School' of Paton, Findlay and Cathcart: Conservative Thought in Chemical Physiology, Nutrition and Public Health." *Social Studies of Science* 19 (1989): 195–238.

Theriot, Nancy M. "Negotiating Illness: Doctors, Patients, and Families in the Nineteenth Century." *Journal of the History of the Behavioral Sciences* 37 (Fall 2001): 349–68.

Vernon-Roberts, Barrie. "Christian Georg Schmorl: Pioneer of Spinal Pathology and Radiology." *Spine* 19 no. 23 (1994): 2724–727.

Warren, Christian. " Northern Chills, Southern Fevers: Race-Specific Mortality in American Cities." *Journal of Southern History* 63 (Feb. 1997).

Wolf, George. "The Discovery of Vitamin D: The Contribution of Adolf Windaus." *The Journal of Nutrition* 34, no. 6 (June 2004): 1299–302.

Woods, Robert. "Lying-In and Laying-Out: Fetal Health and the Contribution of Midwifery." *Bulletin of the History of Medicine* 81 (Winter 2007): 730–59.

Books

Ackeknecht, Erwin. *Rudolf Virchow: The Development of Science*. New York: Arno Press, 1981.
Apple, Rima. *Mothers and Medicine: A Social History of Infant Feeding*. Madison: University of Wisconsin Press, 1987.
Apple, Rima. *Perfect Motherhood: Science and Childrearing in America*. New Brunswick: Rutgers University Press, 2006.
Apple, Rima. *Vitamania: Vitamins in American Culture*. New Brunswick: Rutgers University Press, 1996.
Appleman, Philip, ed. *Darwin: Texts, Backgrounds, Contemporary Opinion, Critical Essays*. New York: W.W. Norton, 1979.
Ashby, LeRoy. *Endangered Children: Dependency, Neglect and Abuse in American History*. New York: Twayne, 1997.
Barrett, Frank R. *Disease and Geography: The History of an Idea*. Toronto: Atkinson College, Department of Geography, 2000.
Beardsley, Edward H. *A History of Neglect: Health Care for Blacks and Mill Workers in the Twentieth Century South*. Knoxville: University of Tennessee Press, 1990.
Beaton, G.H., and J.M. Bengoa, eds. *Nutrition in Preventive Medicine: The Major Deficiency Syndromes, Epidemiology, and Approaches to Control*. Geneva: World Health Organization, 1976.
Berlin, Ira, and Leslie M. Harris. *Slavery in New York*. New York: New Press, 2005.
Black, Edwin. *War Against the Weak: Eugenics and America's Campaign to Create a Master Race*. New York: Thunder's Mouth Press, 2003.
Blight, David. *Race and Reunion: The Civil War in American History*. Cambridge: Harvard University Press, 2001.
Block, Jennifer. *Pushed: The Painful Truth about Childbirth and Modern Maternity Care*. Cambridge: DaCapo Press, 2007.
Bordo, Susan. *Unbearable Weight: Feminism, Western Culture, and the Body*. Berkeley: University of California Press, 1993.
Borst, Charlotte. *Catching Babies: The Professionalization of Childbirth, 1870–1920*. Cambridge: Harvard University Press, 1995.
Bremner, Robert, ed., *Children and Youth in America: A Documentary History*, 2 vols. Cambridge: Harvard University Press, 1971.
Bruinius, Harry. *Better for All the World: The Secret History of Forced Sterilization and America's Quest for Racial Purity*. New York: Alfred A. Knopf, 2006.
Bulmer, Michael. *Francis Galton: Pioneer of Heredity and Biometry*. Baltimore: Johns Hopkins University Press, 2003.
Bynum, W.F. *The Science and Practice of Medicine in the Nineteenth Century*. Cambridge: Cambridge University Press, 1994.
Carter, Jenny, and Thérèse Duriwz. *With Child: Birth Through the Ages*. Edinburgh: Mainstream, 1986.
Cassedy, James. *American Medicine and Statistical Thinking, 1800–1860*. Cambridge: Harvard University Press, 1984.
Cassidy, Tina. *Birth: The Surprising History of How We are Born*. New York: Atlantic Monthly Press, 2006.
Chesney, Alan Mason. *Johns Hopkins Hospital and the Johns Hopkins University School of Medicine: A Chronicle*, vol. 1. Baltimore: Johns Hopkins University Press, 1943.
Crawford, T. Hugh. *Modernism, Medicine and William Carlos Williams*. Norman: University of Oklahoma Press, 1993.
Cule, John, and Terry Turner, eds. *Childcare Through the Centuries*. Cardiff: British Society for the History of Medicine, 1986.
Daniels, Roger. *Coming to America: A History of Immigration and Ethnicity in American Life*. New York: Harper Perennial, 2002.
Davis, Mike. *Late Victorian Holocausts: El Niño Famines and the Making of the Third World*. London: Verso, 2002.
Davis, Philip, ed. *Childbirth: Changing Ideas and Practices in Britain and America: 1600 to the Present*, vol. 5. New York: Garland Press, 1996.
Davis-Floyd, Robbie E. *Birth as an American Rite of Passage*. Berkeley: University of California Press, 1992.
Dowling, Harry. *City Hospitals: The Undercare of the Underprivileged*. Cambridge: Harvard University Press, 1982.
Duden, Barbara. *Disembodying Women:*

Perspectives on Pregnancy and the Unborn. Cambridge: Harvard University Press, 1993.

Duncan, David. *The Life and Times of Herbert Spencer*. Cambridge: Cambridge University Press, 2015.

Ehrenreich, Barbara, and Deirdre English. *For Her Own Good: 150 Years of the Experts' Advice to Women*. Garden City, NY: Anchor Books, 1979.

Fabian, Ann. *The Skull Collectors: Race, Science, and America's Unburied Dead*. Chicago: University of Chicago Press, 2010.

Fagan, Brian. *Floods, Famines, and Emperors: El Niño and the Fate of Civilizations*. New York: Basic Books, 1999.

Fee, Elizabeth. *Disease and Discovery: A History of the Johns Hopkins School of Hygiene and Public Health 1916–1939*. Baltimore: Johns Hopkins University Press, 1987.

Fletcher, Anthony. *Gender, Sex, and Subordination in England 1500–1800*. New Haven: Yale University Press, 1999.

Fogel, Robert, and Stanley L. Engerman. *Time on the Cross: Evidence and Methods, A Supplement*. Boston: Little, Brown, 1974.

Foucault, Michel. *The Birth of the Clinic: An Archaeology of Medical Perception*. New York: Vintage, 1994.

Fraser, Gertrude Jacinta. *African American Midwifery in the South: Dialogues of Birth, Race, and Memory*. Cambridge: Harvard University Press, 1998.

Gamble, Vanessa. *Making a Place for Ourselves: The Black Hospital Movement 1920–1945*. Oxford: Oxford University Press, 1987.

Golden, Janet, ed. *Infant Asylums and Children's Hospitals: Medical Dilemmas and Developments, 1850- 1920: An Anthology of Sources*. New York: Garland, 1989.

Gould, Stephen Jay. *The Mismeasure of Man*. New York: W.W. Norton, 1996.

Gould, Stephen Jay. *The Structure of Evolutionary Theory*. Cambridge: Harvard University Press, 2002.

Grob, Gerald. *The Deadly Truth: A History of Disease in America*. Cambridge: Harvard University Press, 2002.

Haines, Michael, and Richard H. Steckel, eds. *A Population History of North America*. Cambridge: Cambridge University Press, 2000.

Halpern, Stanley A. *American Pediatrics: The Social Dynamics of Professionalism*. Berkeley: University of California Press, 1988.

Hammonds, Evelyn. *Childhood's Deadly Scourge: The Campaign to Control Diphtheria in New York City, 1880–1930*. Baltimore: Johns Hopkins University Press, 1999.

Hareven, Tamare, and Maris Vinovskis, eds. *Family and Population in Nineteenth-Century America*. Princeton: Princeton University Press, 1978.

Harvey, A. McGehee. *Adventures in Medical Research: A Century of Discovery at Johns Hopkins*. Baltimore: Johns Hopkins University Press, 1976.

Holick, Michael F. *The Vitamin D Solution*. New York: Hudson Street Press, 2010.

Horsman, Reginald. *Race and Manifest Destiny: The Origins of American Racial Anglo-Saxonism*. Cambridge: Harvard University Press, 1981.

Jablonski, Nina G. *Living Color: The Biological and Social Meaning of Skin Color*. Berkeley: University of California Press, 2014.

Jackson, John P., and Nadine M. Weidman. *Race, Racism and Science: Social Impact and Interaction*. New Brunswick: Rutgers University Press, 2004.

Jordanova, Ludmilla. *Nature Displayed: Gender, Science and Medicine 1760–1820*. London: Addison Wesley Longman, 1999.

Kevles, Daniel. *In the Name of Eugenics: Genetics and the Uses of Human Heredity*. New York: Alfred A. Knopf, 1985.

Kiple, Kenneth. *The Caribbean Slave: A Biological History*. Cambridge: Cambridge University Press, 2002.

Kiple, Kenneth, and Virginia Himmelsteib King. *Another Dimension to the Black Diaspora: Diet, Disease, and Racism*. Cambridge: Cambridge University Press, 1981.

Kiple, Kenneth, ed. *The Cambridge World History of Human Disease*. Cambridge: Cambridge University Press, 1993.

Kiple, Kenneth, and Krimheld Conee Ornelas, eds. *Cambridge World History of Food*, vol. 1. Cambridge: Cambridge University Press, 2000.

Kohler, Robert E. *From Medical Education to Biochemistry: The Making of a Biomedical Discipline*. Cambridge: Cambridge University Press, 1982.

Bibliography 291

LaQuer, Thomas. *Making Sex: Body and Gender from the Greeks to Freud.* Cambridge: Harvard University Press, 1992.

Larson, Edward. *Evolution: The Remarkable History of a Scientific Theory.* New York: Modern Library, 2006.

Lawless, Jo Murphy. *Reading Birth and Death: A History of Obstetric Thinking.* Bloomington: Indiana University Press, 1999.

Laxton, Edward. *The Famine Ships: The Irish Exodus to America.* New York: Henry Holt, 1998.

Leavitt, Judith. *Brought to Bed: Childbearing in America, 1750–1950,* expanded ed. New Haven: Yale University Press, 1989.

Leavitt, Judith, and Ronald Numbers, eds. *Sickness and Health: Readings in the History of Medicine and Public Health.* Madison: University of Wisconsin Press, 1978.

Lederer, Susan E. *Subjected to Science: Human Experimentation in America Before the Second World War.* Baltimore: Johns Hopkins University Press, 1995.

Lee, Valerie. *Granny Midwives and Black Women Writers: Double-Dutched Readings.* New York: Routledge, 1996.

Leonard, Thomas C. *Illiberal Reformers: Race, Eugenics, and American Economics in the Progressive Era.* Princeton: Princeton University Press, 2016.

Litoff, Judy Barrett, ed. *The American Midwife Debate: A Sourcebook on Its Modern Origins.* Westport, CT: Greenwood Press, 1986.

Loudon, Irvine. *Death in Childbirth: An International Study of Maternal Care and Maternal Mortality, 1800–1950.* Oxford: Clarendon Press, 1993.

Lovejoy, Arthur O. *The Great Chain of Being.* Cambridge: Harvard University Press, 1936 and 1964.

Ludmerer, Kenneth M. *Learning to Heal: The Development of American Medical Education.* Baltimore: Johns Hopkins University Press, 1985.

MacNeill, William H. *Plagues and Peoples.* New York: Doubleday, 1977.

McBride, David. *Integrating the City of Medicine: Blacks in Philadelphia Health Care, 1910–1960.* Philadelphia: Temple University Press, 1989.

McCann, Carole R. *Birth Control Politics in the United States, 1916–1945.* Ithaca: Cornell University Press, 1994.

McDowell, Lee R. *Vitamin History: The Early Years.* Sarasota: Design, 2013.

McGregor, Deborah Kuhn. *From Midwives to Medicine: The Birth of American Gynecology.* New Brunswick: Rutgers University Press, 1998.

McKeown, Thomas. *The Modern Rise of Population.* New York: Academic Press, 1976.

Meckel, Richard. *Save the Babies: American Public Health Reform and the Prevention of Infant Mortality.* Ann Arbor: University of Michigan Press, 1998.

Michel, Sonya. *Children's Interests, Mothers' Rights: The Shaping of America's Child Care Policy.* New Haven: Yale University Press, 1999.

Moran, Gerard. *The History of the Irish Famine: The Exodus.* London: Routledge, 2018.

Morantz-Sanchez, Regina. *Sympathy and Science: Women Physicians in American Medicine.* Oxford: Oxford University Press, 1985.

More, Ellen. *Restoring the Balance: Women Physicians and the Profession of Medicine, 1850–1995.* Cambridge: Harvard University Press, 1995.

Morgan, Jennifer L. *Laboring Women: Reproduction and Gender in New World Slavery.* Philadelphia: University of Pennsylvania Press, 2004.

Muncy, Robin. *Creating a Female Dominion in American Reform, 1890–1935.* New York: Oxford University Press, 1991.

Oliver, Wade. *The Man Who Lived for Tomorrow: A Biography of William Hallock Park, M.S.* New York: E.P. Dutton, 1941.

Owens, Deirdre Cooper. *Medical Bondage: Race, Gender, and the Origins of American Gynecology.* Athens: University of Georgia Press, 2018.

Painter, Nell Irvin. *The History of White People.* New York: W.W. Norton, 2010.

Park, Katharine Park. *Secrets of Women: Gender, Generation, and the Origins of Human Dissection.* New York: Zone Books, 2006.

Pascoe, Peggy. *What Comes Naturally: Miscegenation Law and the Making of Race in America.* New York: Oxford University Press, 2010.

Porter, Roy. *The Greatest Benefit to Mankind: A Medical History of Humanity*. New York: W.W. Norton, 1997.

Pyenson, Lewis, and Susan Sheets-Pyenson. *Servants of Nature: A History of Scientific Institutions, Enterprises and Sensibilities*. New York: W.W. Norton, 1999.

Reagan, Leslie. *When Abortion Was a Crime: Women, Medicine, and Law in the United States, 1867–1973*. Berkeley: University of California Press, 1997.

Reilly, Philip R., M.D., J.D. *The Surgical Solution: A History of Involuntary Sterilization in the United States*. Baltimore: Johns Hopkins University Press, 1991.

Reverby, Susan, ed. *Tuskegee's Truths: Rethinking the Tuskegee Syphilis Study*. Chapel Hill: University of North Carolina Press, 2000.

Roberts, Charlotte, and Keith Dorchester. *The Archeology of Disease*, 3rd ed. Ithaca: Cornell University Press, 2005.

Rock, John, Timothy Johnson, and J. Donald Woodruff, eds. *The First One Hundred Years: Department of Gynecology and Obstetrics, The Johns Hopkins University School of Medicine*. Baltimore: Johns Hopkins University Press, 1991.

Rushton, Philippe. *Race, Evolution and Behavior*. London: Charles Darwin Research Institution, 2000.

Russett, Cynthia. *Sexual Science: The Victorian Construction of Womanhood*. Cambridge: Harvard University Press, 1989.

Sappol, Michael. *A Traffic of Dead Bodies: Anatomy and Embodied Social Identity in Nineteenth-Century America*. Princeton: Princeton University Press, 2002.

Savitt, Todd. *Medicine and Slavery: The Diseases and Health Care of Blacks in Antebellum Virginia*. Urbana: University of Illinois Press, 1978.

Savitt, Todd. *Race and Medicine in Nineteenth- and Early Twentieth-Century America*. Kent: Kent State University Press, 2007.

Schiebinger, Londa. *The Mind Has No Sex: Women in the Origins of Modern Science*. Cambridge: Harvard University Press, 1989.

Scott, Joan Wallach. *Gender and the Politics of History*. New York: Columbia University Press, 1988.

Smith, Susan L. *Sick and Tired of Being Sick and Tired*. Philadelphia: University of Pennsylvania Press, 1995.

Sonnelitter, Karen. *The Great Irish Famine: A History in Documents*. Peterborough: Broadview Press, 2018.

Stanton, William. *The Leopard's Spots: Scientific Attitudes Toward Race in America, 1815–1859*. Chicago: University of Chicago Press, 1960.

Stern, Alexandra Minna, and Harold Merkel, eds. *The Formative Years: Children's Health in the United States, 1880–2000*. Ann Arbor: University of Michigan Press, 2005.

Stocking, George. *Race, Culture, and Evolution: Essays in the History of Anthropology*. New York: Free Press, 1968.

Stocking, George. *Victorian Anthropology*. New York: Free Press, 1987.

Sussman, Robert Wald. *The Myth of Race: The Troubling Persistence of an Unscientific Idea*. Cambridge: Harvard University Press, 2014.

Tada, K., G. Mehta, and N. Murata. *Japanese Style: Architecture and Interiors and Design*. North Clarendon, VT: Tuttle, 2005.

Takaki, Ronald. *A Different Mirror: A History of Multicultural America*. Boston: Little, Brown, 1993.

Tomes, Nancy. *The Gospel of Germs: Men, Women, and the Microbe in American Life*. Cambridge: Harvard University Press, 1998.

Van Gennep, Arnold. *Rites of Passage*. Trans. Monika Vizedom and Gabrielle Caffee. Chicago: University of Chicago, 1960.

Veeder, Borden S. *Pediatric Profiles*. St. Louis: C.V. Mosby Company, 1957.

Wacker, R. Fred. *Ethnicity, Pluralism and Race: Race Relations Theory in America Before Myrdal*. Westport, CT: Greenwood Press, 1983.

Wailoo, Keith. *Dying in the City of the Blues: Sickle Cell Anemia and the Politics of Race and Health*. Chapel Hill: University of North Carolina Press, 2001.

Washington, Harriet A. *Medical Apartheid: The Dark History of Experimentation on Black Americans from Colonial Times to the Present*. New York: Doubleday, 2006.

Wertz, Richard W., and Dorothy C. Wertz, *Lying-In: A History of Childbirth in*

America. New York: Schocken Books, 1979.

Wiebe, Robert H. *The Search for Order 1877-1920*. New York: Hill and Wang, 1966.

Wilkerson, Isabel. *The Warmth of Other Suns: The Epic Story of America's Great Migration*. New York: Random House, 2009.

Wilson, Adrian. *The Making of Man-Midwifery: Childbirth in England, 1660-1770*. Cambridge: Harvard University Press, 1995.

Wilson, Philip K., ed. *Childbirth: Changing Ideas and Practices in Britain and America, 1600 to the Present*, vol. 2: *The Medicalization of Obstetrics: Personnel, Practice, and Instruments*. New York: Garland, 1996.

Wolf, Jacqueline. *Don't Kill Your Baby: Public Health and the Decline of Breast Feeding*. Athens: Ohio University Press, 2001.

Woloff, Milford, and Rachel Caspari. *Race and Human Evolution*. New York: Simon & Schuster, 1997.

Index

Abel, John, pigmentation study 231; see also Davis, Walter
Acker, George, rickets and race 87–89, 91, 92, 93
Agassiz, Louis 58, 59
American Association for the Study and Prevention of Infant Mortality (AASPIM) 202–6, 208, 213, 217
American School of Anthropology 58–61
anesthesia 69, 127, 136, 137, 139, 142, 164, 170–73, 245, 246
antisepsis 69, 138, 139, 245, 246, 249
Australopithecus afarensis (Lucy) 14

Babies Hospital, New York City 149–50, 155
Baltimore 117–18
Bard, Samuel, American obstetrics 19
Barlow, Thomas, scurvy and rickets 38
Baudeloque, Jean-Louis, pelvimetry 21–24, 26, 28, 34, 134, 140, 174
Berzelius, Jons Jacob, calcium research 43
Bettman, Henry Wald, premature birth 136
birth control 213–14
Blackfan, Kenneth, Harriet Lane Home 155, 157
Bland-Sutton, John, lion cub cure 96, 241
Boaz, Franz 89, 186, 196–97
breastfeeding 48, 93, 152, 239
Breus, Carl, rickets anatomy 174, 220, 221; see also Kolisko, Alexander
British Medical Research Committee and Advisory Council 222, 224, 227
Broca, Paul 26, 55, 56, 58, 186, 196
Buchan, William, rickets and exercise 100
Bureau of Contraceptive Advice, Baltimore 214

Caesarean Section 7, 20, 69, 86, 122, 123, 127, 136, 137–38, 139, 142, 143, 175, 177,
178, 201, 205, 216, 217, 218, 222, 246, 248, 249
calcium research 43–44
Chamberlin family, forceps development 18, 34
chemistry of light 100–1
Chick, Dame Harriet, Vienna rickets study 224–25
Chinese Exclusion Act 80
Cock, Thomas F., American obstetrics 26–27, 28
cod liver oil 8, 46–47, 69, 83, 92, 96, 107, 147, 157–58, 159, 192–94, 197, 224, 225, 228, 229, 230, 234, 238, 241, 242
Columbus Hill Study, New York City 192–197, 227
contracted pelvis: analysis, Outdoor Obstetrical Service, Johns Hopkins 164–70; defined 5, 17, 128, 130–34
craniotomy 20, 128, 135, 136, 137, 168, 177, 246
Crowell, Elisabeth, midwifery study, New York City 206
Cuvier, Georges 52–53, 55, 179

Darwin, Charles 63–65, 67–68
Davenport, Charles B. eugenics 198, 203
Davis, Edward, pelvimetry 131, 134, 140, 143
Davis, Effa V. (obstetrician) 132–33, 143
Davis, Walter: pigmentation study 231; see also Abel, John
DeBow, J.D.B., Seventh Census of the U.S. 42
DeLee, Joseph B., obstetrics 136–37, 141, 144–45, 201, 206, 246–47
Deventer, Hendrick van, rickets and birth 17–19, 21, 22, 26, 34, 122, 174
DeWees, William, pelvimetry 26, 28
diathesis defined (hereditary disease) 48, 62, 66

295

Dick, J. Lawson, rickets and civilization, 20th century 232–33
dispensaries, function described 118, 148
Dobbin, George W., Outdoor Obstetrical Service 130–31, 178, 180
domestication, human, theory of 103–5
DuBois, W.E.B. 78, 89–90, 215
dystocia, defined 14, 128

Edgar, James Clifton, pelvimetry 131–32, 134
Eliot, Martha May, New Haven study 219, 233–35
embryotomy 20
Emmett, Thomas Addis, gynecology research 70–74, 174
Engelmann, George, obstetrician 74
Engerman, Stanley, cliometric historian 88, 183
episiotomy 136, 247, 248
ergot, obstetrical use 171, 173
eugenics 67, 176, 182–83, 198, 203–4, 213, 214–17, 250
evolution and race 64

Ferguson, Margaret, Glasgow rickets study 222–25
Findlay, Leonard, etiology of rickets 101–2, 104, 108–9, 220, 222–23, 230, 242
Forceps 7, 18–20, 128, 135, 136, 168, 170, 171, 173, 174, 177, 246, 247, 248
Fruitnight, J. Henry, ethnicity and rickets 92, 93–94, 107
Funk, Casimer discovery of vitamin A 191–92, 223, 226
funnel pelvis 174–75

Galton, Francis, eugenics 67, 203, 215
gender roles 16–17
germ theory 68, 76, 200
Glisson, Francis, early rickets research 33–34, 43, 198
Goldblatt, Harry, ultraviolet research 235, 236, 238; *see also* Soames, Katharine Marjorie
Gould, Stephen Jay 58
Great Chain of Being 6, 50–51, 54, 65, 75
Great Migration 79, 88
gynecology, origins 69–70

Haeckel, Ernst 65
Hansemann, David Paul von, theory of human domestication 103–5, 197, 232, 233, 241
Harriet Lane Home for Invalid Children,

Johns Hopkins, origin 152–56, 188, 190, 225, 226
Harris, Robert, Caesarean Section study 20, 86, 128
Hebrew Infant Asylum, experimentation 189–90, 227, 228
Hess, Alfred F., pediatric research 188–99, 218, 225, 227–29, 231–33, 236, 237–39
Higginbotham, Evelyn Brooks, metalanguage of race 78
Hirsch, August, geography of disease 39–40, 45, 80, 91, 97–98, 100, 220, 241
Hodge, Hugh, childbirth 28–30, 36, 57, 85, 125, 142
Holt, L. Emmett, pediatrics 92, 107, 149–52, 154–55, 156, 158, 159, 188, 189, 197, 204
Hopkins, Frederick Gowland, biochemist 223–24, 225, 229
hospital mortality in birth 143–45
Hottentot Venus (Saartjie Baartman) 52–53, 179
Howland, John, Harriet Lane Home 154–59, 188, 190, 197, 226, 230
Huldschinsky, Kurt, ultraviolet light 224, 228
human evolution, stages 14
Hume, Eleanor Margaret, ultraviolet study 236; *see also* Smith, Hannah Henderson
Hunter, William, female anatomy 15–16, 22
Huntly, William, rickets in Rajputama 99
Hutchinson, H.S., rickets in Bombay 225–26, 230
hygiene, concept 93, 108, 109, 137
hysteria, birth related 171–73

India, famine 97–99
Irish, separate race 51–52
Irish famine 71–72, 243, 245
Italian migration, incidence of rickets 90–92

Jacobi, Abraham, pediatrics 36, 37, 146–48, 149, 154, 159, 189, 202
Jenner, William, description of rickets 35, 37, 38, 44, 48, 62, 66, 83, 96, 147
Johns Hopkins Medical School 115–16, 118–25
Johns Hopkins dispensary 118–19
Johnson, Joseph Tabor, rickets and race 81, 85, 134

Kassowitz, Max, rickets as congenital disease 102, 220

Kelly, Howard, Johns Hopkins 115, 120, 122, 123, 164
Kerr, J.M. Munro, Caesarean Section 138, 142
King, Alfred Freeman Africanus, pelvimetry 134, 140
Knox, J.H. Mason (AASPIM) 202-3, 218
Koch, Robert, germ theory 68
Kolisko, Alexander, rickets anatomy 174, 220, 221; *see also* Breus, Carl
Kramer, Benjamin, Harriet Lane Home 155, 157, 158, 227

Lane, Clayton Arbuthnot, childbirth in India 184, 186
Liebig, Justus von, chemistry of nutrition 43-44
Linneaus, Carl, taxonomy 51, 63-64
Litzmann, Carl, pelvimetry 23-26, 28, 72, 85, 122, 128, 163, 164, 165, 166, 170, 174, 181, 220, 246
Loudon, Irvine, medical historian 6, 144

Marriot, W. McKim, Harriet Lane Home 155, 157
maternal mortality 200-1
McCullom, Elmer, biochemist 226, 228, 229-30, 236, 239
Meigs, Charles, obstetrics, forceps use 19-20, 27, 28, 57, 59
Meigs, J. Forsyth, childhood sickness 83; *see also* Pepper, William
Mellanby, Edward, rickets research 224-25, 227
Michaelis, Gustav, pelimetry 23-26, 28, 122, 163, 165, 220
midwifery 117, 119, 120, 201-2, 204-6, 247, 248
military draft, U.S. (Great War), 1917 197-98
Morse, John Lovett, pediatrics 105-7, 108
Morton, Samuel George, American School of Anthropology 58-60, 186

Naegele, Franz Carl, pelvimetry 23
New Immigration, U.S. 79-80
newspaper advice on rickets 109-10
Nihell, Elizabeth, English midwife 19
"normal pelvis" 134, 139-41
nutrition, theories 93, 97, 151-52, 156, 158-59

obstetrics, development 120-21, 127-33, 205, 245
Osler, William, Johns Hopkins 115, 116, 119

osteomalacia (confused with rickets) 38
Outdoor Obstetrical Service (OOS), Johns Hopkins 119-26, 129, 130, 161, 162, 205, 208; case records 160-77; patient forms 161-68; publications from records 180-86

Palm, Theobald A., rickets in Japan 98-101, 104, 110, 241
Park, Edwards A. obstetrics 103, 156, 218, 227-33, 235, 239, 243
Parry, John, Caesarean research 82-86, 96, 128
Pasteur, Louis 68
Pearl, Raymond, eugenics 213
pediatrics, development 75-77, 146
pelvic anatomy and race 50-54
pelvic disproportion defined 21
pelvimetry 7, 11, 21-25, 55, 122, 131-34, 139, 161-78, 221, 245-46
Pepper, William childhood sickness 83; *see also* Meigs, J. Forsyth
phosphorous, rickets treatment 47, 92, 96, 102, 108, 157, 159, 230
pigmentation 100, 108, 231
Pinard, Adolphe, French obstetrician 135, 136, 139
Pirquit, Clement von, Harriet Lane Home 153, 225
polygenesis 58, 203
Porro, Eduardo, Caesarean section 138
Progressive Era (Age of Reform) 7, 113-15, 202, 203, 219, 249, 250
prone birth position 171
pubiotomy 138, 139, 175

race: definition of concept 51; metalanguage of 78, 244; obstetrical definition 178-187; suicide 7, 88, 135, 199, 203-4, 249
racial degeneration, concept 73, 80, 87-89, 94
rats as experimental subjects 226, 228, 235-36
Reynolds, Edward, pelvimetry 128-30
rickets: African Americans, 19th century 41-42; archaeological evidence 31-32; defined 5-6; early medical studies 33-38; effects on childbirth 34-35
Riggs, Theodore F., Outdoor Obstetrical Service 134, 183-87
Rochester, Anna, infant mortality, Baltimore 208-10
Roosevelt, Theodore 124
Rotch, Thomas Morgan, infant formula 107

298 Index

Routh, Amand, Caesarean Section in Great Britain 222

Saenger, Max, Caesarean Section 138
Sanger, Margaret 214, 215
Schmorl, Georg, pathology of rickets 220–21, 222
scurvy 190, 227
Sherwood, Mary, midwifery study, Baltimore 206–8; *see also* Walsh, Lilian
Shipley, Paul G., pathology at Harriet Lane Home 227, 228
Simmelweis, Ignaz, childbed fever 24
Simmonds, Nina, chemistry of hygiene 227, 229–30
Sims, J. Marion, origins of gynecology 70, 72, 180
slavery and health 60–61
Smellie, William, childbirth 19, 22, 23, 26, 28, 122
Smith, Hannah Henderson, ultraviolet study 236; *see also* Hume, Eleanor Margaret
Snow, Irving M., Italian immigration and rickets 90–92
Snow, John, rickets and nutrition 44, 68
Soames, Katharine Marjorie, ultraviolet research 235, 236, 238; *see also* Goldblatt, Harry
Southworth, Thomas, infant formula 107–8
Spencer, Herbert, Social Darwinism 67
spondylolisthesis 166, 178–80
Standards of Child Welfare, White House Conference, 1919 211
Steckel, Richard, cliometrician 61, 88
Steenbock, Harry, Vitamin D in foods 236, 239
sterilization 214–16
symphysiotomy 138–39, 168, 171, 177, 178, 246

tetany, confused with rickets 38, 96, 157
toxin, as source of rickets 102

Turner, William, pelvic classification 56, 174
twilight sleep 139

ultraviolet light (heliotherapy) 8, 224, 225, 228, 230, 235
Unger, Lester, Columbus Hill study 192, 193, 195

Verneau, Renee, pelvimetry 55–56
version, defined 17, 135
Vesalius, Andreas, human anatomy 15, 21
vesico-vaginal fistula 69–72
Virchow, Rudolf, pelvimetry 36–37, 65–66, 72, 103, 116, 146, 220
Vitamin D, identified 8, 229; cure for rickets 230–39
vitamins, discovery 191–92
Vrolik, Gerardus, pelvic classification 54

Walsh, Lilian, midwifery study, Baltimore 206–8; *see also* Sherwood, Mary
Washington, Booket T. 90
Weber, Moritz Ignaz, pelvic classification 54
Welch, William H., Johns Hopkins 115, 116, 119, 120, 152, 202, 204
Whistler, Daniel, rickets named 33
Williams, Daniel Hale, physician and Black leader 89
Williams, J. Whitridge, Johns Hopkins 119–24, 126, 128–31, 134–40, 143, 145, 161–68, 170–88, 196, 201–6, 212–18, 247, 248
Williams, William Carlos 127
Windaus, Adolf, ergosterol research 237–38
Wisconsin Alumni Research Foundation, Vitamin D licensing 239
Woodbury, Robert Morse, statistician 144, 196, 200

X-rays (Roentgen rays) 159, 221, 228, 234

www.ingramcontent.com/pod-product-compliance
Ingram Content Group UK Ltd.
Pitfield, Milton Keynes, MK11 3LW, UK
UKHW041925140426
5217IPUK00014B/327